The Ethics of
Organ Transplants

Edited by
ARTHUR L. CAPLAN
and DANIEL H. COELHO

The Ethics of
Organ Transplants

THE CURRENT DEBATE

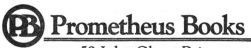

Prometheus Books

59 John Glenn Drive
Amherst, New York 14228-2197

Published 1998 by Prometheus Books

02 01 00 99   5 4 3 2

Library of Congress Cataloging-in-Publication Data

The ethics of organ transplants : the current debate / edited by Arthur L. Caplan and
    Daniel H. Coelho.
        p.   cm.
    Includes bibliographical references.
    ISBN 1–57392–224–2 (alk. paper)
    1. Transplantation of organs, tissues, etc.—Moral and ethical aspects.
2. Medical ethics. I. Caplan, Arthur L. II. Coelho, Daniel H.
RD120.7.E86   1998
174'.25—dc21   98–31722
                                                                                   CIP

Printed in the United States of America on acid-free paper

Contents

PART TWO: POLICY

PART THREE: COMMODIFICATION

PART FOUR: ALLOCATION AND RATIONING

PART FIVE: VALUE

Introduction

Arthur L. Caplan and Daniel H. Coelho

Recent advances in medical technology and research have made possible an unprecedented level of health care for those living in economically advanced nations like the United States. Antibiotics, chemotherapy, functional imaging, telemedicine, reproductive technology, artificial organs, and transplantation are just a few of the weapons in our medical arsenal today that simply did not exist only fifty years ago. Not coincidentally, the field of bioethics has also grown over the same time span. Much of the concern about ethics is driven by the power of our new technological medical prowess. All too often it seems as though medicine asks "Can we?" before asking "Should we?" and thus many Americans are doubtful that ethics can ever keep pace with rapidly changing technologies.

However, technology need not be our master. If we think hard about the ethical implications of what a particular technology might permit us to do, if thinking about the ethical consequences of technological innovation becomes an essential part of research in biomedicine, and if we realize that as citizens and patients it is up to each of us to attend to the ethical and social ramifications of what biomedicine does to our lives, our pocketbooks, and our society, then we may be able to shape biomedical progress to best suit our values. Organ transplantation is one area where progress has been astounding but where ethical reflection has done a reasonably good job of keeping pace.

Ever since its inception in the 1950s, organ transplantation has been accompanied by many hard questions about the ethics of taking organs from the dead and the living and giving them to others. It has been one of the most fertile sources of discussion among physicians, ethicists, policy makers, and lay people. Some go so far as to claim that bioethics was born out of the attempt to treat organ failure with technologies such as kidney transplantation and renal dialysis.

Shortage has been a driving force behind the attention that the ethics of transplantation has received. The huge and frustrating shortage in the supply of transplantable organs and tissues for those who might benefit from them has prodded society to search for new sources of organs, new methods of procurement, new ways of managing dying, and innovative strategies for fairly distributing this scarce life-saving resource. Scarcity is an ever-present reality of transplantation so there is no avoiding tough questions about rationing, distribution, and what to do when someone must be told "no."

But scarcity is not the sole basis for interest in the ethics of organ transplantation. Even if the shortage of organs for transplant were somehow, miraculously, to disappear, there are still many other ethical questions that surround transplantation. Some argue that there is something wholly unnatural about taking a body part from one person and putting into another living human being. Despite the macabre aspect of using the dead to help the living, and the reality of using a tragedy for one person to help another, tens of thousands of transplantations are performed every year in the United States alone. In Part One we examine the moral complexities of using diverse organ sources. At first living and willing relatives were used as organ sources for transplantation, since there was no way to overcome biological differences between unrelated persons. But with the development of prednisone and later cyclosporin A came a huge increase in cadaveric grafts. As the success rate improved there was an increased demand for its benefits and for more transplant surgeons, centers, and programs. Organ shortages worsened and new sources began to be explored. Non-biologically related but emotionally related family members such as in-laws, altruistic not emotionally related donors such as friends, fetuses, anencephalic infants, patients in vegetative states, prisoners, and animals have all come under close ethical scrutiny for their "appropriateness" as donor sources. Within the coming years the transplant community may even find itself wrestling with the moral implications of cloning organs for transplant. In this section we discuss definitions of death and whether there are moral prohibitions or considerations that ethically compromise the use of certain potential sources, even in the face of profound organ shortages.

In Part Two we look at various proposals to increase the donor pool by maximizing the efficiency of the procurement system rather than expanding into marginal or new donor populations. Clearly, existing policy and law based on education, altruism, individual autonomy, and voluntarism has failed to alleviate our nation's organ shortages. So should this well entrenched moral and legal framework be changed? To answer this question we need to examine such issues as What role does the family play after death? How obligatory is it to follow an organ donor card? What are the ethical ramifications of an "opting in" or "opting out" system? Can we assume that people would want to donate their organs? Can the rights of the deceased, if any, be overridden by the need to advance the good of others or the good of society as a whole? This section includes many opposing viewpoints on alternative proposals to mitigate organ shortages.

In Part Three we see how others in the transplant community have pushed the moral envelope even further, suggesting the beneficial role of financial incentives and markets in body parts in increasing the supply of organs. The proponents of such monetary agreements argue that commodification does not contradict altruism, and even encourages it. Proposals of compensation and calls for the establishment of free organ markets have proven to be a tough pill to swallow for many in the transplant community. Opponents of commodification staunchly denounce the gross violation of fundamental ethical principles, including informed consent and the dignity of the human body. Recently, however, more and more are beginning to believe that money and morals can mix. Also in this section we begin to shift away from issues of commodification in procurement and focus more on commodification in the allocation and distribution of scarce organs. Proposals for outright organ sales are suggested by authors who only years earlier had summarily dismissed any commodification of organs. Such articles are clear examples of the evolution (or regression, depending how one looks at it) of transplant morality. This section closes with an analysis of the role money plays in gaining access to transplantation. It is a debate that exemplifies the critical issues of economics, values, and allocation in a system of limited resources. It should also remind us that there are ethical issues generated for a system that uses altruism to obtain organs but the ability to pay to distribute them.

Deficiencies in the supply of transplantable organs have forced the transplant community to think about how to allocate scarce resources. In Part Four the issues of life and death become terribly apparent, as policy makers must decide the ultimate question—"Who lives and who dies?" Here ethical analysis brings up fundamental questions of distributive justice. Should those in most urgent need of an organ be given priority over those who stand to have the best chance at life? Should we take into account the fact that someone has already had a chance at a transplant in deciding what priority to give those on lists when a transplant fails? What about people who are directly responsible for their organ failure—a smoker in need of a lung transplant or an alcoholic in need of a new liver—should personal responsibility weigh in the mind of the surgeon or the insurance company in deciding who will live? Is a transplant to be considered a part of the health care that constitutes a fundamental right?

There are still much larger questions—many of which members of the transplant community have been less willing to address. Why do transplants at all? What is the benefit of spending much to save a few? Is this a fair practice? Is it just? How much are we willing to let our values shift before we say "enough is enough"? These are the more fundamental moral issues addressed in Part Five.

The answers to the ethical challenges posed by transplant involve complex scientific, sociological, philosophical, political, legal, economic, and religious themes that interplay with each other. But that is what makes them so interesting and compelling. To understand transplant requires you to understand many different dimensions of an issue.

In that sense transplantation is a wonderful case study for understanding many ethical problems in biomedicine. Close examination of the ethical debates that accompany transplantation is valuable not only in understanding this particular technology and the formation of specific policies, but also because it helps us to better understand and respond to greater issues involved in American health care.

PART ONE

Sources

Where do organs come from? What kind of organs and tissues are used? What sorts of people are they coming from? Are people the only sources of organs and tissues used in transplantation? Fifty years ago these questions would be science fiction, not science. Advances in surgery, immunology, and pharmacology have made possible the transplantation of hearts, livers, kidneys, lungs, pancreases, bone marrow, skin, and corneas. Yet, along with these technological advances, society has had to explore new and often controversial sources to alleviate a scarcity of useable organs and tissues.

New technologies like transplantation force society to continually reexamine the value and boundaries of life and death. The procurement of organs from deceased individuals (with their prior permission) to be used for transplantation would appear to be straightforward and ethically uncontroversial. But how do we define "deceased"? Is death an event or a process? Is it when your heart stops? Is it brain death? If so, how do you define "brain death"? Barbara Ott addresses precisely these issues in her analysis of theoretical perspectives on defining death. Robert Truog asserts that the current definitions of death may not make either ethical or practical sense, especially with respect to organ procurement. Both of these articles provoke the reader to understand that where the line is drawn between life and death is not simply a matter of biological or medical facts.

Certain organs need not always come from the deceased. In fact, for reasons of histocompatibility, organs from living donors are often preferred. Usually, these organs are donated by a relative, e.g., a mother donating a kidney to her child, a brother donating bone marrow to his twin, a cousin donating a lobe of her lung to her baby niece. However, living related transplants themselves have come under close scrutiny from the medical and

13

bioethical fields. In one such analysis, R. W. Strong and S. V. Lynch examine the difficulties of gauging familial pressures on the potential donor, real or perceived, and their effect on outcome. Is it really possible to give voluntary consent to donate your organ to a family member? What about unrelated living donors? Andrew S. Levey and his colleagues provide an excellent analysis, both practical and ethical, of the pros and cons of expanding the potential organ pool.

Even greater controversy arises when considering the sources that do not or cannot give informed consent to donate their organs. For example, when President Clinton lifted the moratorium on fetal tissue research and transplantation in 1993, he opened the door to huge advances in the treatment of Parkinson's, Alzheimer's, and other neurodegenerative diseases. However, the lifting of the ban came under immediate and intense criticism, bringing the debate over fetal rights and abortion to an unprecedented level. (There is still no federal funding for any form of human fetal tissue transplantation research.) John Robertson's article on fetal tissue transplants presents some compelling justification for this practice, concluding that ethical concerns should not bar procurement as a therapy for serious illness. However, citing serious problems in using fetal tissues from non-elective abortions, Daniel J. Garry and his colleagues assert that the risks imposed on human subjects from these sources could only result in hindering scientific progress itself.

Akin to the debate over fetal tissue use, the use of anencephalic infants as sources of transplantable organs has created much controversy in the medical, ethical, political, and religious arenas. In the two articles presented, the AMA's Council on Ethical and Judicial Affairs and D. Alan Shewmon et al. come to different conclusions about the moral and practical sense of using anencephalic infants as sources of transplantable organs. This issue proved so controversial that the AMA committee abandoned its attempt to change public policy in the United States with respect to donation. However, anencephalic infants have been used as donors in European nations such as Germany and Italy. Here, the issues of defining death once again are shown to involve moral as well as biological factors.

Some have suggested expanding the pool of potential donors to patients in permanent vegetative states. Members of the International Forum for Transplant Ethics analyzed the moral and practical advantages and disadvantages of using these organs once a decision has been made to withdraw treatment and allow the patient to die.

Although there have been only scattered reports over the past decade about the use of animal organs in human transplant therapy, the possibility of this becoming a widespread practice is becoming very real indeed. Huge advances in animal molecular and genetic engineering may soon eliminate the need for any human donor, alive or dead. Given our current desperate shortage of organs, Arthur L. Caplan asserts that xenografting can be morally justified. However, James Lindemann Nelson believes that the difficulty in determining the moral equivalence of animals with respect to humans is reason enough to redirect our efforts from xenografting research and therapy to human effort and resources.

Today, efforts to develop artificial organs have been largely unsuccessful. While development and use of these devices would no doubt alleviate much of the moral ambiguity of organ procurement, it does not seem likely that this technology will be available (or even affordable) for many years. However, an even more fantastic and terrifying scientific reality has emerged that may forever change the way we think about organ procurement. Advances in the cloning of animals from fetal and adult cells make it likely that someday this technology could be used to make animal donors that are more compatible with human biology. Perhaps, too, cloning could be used to make human tissues or even human organs.

Clearly, the shortage of transplantable organs drives the search for new sources of organs. Yet, will the demand for organs become so overwhelming that society will shift its values? What will be the ultimate social cost of meeting the need of those facing death unless a transplantable organ or tissue can be found for them? As research advances pave the way for new sources of organs, we must carefully weigh the potential alleviation of shortage against the ethical permissibility of using these new sources. One thing is for sure: the demand for transplantable organs must be balanced against a framework of acceptable values. What that framework should be will continue to be the subject of much discussion, debate, and legislative attention.

Arthur L. Caplan
Daniel H. Coelho

1. Defining and Redefining Death
Barbara B. Ott

The death of a critically ill patient is sad and stressful but not uncommon: consequently, critical care nurses are often confronted with the possibility of a patient's death. Technological advances have enabled nurses, physicians, and other healthcare professionals to rally around a patient to postpone death. This experience is stressful to all involved because personal philosophy, spirituality, and values are entangled within it. Death evokes universal feelings of fear, loss, and grief. Largely because of these universal feelings, society permits vast sums of money to be expended to prevent or postpone death. Yet a clear definition of death has not been determined.

The boundaries of life and death are not as clear today as in the past. ICU patients may be physiologically dependent on a left ventricular assist device, a pacemaker, a ventilator, dialysis, and vasoactive drugs. Some are immunosuppressed, have a donated liver, paralyzed musculoskeletal system, and non-functioning gastrointestinal tract, and show no evidence of cerebral activity. What criteria will be used to determine their death?

The determination of death is important for personal, social, religious, legal, moral, and medical reasons. Certain rights, roles, and duties surround death. It would be ideal if there were consensus among healthcare professionals and society as a whole concerning the definition of death. The various definitions of death can cause distrust of healthcare professionals and an uneasiness in the community.

Reprinted with permission of *Alternative Therapies in Health and Medicine, American Journal of Critical Care,* 4, no. 6 (November 1995): 476–80.

CURRENT DEFINITIONS

In the United States there are essentially three definitions of death from a theoretical perspective: the traditional heart-lung definition, the whole-brain definition, and the higher-brain definition. Each definition uses differing underlying assumptions within its own theoretical framework.

Heart-Lung Death

The traditional heart-lung definition, the standard for centuries, is the irreversible cessation of spontaneous respiration and circulation. The accepted criterion for death until the 1960s, this definition emerged from the historical idea that the flow of body fluids was essential for life. Usually, when the heart stopped beating, respiration ceased, so that it was unnecessary to describe the practical or clinical considerations of one stopping before the other.

However, the rapid advancement of medical technology in this century led to the ability to sustain body functions with machines and medications. Diseased lungs continued to function with the aid of mechanical ventilators, and damaged hearts continued to beat with medications and pacemakers. Advances in medical technology also made possible the successful transplantation of vital organs. The developing transplantation programs needed a standard definition of death. The programs also needed criteria or tests of death that would allow for the rapid procurement of organs before their deterioration.

Whole-Brain Death

In 1968 the Ad Hoc Committee of the Harvard Medical School[1] defined brain death in the first published work aimed at changing societal as well as legal definitions of death. Much scholarly discussion followed in the philosophical and ethical literature. Fletcher[2] examined the qualities necessary to be alive and human, and in 1973 he stated that a consensus on humanness may be difficult to achieve. He proposed twelve indicators of humanness and invited comments and suggestions from others. He asked others to select one essential trait that held the essence of humanness. This request generated a debate, with several noted scholars responding to his call. The resulting paper described neocortical functioning as the key to the definition of a human being.[3] This idea had many supporters, but it was not adopted theoretically by the healthcare community or operationally by law.

In 1980 the President's Commission for the Study of Ethical Problems in Medicine and Biomedical and Behavioral Research[4] drafted the United States Uniform Determination of Death Act, which allowed brain death to become part of the legal standard. This definition was in addition to the cardiorespiratory standard from the past. Brain death was defined "the irreversible cessation of all functions of the entire brain, including the brain stem."[4] This theoretical definition did not include specific neurological criteria for determining death at the bedside: the operational definition was to be decided by clinicians at the bedside using accepted medical standards.[4]

In 1981 the operational definition and criteria needed to diagnose brain death were provided by medical consultants to the President's Commission.[5] In the "Guidelines for Determination of Death" it was proposed that standard medical practice should be used when testing for brain death; several common standards have emerged. Most protocols require two separate clinical examinations including induction of painful stimuli, pupillary responses to light, oculovestibular testing, and apnea testing. Confirmatory examinations are not mandatory, but electroencephalographic testing, cerebral bloodflow studies, and brainstem auditory evoked responses may be part of the evaluation.[6] Although agreement on the criteria to be used in determining whole-brain death is fairly standard, variations occur. Most hospitals have a printed protocol or standard that specifies brain death criteria at that institution.

Great care is taken in the measurement of whole-brain death. To enhance accuracy, standard practice is not to perform brain death testing while a patient is hypothermic, hypotensive, or under the influence of neuromuscular blocking agents or barbiturates. Norton[6] has provided a detailed description of the procedures for testing the criteria of brain death.

One of the advantages of the whole-brain concept of death is that patients pronounced dead by the whole-brain definition look much like those pronounced dead by the traditional definition. They do not breathe spontaneously, do not have spontaneous movement, and do not respond to the environment. Moreover, if there is no emergency intervention to breathe for them, their hearts will stop.

The whole-brain definition, reasonably well-accepted by the US public and healthcare professionals, has permitted transplant teams to procure organs and physicians to withdraw treatment from brain-dead patients. However, considerable controversy surrounds the whole-brain definition, both from people who support the heart-lung definition and those who support the higher-brain definition. Much of the problem stems from the physiological status of the brain-dead patients. Patients who lack whole-brain functioning still have a heartbeat; they can digest food and excrete waste products, and they may even bear children.[7] These attributes can be disquieting to the family, caregivers, and those supporting the traditional heart-lung definition. People who support the higher-brain definition have proposed that these attributes do not count, because they do not show integrative function.[7]

Veatch[8] and Troug and Fackler[9] have challenged the internal consistency of the operational definition of whole-brain death. They questioned if patients who are brain-dead by the current standard criteria actually have irreversible cessation of all functions of the brain. Studies have shown that about 20 percent of patients who are brain-dead, using standard criteria, demonstrate cerebral electrical activity on the electroencephalogram.[10-12] Consequently, in these patients some amount of brain function remains. Bernat,[13] who supports the whole-brain definition, acknowledged this brain activity but stated that isolated nests of neurons may remain functioning, but that "they no longer contribute to the functioning of the organism as a whole; their continued functioning is now irrelevant to the dead organism."[13(p 25)]

Another physiologic question surrounding whole-brain death criteria concerns the endocrine function of the hypothalamus.[9,13] The hormone arginine vasopressin is synthesized in the hypothalamus and regulates serum osmolality. Lack of regulated arginine vasopressin secretion causes diabetes insipidus, a condition familiar to critical care personnel. Investigators[14,15] have shown that diabetes insipidus did not occur in about 20 percent of patients who were clinically brain-dead. In studies of other endocrine functions in brain-dead patients, researchers supported the claim that not all functions of the entire brain had ceased.[16,17] Therefore, enough scientific evidence exists to cast doubt on the standard definition of whole-brain death that includes irreversible cessation of all functions of the entire brain.

Troug and Fackler[9] suggested that the President's Commission intended brain death to mean the irreversible loss of essential functions. However, no standard criteria exist for evaluating what activities represent essential or significant functioning.

Higher-Brain Death

In 1975, early in the brain-death debate. Veatch[8] challenged the whole-brain death definition. He doubted that the entire brain had to be dead for the individual to be considered dead, defining death in this manner: "One is dead when there is irreversible loss of all 'higher' brain functions."[18(p19)] Veatch[19] and Youngner and Arnold[20] advocated a higher-brain definition of death—the irreversible loss of cognitive function—arguing that the permanent loss of cognition should be the criterion for death. Beecher,[21] explaining why the brain is more important than the spinal cord, stated that the critical functions are "the individual's personality, his conscious life, his uniqueness, his capacity for remembering, judging, reasoning, acting, enjoying, worrying, and so on." All these activities require cerebral functioning.

This higher-brain concept must be seriously evaluated. As medical technology advances, there seems to be no limit to finding "replacement parts" for much of our physical being. Can replacing parts of the brain be far off? Because of this, the capacity for consciousness and the ability to relate to others may become more relevant. The activities of our higher brains may come to be viewed as the defining portion of our humanness. Pellegrino and

Thomasma[22] questioned whether a being that is permanently unconscious and unable to interact with its environment is a person or merely a subjugation of human life to machinery that should be avoided. Jonsen[23] questioned what kind of life is supported by life support and suggested that it is the perpetuation of personhood that is important.

Green and Winkler[24] supported the higher brain-death definition, stating it is personal identity that dies with brain death and that the person thus ceases to exist. When the body has been stripped of all its psychological traits by brain death, the person ceases to exist. Therefore, irreversible cessation of higher-brain function is the death of that person. Green and Winkler also asserted that "the discontinuation of medical care of brain-dead patients is morally acceptable, even mandatory."[24(p129)]

DISAGREEMENT

It is not surprising that there is disagreement about the appropriateness of the higher-brain concept of death. Those who disagree with this argument have stated that even though an individual who is in a persistent vegetative state "might as well be dead," it is much different from actually "being dead." The human being may be dead, but the biological organism is not dead. Many people describe an uncomfortable psychological response to individuals who would be labeled whole-brain dead that is different from their response to a traditionally dead individual. Societal consensus on this definition may be difficult.

Also, some argue that patients who meet the criteria of higher-brain death may not look dead. For instance, a patient in a persistent vegetative state would be considered dead using the higher-brain death definition. However, because they are still breathing, it is emotionally uncomfortable to consider them dead. If the higher-brain death definition were adopted, it would have to be permissible to wait until spontaneous respirations had ceased before sending this individual to the morgue. This is now done with patients pronounced dead by the whole-brain death definition. Caregivers wait until the heart has stopped before sending them to the morgue.

The slippery slope argument has been used as an objection to the higher-brain definition of death. It is feared that if the higher-brain formula for death were implemented, eventually those who are severely mentally retarded would be labeled dead. Even those with severe mental illness who do not interact with others or their environment might be considered dead. Other scholars[24] argue that it is highly unlikely that a public that is quite accepting of whole-brain death would ever come to believe that the profoundly retarded or the senile are dead.

A NEW APPROACH

An entirely different proposal came from Morrison,[25] who stated that there is no sharp dichotomy between life and death. He asserted that death is a process, not an event, and that we should stop worrying about a single answer to the question of death. Likewise, Halevy and Brody[26] recommended that we not struggle with the impossible task of creating a single theoretically satisfactory and practically relevant criterion of death. They suggested that three clinically significant questions should be answered separately:

> When can care be unilaterally withheld (as opposed to stopping support at the request of a patient or surrogate)? Answer: With irreversible cessation of conscious functioning. When can organs be procured? Answer: When current clinical tests for brain death are satisfied. When is a patient ready for the services of the undertaker rather than those of the clinician? Answer: With asystole.[26(p523)]

The debate continues in many disciplines over which definition of death should be used. Some cultural and religious groups have a conscientious objection to any definition of brain death. Their views could be reflected in any ensuing public policy, with an exemption clause. For instance, in New Jersey law[27] the declaration of death contains an exemption clause stating that an individual will not be declared dead on the basis of neurological criteria if this would violate the individual's religious beliefs. This type of exemption could allow a legal alternative for people who reject brain death on philosophical or religious grounds.

The inconsistencies of clinical diagnosis and clinical criteria for brain death, as well as differing philosophical, cultural, and spiritual definitions of death, have lead to confusion among healthcare professionals. Youngner et al.[28] studied 115 physicians and 80 nurses who were involved in the care of patients who could be declared brain dead. In the study 63 percent of respondents were able to answer correctly that irreversible loss of all brain function was required for a patient to be declared brain dead. Most of the other respondents thought that only loss of all cortical function was required for a patient to be declared dead. When applying their knowledge of brain death criteria, only 35 percent were able to correctly identify the legal death status of patients in the two hypothetical case scenarios that were presented.

Confusion also surrounds the concept of irreversibility as applied to the definition of death. Both the conceptual and operational definitions of irreversibility should be clarified. What does "irreversible loss of consciousness" mean? Is loss of consciousness irreversible because it is physiologically impossible to revive an individual despite the use of current information and technology? Or is loss of consciousness irreversible because we do not want to subject an individual to the assault associated with cardiopulmonary resuscitation and emergency life-supporting technology? We need further clarification of the difference between these two concepts of irreversibility and more specific usage in the literature.

CONCLUSION

Although moral, philosophical, and spiritual aspects of the brain death debate may preclude clear empirical answers, the debate must continue and we must strive for public and professional consensus. Continuation of the dialogue surrounding brain death is important. Critical care professionals are in a unique position to encourage the discussion and debate. We must contribute to the public and professional education processes and the formulation of sensitive public policy.

Is the difficulty we face in this discussion really the challenge of theoretically or operationally defining death? Or defining life? Or is the fundamental difficulty really in defining . . . person?

REFERENCES

1. Report of the Ad Hoc Committee of the Harvard Medical School to examine the definition of brain death: a definition of irreversible coma. *JAMA*. 1968;205:337-340.

2. Fletcher JF. Medicine and the nature of man. In: Veatch RM, Gaylin W, Morgan C, eds. *The Teaching of Medical Ethics*. Hastings-on-Hudson, NY: Institute of Science, Ethics and the Life Sciences; 1973:47-58.

3. Fletcher JF. Four indicators of humanhood: the enquiry matures. *Hastings Cent Rep*. 1974;4(6):4-7.

4. President's Commission for the Study of Ethical Problems in Medicine and Biomedical and Behavioral Research. *Defining Death: Medical, Ethical, and Legal Issues in the Definition of Death*. Washington DC: US Government Printing Office; 1981.

5. Medical Consultants on the Diagnosis of Death to the President's Commission for the Study of Ethical Problems in Medicine and Biomedical and Behavioral Research. Guidelines for the determination of death. *JAMA*. 1981;246:2184-2186.

6. Norton DJ. Clinical applications of brain death protocols. *J Neurosci Nurs*. 1992;24:354-358.

7. Botkin JR, Post SG. Confusion in the determination of death: distinguishing philosophy from physiology. *Perspect Biol Med*. 1992;36:129-138.

8. Veatch RM. The whole-brain-oriented concept of death: an outmoded philosophical formulation. *J Thanatol*. 1975;3(1):13-30.

9. Troug RD, Fackler JC. Rethinking brain death. *Crit Care Med*. 1992;20(12):1705-1713.

10. Pallis C. ABCs of brain stem death: prognostic significance of a dead brain stem. *Br Med J*. 1983;286:123-124.

11. Walker AF. *Cerebral Death*. Baltimore, Md: Urban & Schwarzenberg; 1981:89-90.

12. Grigg MM, Kelly MA, Celesia GG, et al. Electroencephalographic activity after brain death. *Arch Neurol*. 1987;44:948-954.

13. Bernat JL. How much of the brain must die in brain death? *J Clin Ethics.* 1992;3(1):21-26.

14. Howlett TA, Keogh AM, Perry L, et al. Anterior and posterior pituitary function in brain-stem dead donors: a possible role for replacement therapy. *Transplantation.* 1989;47:828-834.

15. Outwater KM, Rockhoff MA. Diabetes insipidus accompanying brain death in children. *Neurology.* 1984;34:1243-1246.

16. Anthony GJ, Van Wyk JJ, French FS, et al. Influence of pituitary stalk section on growth hormone, insulin and TSH secretion in women with metastatic breast cancer. *J Clin Endocrinal Metab.* 1969;29:1238-1250.

17. Hall GM, Mashiter K, Lumley J, et al. Hypothalamic-pituitary function in the "brain dead" patient. *Lancet.* 1980;2:1259. Letter.

18. Veatch RM. The impending collapse of the whole-brain definition of death. *Hastings Cent Rep.* 1993;23(4):18-24.

19. Veatch RM. Brain death and slippery slopes. *J Clin Ethics.* 1992;3:181-187.

20. Youngner SJ, Arnold RM. Ethical, psychosocial, and public policy implications of procuring organs from non-heart beating cadaver donors. *JAMA.* 1993;269:2769-2774.

21. Beecher HK. The new definition of death: some opposing views. Presented at the meeting of the American Association for the Advancement of Science. Chicago, Ill: December 1970.

22. Pellegrino ED, Thomasma DC. *The Virtues in Medical Practice.* New York, NY: Oxford University Press; 1993:124.

23. Jonsen AR. What does life support support? In: Winsdale W, ed. *Personal Choices and Public Commitments: Perspectives on the Humanities.* Galveston, Tex: Institute for the Medical Humanities; 1988:66-67.

24. Green MB, Wikler D. Brain death and personal identity. *Philosophy and Public Affairs.* 1980;9(2):105-133.

25. Morrison RS. Death: Process or event? *Science.* 1971;173:694-698.

26. Halevy A, Brody B. Brain death: reconciling definitions, criteria, and tests. *Ann Intern Med.* 1993;119:519-525.

27. New Jersey Statutes. Annotated. *Declaration of Death.* 26:6A-5. St. Louis, Mo: West Publishing; 1991:232-235.

28. Youngner SJ, Landefeld S, Coulton CJ, Juknialis BW, Leary M. Brain death and organ retrieval: a cross-sectional survey of knowledge and concepts among health professionals. *JAMA.* 1989;261:2205-2210.

2. Is It Time to Abandon Brain Death?

Robert D. Truog

Over the past several decades, the concept of brain death has become well entrenched within the practice of medicine. At a practical level, this concept has been successful in delineating widely accepted ethical and legal boundaries for the procurement of vital organs for transplantation. Despite this success, however, there have been persistent concerns over whether the concept is theoretically coherent and internally consistent.[1] Indeed, some have concluded that the concept is fundamentally flawed, and that it represents only a "superficial and fragile consensus."[2] In this analysis I will identify the sources of these inconsistencies, and suggest that the best resolution to these issues may be to abandon the concept of brain death altogether.

DEFINITIONS, CONCEPTS, AND TESTS

In its seminal work "Defining Death," the President's Commission for the Study of Ethical Problems in Medicine and Biomedical and Behavioral Research articulated a formulation of brain death that has come to be known as the "whole-brain standard."[3] In the Uniform Determination of Death Act, the President's Commission specified two criteria for determining death: (1) irreversible cessation of circulatory and respiratory functions, or (2) irreversible cessation of all functions of the entire brain, including the brainstem."

Neurologist James Bernat has been influential in defending and refining this standard. Along with others, he has recognized that analysis of the con-

---

Originally published in *Hastings Center Report* 27, no.1 (1997): 29–37. Reproduced by permission. © The Hastings Center.

cept of brain death must begin by differentiating between three distinct levels. At the most general level, the concept must involve a *definition.* Next, *criteria* must be specified to determine when the definition has been fulfilled. Finally, *tests* must be available for evaluating whether the criteria have been satisfied.[4] As clarified by Bernat and colleagues, therefore, the concept of death under the whole-brain formulation can be outlined as follows:[5]

> *Definition of Death:* The "permanent cessation of functioning of the organism as a whole."

> *Criterion for Death:* The "permanent cessation of functioning of the entire brain.

> *Tests for death:* Two distinct sets of tests are available and acceptable for determining that the criterion is fulfilled:
> (1) The cardiorespiratory standard is the traditional approach for determining death and relies upon documenting the prolonged absence of circulation or respiration. These tests fulfill the criterion, according to Bernat, since the prolonged absence of these vital signs is diagnostic for the permanent loss of all brain function.
> (2) The neurological standard consists of a battery of tests and procedures, including establishment of an etiology sufficient to account for the loss of all brain functions, diagnosing the presence of coma, documenting apnea and the absence of brain-stem reflexes, excluding reversible conditions, and showing the persistence of these findings over a sufficient period of time.[6]

CRITIQUE OF THE CURRENT FORMULATION OF BRAIN DEATH

Is this a coherent account of the concept of brain death? To answer this question, one must determine whether each level of analysis is consistent with the others. In other words, individuals who fulfill the tests must also fulfill the criterion, and those who satisfy the criterion must also satisfy the definition.[7]

First, regarding the tests-criterion relationship, there is evidence that many individuals who fulfill all of the tests for brain death do not have the "permanent cessation of functioning of the entire brain." In particular, many of these individuals retain clear evidence of integrated brain function at the level of the brainstem and midbrain, and may have evidence of cortical function.

For example, many patients who fulfill the tests for the diagnosis of brain death continue to exhibit intact neurohumoral function. Between 22 percent and 100 percent of brain-dead patients in different series have been found to retain free-water homeostasis through the neurologically mediated secretion of arginine vasopressin, as evidenced by serum hormonal levels and the absence of diabetes insipidus.[8] Since the brain is the only source of the regulated secretion of arginine vasopressin, patients without diabetes insipidus do not have the loss of all brain function. Neurologically regulated secretion of other hormones is also quite common.[9]

In addition, the tests for the diagnosis of brain death require the patient not to be hypothermic.[10] This caveat is a particularly confusing Catch 22, since the absence of hypothermia generally indicates the continuation of neurologically mediated temperature homeostasis. The circularity of this reasoning can be clinically problematic, since hypothermic patients cannot be diagnosed as brain-dead but the absence of hypothermia is itself evidence of brain function.

Furthermore, studies have shown that many patients (20 percent in one series) who fulfill the tests for brain death continue to show electrical activity on their electroencephalograms.[11] While there is no way to determine how often this electrical activity represents true "function" (which would be incompatible with the criterion for brain death), in at least some cases the activity observed seems fully compatible with function.[12]

Finally, clinicians have observed that patients who fulfill the tests for brain death frequently respond to surgical incision at the time of organ procurement with a significant rise in both heart rate and blood pressure. This suggests that integrated neurological function at a supraspinal level may be present in at least some patients diagnosed as brain-dead.[13] This evidence points to the conclusion that there is a significant disparity between the standard tests used to make the diagnosis of brain death and the criterion these tests are purported to fulfill. Faced with these facts, even supporters of the current statutes acknowledge that the criterion of "whole-brain" death is only an "approximation."[14]

If the tests for determining brain death are incompatible with the current criterion, then one way of solving the problem would be to require tests that always correlate with the "permanent cessation of functioning of the entire brain." Two options have been considered in this regard. The first would require tests that correlate with the actual destruction of the brain, since complete destruction would, of course, be incompatible with any degree of brain function. Only by satisfying these tests, some have argued, could we be assured that all functions of the entire brain have totally and permanently ceased.[15] But is there a constellation of clinical and laboratory tests that correlate with this degree of destruction? Unfortunately, a study of over 500 patients with both coma and apnea (including 146 autopsies for neuropathologic correlation) showed that "it was not possible to verify that a diagnosis made prior to cardiac arrest by any set or subset of criteria would invariably correlate with a diffusely destroyed brain."[16] On the basis of these data, a definition that required total brain destruction could only be confirmed at autopsy. Clearly, a condition that could only be determined after death could never be a requirement for declaring death.

Another way of modifying the tests to conform with the criterion would be to rely solely upon the cardiorespiratory standard for determining death. This standard would certainly identify the permanent cessation of all brain function (thereby fulfilling the criterion), since it is well established by common knowledge that prolonged absence of circulation and respiration results in the death of the entire brain (and every other organ). In addition, fulfillment of these tests would also convincingly demonstrate the cessation of function of the organism as a whole (thereby fulfilling the definition). Unfortunately, this approach for resolving the problem would also make it virtually impossible to obtain vital organs in a viable condition for transplantation, since under current laws it is generally necessary for these organs to be removed from a heart-beating donor.

These inconsistencies between the tests and the criterion are therefore not easily resolvable. In addition to these problems, there are also inconsistencies between the criterion and the definition. As outlined above, the whole-brain concept assumes that the "permanent cessation of functioning of the entire brain" (the criterion) necessarily implies the "permanent cessation of functioning of the organism as a whole" (the definition). Conceptually, this relationship assumes the principle that the brain is responsible for maintaining the body's homeostasis, and that without brain function the organism rapidly disintegrates. In the past, this relationship was demonstrated by showing that individuals who fulfilled the tests for the diagnosis of brain death inevitably had a cardiac arrest within a short period of time, even if they were provided with mechanical ventilation and intensive care.[17] Indeed, this assumption had been considered one of the linchpins in the ethical justification for the concept of brain death.[18] For example, in the largest empirical study of brain death ever performed, a collaborative group working under the auspices of the National Institutes of Health sought to specify the necessary tests for diagnosing brain death by attempting to identify a constellation of neurological findings that would inevitably predict the development of a cardiac arrest within three months, regardless of the level or intensity of support provided.[19]

This approach to defining brain death in terms of neurological findings that predict the development of cardiac arrest is plagued by both logical and scientific problems, however. First, it confuses a prognosis with a diagnosis. Demonstrating that a certain class of patients will suffer a cardiac arrest within a defined period of time certainly proves that they are *dying*, but it says nothing about whether they are *dead*.[20] This conceptual mistake can be clearly appreciated if one considers individuals who are dying of conditions not associated with severe neurological impairment. If a constellation of tests could identify a subgroup of patients with metastatic cancer who invariably suffered a cardiac arrest within a short period of time, for example, we would certainly be comfortable in concluding that they were dying, but we clearly could not claim that they were already dead.

Second, this view relies upon the intuitive notion that the brain is the principal organ of the body, the "integrating" organ whose functions cannot be replaced by any other organ or by artificial means. Up through the early 1980s, this view was supported by numerous studies showing that almost all patients who fulfilled the usual battery of tests for brain death suffered a cardiac arrest within several weeks.[21]

The loss of homeostatic equilibrium that is empirically observed in brain-dead patients is almost certainly the result of their progressive loss of integrated neurohumoral and autonomic function. Over the past several decades, however, the intensive care units (ICUs) have become increasingly sophisticated "surrogate brainstems," replacing both the respiratory functions as well as the hormonal and other regulatory activities of the damaged neuraxis.[22] This technology is presently utilized in those tragic cases in which a pregnant woman is diagnosed as brain-dead and an attempt is made to maintain her somatic existence until the fetus reaches a viable gestation, as well as for prolonging the organ viability of brain-dead patients awaiting organ procurement.[23] Although the functions of the brainstem are considerably more complex than those of the heart or the lungs, in theory (and increasingly in practice) they are entirely replaceable by modern technology. In terms of maintaining homeostatic functions, therefore, the brain is no more irreplaceable than any of the other vital organs. A definition of death predicated upon the "inevitable" development of a cardiac arrest within a short period of time is therefore inadequate, since this empirical "fact" is no longer true. In other words, cardiac arrest is inevitable only if it is allowed to occur, just as respiratory arrest in brain-dead patients is inevitable only if they are not provided with mechanical ventilation. This gradual development in technical expertise has unwittingly undermined one of the central ethical justifications for the whole-brain criterion of death.

In summary, then, the whole-brain concept is plagued by internal inconsistencies in both the tests-criterion and the criterion-definition relationships, and these problems cannot be easily solved. In addition, there is evidence that this lack of conceptual clarity has contributed to misunderstandings about the concept among both clinicians and laypersons. For example, Stuart Youngner and colleagues found that only 35 percent of physicians and nurses who were likely to be involved in organ procurement for transplantation correctly identified the legal and medical criteria for determining death.[24] Indeed, most of the respondents used inconsistent concepts of death, and a substantial minority misunderstood the criterion to be the permanent loss of consciousness, which the President's Commission had specifically rejected, in part because it would have classified anencephalic newborns and patients in a vegetative state as dead. In other words, medical professionals who were otherwise knowledgeable and sophisticated were generally confused about the concept of brain death. In an editorial accompanying this study, Dan Wikler and

Alan Weisbard claimed that this confusion was "appropriate," given the lack of philosophical coherence in the concept itself.[25] In another study, a survey of Swedes found that laypersons were more willing to consent to autopsies than to organ donation for themselves or a close relative. In seeking an explanation for these findings, the authors reported that "the fear of not being dead during the removal of organs, reported by 22 percent of those undecided toward organ donation, was related to the uncertainty surrounding brain death."[26]

On one hand, these difficulties with the concept might be deemed to be so esoteric and theoretical that they should play no role in driving the policy debate about how to define death and procure organs for transplantation. This has certainly been the predominant view up to now. In many other circumstances, theoretical issues have taken a back seat to practical matters when it comes to determining public policy. For example, the question of whether tomatoes should be considered a vegetable or a fruit for purposes of taxation was said to hinge little upon the biological facts of the matter, but to turn primarily upon the political and economic issues at stake.[27] If this view is applied to the concept of brain death, then the best public policy would be that which best served the public's interest, regardless of theoretical concerns.

On the other hand, medicine has a long and respected history of continually seeking to refine the theoretical and conceptual underpinnings of its practice. While the impact of scientific and philosophical views upon social policy and public perception must be taken seriously, they cannot be the sole forces driving the debate. Given the evidence demonstrating a lack of coherence in the whole-brain death formulation and the confusion that is apparent among medical professionals, there is ample reason to prompt a look at alternatives to our current approach.

ALTERNATIVE APPROACHES TO THE WHOLE-BRAIN FORMULATION

Alternatives to the whole-brain death formulation fall into two general categories. One approach is to emphasize the overriding importance of those functions of the brain that support the phenomenon of consciousness and to claim that individuals who have permanently suffered the loss of all consciousness are dead. This is known as the "higher-brain" criterion. The other approach is to return to the traditional tests for determining death, that is, the permanent loss of circulation and respiration. As noted above, this latter strategy could fit well with Bernat's formulation of the definition of death, since adoption of the cardiorespiratory standard as the test for determining death is consistent with both the criterion and the definition. The problem with this potential solution is that it would virtually eliminate the possibility of procuring vital organs from heart-beating donors under our present system of law and ethics, since current requirements insist that organs be removed only from individuals who have been declared dead (the "dead-donor rule").[28] Consideration of this latter view would therefore be feasible only if it could be linked to fundamental changes in the permissible limits of organ procurement.

The Higher-Brain Formulation

The higher-brain criterion for death holds that maintaining the potential for consciousness is the critical function of the brain relevant to questions of life and death. Under this definition, all individuals who are permanently unconscious would be considered to be dead. Included in this category would be (1) patients who fulfill the cardiorespiratory standard, (2) those who fulfill the current tests for whole-brain death, (3) those diagnosed as being in a permanent vegetative state, and (4) newborns with anencephaly. Various versions of this view have been defended by many philosophers, and arguments have been advanced from moral as well as ontological perspectives.[29] In addition, this view correlates very well with many common-sense opinions about personal identity. To take a stock philosophical illustration, for example, consider the typical reaction of a person who has undergone a hypothetical "brain switch" procedure, where one's brain is transplanted into another's body, and vice versa. Virtually anyone presented with this scenario will say that "what matters" for their existence now resides in the new body, even though an outside observer would insist that it is the person's old body that "appears" to be the original person. Thought experiments like this one illustrate that we typically identify ourselves with our experience of consciousness, and this observation forms the basis of the claim that the permanent absence of consciousness should be seen as representing the death of the person.

Implementation of this standard would present certain problems, however. First, is it possible to diagnose the state of permanent unconsciousness with the high level of certainty required for the determination of death? More specifically, is it currently possible to definitively diagnose the permanent vegetative state and anencephaly? A Multi-Society Task Force recently outlined guidelines for diagnosis of permanent vegetative state and claimed that sufficient data are now available to make the diagnosis of permanent vegetative state in appropriate patients with a high degree of certainty.[30] On the other hand, case reports of patients who met these criteria but who later recovered a higher degree of neurological functioning suggest that use of the term "permanent" may be overstating the degree of diagnostic certainty that is currently possible. This would be an especially important issue in the context of diagnosing death, where false positive diagnoses would be particularly problematic.[31] Similarly, while the Medical Task Force on Anencephaly has concluded that most cases of anencephaly can be diagnosed by a competent clinician without significant uncertainty, others have emphasized the ambiguities inherent in evaluating this condition.[32]

Another line of criticism is that the higher-brain approach assumes the definition of death should reflect the death of the *person,* rather than the death of the *organism.*[33] By focusing on the person, this theory does not account for what is common to the death of all organisms, such as humans, frogs, or trees. Since we do not know what it would mean to talk about the permanent loss of consciousness of frogs or trees, then this approach to death may appear to be idiosyncratic. In response, higher-brain theorists believe that it is critical to define death within the context of the specific subject under consideration. For example, we may speak of the death of an ancient civilization, the death of a species, or the death of a particular system of belief. In each case, the definition of death will be different, and must be appropriate to the subject in order for the concept to make any sense. Following this line of reasoning, the higher-brain approach is correct precisely because it seeks to identify what is uniquely relevant to the death of a person.

Aside from these diagnostic and philosophical concerns, however, perhaps the greatest objections to the higher brain formulation emerge from the implications of treating breathing patients as if they are dead. For example, if patients in a permanent vegetative state were considered to be dead, then they should logically be considered suitable for burial. Yet all of these patients breathe, and some of them "live" for many years.[34] The thought of burying or cremating a breathing individual, even if unconscious, would be unthinkable for many people, creating a significant barrier to acceptance of this view into public policy.[35]

One way of avoiding this implication would be to utilize a "lethal injection" before cremation or burial to terminate cardiac and respiratory function. This would not be euthanasia, since the individual would be declared dead before the injection. The purpose of the injection would be purely "aesthetic." This practice could even be viewed as simply an extension of our current protocols, where the vital functions of patients diagnosed as brain-dead are terminated prior to burial, either by discontinuing mechanical ventilation or by removing their heart and/or lungs during the process of organ procurement. While this line of argumentation has a certain logical persuasiveness, it nevertheless fails to address the central fact that most people find it counterintuitive to perceive a breathing patient as "dead." Wikler has suggested that this attitude is likely to change over time, and that eventually society will come to accept that the body of a patient in a permanent vegetative state is simply that person's "living remains."[36] This optimism about higher-brain death is reminiscent of the comments by the President's Commission regarding whole-brain death: "Although undeniably disconcerting for many people, the confusion created in personal perception by a determination of 'brain death' does not . . . provide a basis for an ethical objection to discontinuing medical measures on these dead bodies any more than on other dead bodies."[37] Nevertheless, at the present time any inclination toward a higher-brain death standard remains primarily in the realm of philosophers and not policymakers.

Return to the Traditional Cardiorespiratory Standard

In contrast to the higher-brain concept of death, the other main alternative to our current approach would involve moving in the opposite direction and abandoning the diagnosis of brain death altogether. This would involve returning to the traditional approach to determining death, that is, the cardiorespiratory standard. In evaluating the wisdom of "turning back the clock," it is helpful to retrace the development of the concept of brain death back to 1968 and the conclusions of the ad hoc committee that developed the Harvard Criteria for the diagnosis of brain death. They began by claiming:

> There are two reasons why there is need for a definition [of brain death]: (1) Improvements in resuscitative and supportive measures have led to increased efforts to save those who are desperately injured. Sometimes these efforts have only partial success so that the result is an individual whose heart continues to beat but whose brain is irreversibly damaged. The burden is great on patients who suffer permanent loss of intellect, on their families, and on those in need of hospital beds already occupied by these comatose patients. (2) Obsolete criteria for the definition of death can lead to controversy in obtaining organs for transplantations.[38]

These two issues can be subdivided into at least four distinct questions:

1) When is it permissible to withdraw life support from patients with irreversible neurological damage for the benefit of the patient?

2) When is it permissible to withdraw life support from patients with irreversible neurological damage for the benefit of society, where the benefit is either in the form of economic savings or to make an ICU bed available for someone with a better prognosis?

3) When is it permissible to remove organs from a patient for transplantation?

4) When is a patient ready to be cremated or buried?

The Harvard Committee chose to address all of these questions with a single answer, that is, the determination of brain death. Each of these questions involves unique theoretical issues, however, and each raises a different set of concerns. By analyzing the concept of brain death in terms of the separate questions that led to its development, alternatives to brain death may be considered.

Withdrawal of Life Support

The Harvard Committee clearly viewed the diagnosis of brain death as a necessary condition for the withdrawal of life support: "It should be emphasized that we recommend the patient be declared dead before any effort is made to take him off a respirator... [since] otherwise, the physicians would be turning off the respirator on a person who is, in the present strict, technical application of law, still alive" (p. 339).

The ethical and legal mandates that surround the withdrawal of life support have changed dramatically since the recommendations of the Harvard Committee. Numerous court decisions and consensus statements have emphasized the rights of patients or their surrogates to demand the withdrawal of life-sustaining treatments, including mechanical ventilation. In the practice of critical care medicine today, patients are rarely diagnosed as brain-dead solely for the purpose of discontinuing mechanical ventilation. When patients are not candidates for organ transplantation, either because of medical contraindications or lack of consent, families are informed of the dismal prognosis, and artificial ventilation is withdrawn. While the diagnosis of brain death was once critical in allowing physicians to discontinue life-sustaining treatments, decisionmaking about these important questions is now appropriately centered around the patient's previously stated wishes and judgments about the patient's best interest. Questions about the definition of death have become virtually irrelevant to these deliberations.

Allocation of Scarce Resources

The Harvard Committee alluded to its concerns about having patients with a hopeless prognosis occupying ICU beds. In the years since that report this issue has become even more pressing. The diagnosis of brain death, however, is of little significance in helping to resolve these issues. Even considering the unusual cases where families refuse to have the ventilator removed from a brain-dead patient, the overall impact of the diagnosis of brain death upon scarce ICU resources is minimal. Much more important to the current debate over the just allocation of ICU resources are patients with less severe degrees of neurological dysfunction, such as patients in a permanent vegetative state or individuals with advanced dementia. Again, the diagnosis of brain death is of little relevance to this central concern of the Harvard Committee.

Organ Transplantation

Without question, the most important reason for the continued use of brain death criteria is the need for transplantable organs. Yet even here, the requirement for brain death may be doing more harm than good. The need for organs is expanding at an ever-increasing rate, while the number of available organs has essentially plateaued. In an effort to expand the limited pool of organs, several attempts have been made to circumvent the usual restrictions of brain death on organ procurement.

At the University of Pittsburgh, for example, a new protocol allows critically ill patients or their surrogates to offer their organs for donation after the withdrawal of life-support, even though the patients never meet brain death criteria.[39] Suitable patients are taken to the operating room, where intravascular monitors are placed and the patient is "prepped and draped" for surgical incision. Life-support is then withdrawn, and the patient is monitored for the development of cardiac arrest. Assuming this occurs within a short period of time, the attending physician waits until there has been two minutes of pulselessness, and then pronounces the patient dead. The transplant team then enters the operating room and immediately removes the organs for transplantation.

This novel approach has a number of problems when viewed from within the traditional framework. For example, after the patient is pronounced dead, why should the team rush to remove the organs? If the Pittsburgh team truly believes that the patient is dead, why not begin chest compressions and mechanical ventilation, insert cannulae to place the patient on full cardiopulmonary bypass, and remove the organs in a more controlled fashion? Presumably, this is not done because two minutes of pulselessness is almost certainly not long enough to ensure the development of brain death.[40] It is even conceivable that patients managed in this way could regain consciousness during the process of organ procurement while supported with cardiopulmonary bypass, despite having already been diagnosed as "dead." In other words, the reluctance of the Pittsburgh team to extend their protocol in ways that would be acceptable for dead patients could be an indication that the patients may really not be dead after all.

A similar attempt to circumvent the usual restrictions on organ procurement was recently attempted with anencephalic newborns at Loma Linda University. Again, the protocol involved manipulation of the dying process, with mechanical ventilation being instituted and maintained solely for the purpose of preserving the organs until criteria for brain death could be documented. The results were disappointing, and the investigators concluded that "it is usually not feasible, with the restrictions of current law, to procure solid organs for transplantation from anencephalic infants."[41]

Why do these protocols strike many commentators as contrived and even somewhat bizarre? The motives of the individuals involved are certainly commendable: they want to offer the benefits of transplantable organs to individuals who desperately need them. In addition, they are seeking to obtain organs only from individuals who cannot be harmed by the procurement and only in those situations where the patient or a surrogate requests the donation. The problem with these protocols lies not with the motive, but with the method and justification. By manipulating both the process and the definition of death, these protocols give the appearance that the physicians involved are only too willing to draw the boundary between life and death wherever it happens to maximize the chances for organ procurement.

How can the legitimate desire to increase the supply of transplantable organs be reconciled with the need to maintain a clear and simple distinction between the living and the dead? One way would be to abandon the requirement for the death of the donor prior to organ procurement and, instead, focus upon alternative and perhaps more fundamental ethical criteria to constrain the procurement of organs, such as the principles of consent and nonmaleficence.[42]

For example, policies could be changed such that organ procurement would be permitted only with the consent of the donor or appropriate surrogate and only when doing so would not harm the donor. Individuals who could not be harmed by the procedure would include those who are permanently and irreversibly unconscious (patients in a persistent vegetative state or newborns with anencephaly) and those who are imminently and irreversibly dying.

The American Medical Association's Council on Ethical and Judicial Affairs recently proposed (but has subsequently retracted) a position consistent with this approach.[43] The council stated that, "It is ethically permissible to consider the anencephalic as a potential organ donor, although still alive under the current definition of death," if, among other requirements, the diagnosis is certain and the parents give their permission. The council concluded, "It is normally required that the donor be legally dead before removal of their life-necessary organs. . . . The use of the anencephalic neonate as a live donor is a limited exception to the general standard because of the fact that the infant has never experienced, and will never experience, consciousness" (pp. 1617–18).

This alternative approach to organ procurement would require substantial changes in the law. The process of organ procurement would have to be legitimated as a form of justified killing, rather than just as the dissection of a corpse. There is certainly precedent in the law for recognizing instances of justified killing. The concept is also not an anathema to the public, as evidenced by the growing support for euthanasia, another practice that would have to be legally construed as a form of justified killing. Even now, surveys show that one-third of physicians and nurses do not believe brain-dead patients are actually dead, but feel comfortable with the process of organ procurement because the patients are permanently unconscious and/or imminently dying.[44] In other words. many clinicians already seem to justify their actions on the basis of nonmaleficence and consent, rather than with the belief that the patients are actually dead.

This alternative approach would also eliminate the need for protocols like the one being used at the University of Pittsburgh, with its contrived and perhaps questionable approach to declaring death prior to organ procurement. Under the proposed system, qualified individuals who had given their consent could simply have their organs removed under general anesthesia, without first undergoing an orchestrated withdrawal of life support. Anencephalic newborns whose parents requested organ donation could likewise have the organs removed under general anesthesia without the need to wait for the diagnosis of brain death.

The Diagnosis of Death

Seen in this light, the concept of brain death may have become obsolete. Certainly the diagnosis of brain death has been extremely useful during the last several decades, as society has struggled with a myriad of issues that were never encountered before the era of mechanical ventilation and organ transplantation. As society emerges from this transitional period, and as many of these issues are more clearly understood as questions that are inherently unrelated to the distinction between life and death, then the concept of brain death may no longer be useful or relevant. If this is the case, then it may be preferable to return to the traditional standard and limit tests for the determination of death to those based solely upon the permanent cessation of respiration and circulation. Even today we uniformly regard the cessation of respiration and circulation as the standard for determining when patients are ready to be cremated or buried.

Another advantage of a return to the traditional approach is that it would represent a "common denominator" in the definition of death that virtually all cultural groups and religious traditions would find acceptable.[45] Recently both New Jersey and New York have enacted statutes that recognize the objections of particular religious views to the concept of brain death. In New Jersey, physicians are prohibited from declaring brain death in persons who come from religious traditions that do not accept the concept.[46] Return to a cardiorespiratory standard would eliminate problems with these objections.

Linda Emanuel recently proposed a "bounded zone" definition of death that shares some features with the approach outlined here.[47] Her proposal would adopt the cardiorespiratory standard as a "lower bound" for determining death that would apply to all cases, but would allow individuals to choose a definition of death that encompassed neurologic dysfunction up to the level of the permanent vegetative state (the "higher bound"). The practical implications of such a policy would be similar to some of those discussed here, in that it would (1) allow patients and surrogates to request organ donation when and if the patients were diagnosed with whole-brain death, permanent vegetative state, or anencephaly, and (2) it would permit rejection of the diagnosis of brain death by patients and surrogates opposed to the concept.

Emanuel's proposal would not permit organ donation from terminal and imminently dying patients, however, prior to the diagnosis of death.

Despite these similarities, these two proposals differ markedly in the justifications used to support their conclusions. Emanuel follows the President's Commission in seeking to address several separate questions by reference to the diagnosis of death, whereas the approach suggested here would adopt a single and uniform definition of death, and then seek to resolve questions around organ donation on a different ethical and legal foundation.

Emanuel's proposal also provides another illustration of the problems encountered when a variety of diverse issues all hinge upon the definition of death. Under her scheme, some individuals would undoubtedly opt for a definition of death based on the "higher bound" of the permanent vegetative state in order to permit the donation of their vital organs if they should develop this condition. However, few of these individuals would probably agree to being cremated while still breathing, even if they were vegetative. Most likely, they would not want to be cremated until after they had sustained a cardiorespiratory arrest. Once again, this creates the awkward and confusing necessity of diagnosing death for one purpose (organ donation) but not for another (cremation). Only by abandoning the concept of brain death is it possible to adopt a definition of death that is valid for all purposes, while separating questions of organ donation from dependence upon the life/death dichotomy.

TURNING BACK

The tension between the need to maintain workable and practical standards for the procurement of transplantable organs and our desire to have a conceptually coherent account of death is an issue that must be given serious attention. Resolving these inconsistencies by moving toward a higher-brain definition of death would most likely create additional practical problems regarding accurate diagnosis as well as introduce concepts that are highly counterintuitive to the general public. Uncoupling the link between organ transplantation and brain death, on the other hand, offers a number of advantages. By shifting the ethical foundations for organ donation to the principles of nonmaleficence and consent, the pool of potential donors may be substantially increased. In addition, by reverting to a simpler and more traditional definition of death, the long-standing debate over fundamental inconsistencies in the concept of brain death may finally be resolved.

The most difficult challenge for this proposal would be to gain acceptance of the view that killing may sometimes be a justifiable necessity for procuring transplantable organs. Careful attention to the principles of consent and nonmaleficence should provide an adequate bulwark against slippery slope concerns that this practice would be extended in unforeseen and unacceptable ways. Just as the euthanasia debate often seems to turn less upon abstract theoretical concerns and more upon the empirical question of whether guidelines for assisted dying would be abused, so the success of this proposal could also rest upon factual questions of societal acceptance and whether this approach would erode respect for human life and the integrity of clinicians. While the answers to these questions are not known, the potential benefits of this proposal make it worthy of continued discussion and debate.

REFERENCES

1. Some of the more notable critiques include Robert M. Veatch, "The Whole Brain-Oriented Concept of Death. An Outmoded Philosophical Formulation," *Journal of Thanatology* 3 (1975): 13-30; Michael B. Green and Daniel Wikler, "Brain Death and Personal Identity," *Philosophy and Public Affairs* 9 (1980): 105-33; Stuart J. Youngner and Edward T. Bartlett, "Human Death and High Technology: The Failure of the Whole-Brain Formulations," *Annals of Internal Medicine* 99 (1983): 252–58; Amir Halevy and Baruch Brody, "Brain Death: Reconciling Definitions, Criteria, and Tests," *Annals of Internal Medicine* 119 (1993): 519-25.

2. Stuart J. Youngner, "Defining Death: A Superficial and Fragile Consensus," *Archives of Neurology* 49 (1992): 570-72.

3. President's Commission for the Study of Ethical Problems in Medicine and Biomedical and Behavioral Research, *Defining Death* (Washington, D.C.: Government Printing Office, 1981).

4. Karen Gervais has been especially articulate in defining these levels. See Karen G. Gervais, *Redefining Death* (New Haven: Yale University Press, 1986); "Advancing the Definition of Death: A Philosophical Essay," *Medical Humanities Review* 3, no. 2 (1989): 7-19.

5. James L. Bernat, Charles M. Culver, and Bernard Gert, "On the Definition and Criterion of Death," *Annals of Internal Medicine* 94 (1981): 389-94; James L Bernat, "How Much of the Brain Must Die in Brain Death?" *Journal of Clinical Ethics* 3 (1992): 21-26.

6. Report of the Medical Consultants on the Diagnosis of Death, "Guidelines for the Determination of Death," *JAMA* 246 (1981): 2184-86.

7. Aspects of this analysis have been explored previously in, Robert D. Truog and James C. Fackler, "Rethinking Brain Death," *Critical Care Medicine* 20 (1992): 1705-13; Halevy and Brody, "Brain Death."

8. H. Schrader et al., "Changes of Pituitary Hormones in Brain Death," *Acta Neurochirurgica* 52 (1980): 239-48; Kristen M. Outwater and Mark A. Rockoff, "Diabetes Insipidus Accompanying Brain Death in Children," *Neurology* 34 (1984): 1243-46; James C. Fackler, Juan C. Troncoso, and Frank R. Gioia, "Age-Specific Characteristics of Brain Death in Children," *American Journal of Diseases of Childhood* 142 (1988): 999-1003.

9. Schrader et al., "Changes of Pituitary Hormones in Brain Death"; H. J. Gramm et al.,"Acute Endocrine Failure after Brain Death," *Transplantation* 54 (1992): 851-57.

10. Report of Medical Consultants on the Diagnosis of Death, "Guidelines for the Determination of Death": 339.

11. Madeleine M. Grigg et al., "Electroencephalographic Activity after Brain Death," *Archives of Neurology* 44 (1987): 948-54; A. Earl Walker, *Cerebral Death*, 2nd ed. (Baltimore: Urban & Schwarzenberg, 1981), pp. 89-90; and Christopher Pallis, "ABC of Brain Stem Death. The Arguments about the EEG," *British Medical Journal [Clinical Research]* 286 (1983): 284-87.

12. Ernst Rodin et al., "Brainstem Death," *Clinical Electroencephalography* 16 (1985): 63-71.

13. Randall C. Wetzel et al., "Hemodynamic Responses in Brain Dead Organ Donor Patients," *Anesthesia and Analgesia* 64 (1985): 125–28; S. H. Pennefather, J. H. Dark, and R. E. Bullock, "Haemodynamic Responses to Surgery in Brain-Dead Organ Donors," *Anaesthesia* 48 (1993): 1034–38; and D. J. Hill, R. Munglani, and D. Sapsford, "Haemodynamic Responses to Surgery in Brain-Dead Organ Donors," *Anaesthesia* 49 (1994): 835-36.

14. Bernat, "How Much of the Brain Must Die in Brain Death?"

15. Paul A. Byrne, Sean O'Reilly, and Paul M. Quay, "Brain Death—An Opposing Viewpoint," *JAMA* 242 (1979): 1985–90.

16. Gaetano F. Molinari, "The NINCDS Collaborative Study of Brain Death: A Historical Perspective," in U.S. Department of Health and Human Services, *NINCDS monograph No. 24, NIH publication No. 81-2286* (1980): 1-32.

17. Pallis, "ABC of Brain Stem Death," pp. 123-24; Bryan Jennett and Catherine Hessett, "Brain Death in Britain as Reflected in Renal Donors," *British Medical Journal* 283 (1981): 359-62; Peter M. Black, "Brain Death (first of two parts)," *NEJM* 299 (1978): 338-44.

18. President's Commission, *Defining Death*.

19. "An Appraisal of the Criteria of Cerebral Death, A Summary Statement: A Collaborative Study," *JAMA* 237 (1977): 982-86.

20. Green and Wikler, "Brain Death and Personal Identity."

21. President's Commission, *Defining Death*.

22. Green and Wikler, "Brain Death and Personal Identity"; Daniel Wikler, "Brain Death: A Durable Consensus?" *Bioethics* 7 (1993): 239-46.

23. David R. Field et al., "Maternal Brain Death During Pregnancy: Medical and Ethical issues," *JAMA* 260 (1988): 816–22; Masanobu Washida et al., "Beneficial Effect of Combined 3,5,3'-Triiodothyronine and Vasopressin Administration on Hepatic Energy Status and Systemic Hemodynamics after Brain Death," *Transplantation* 54 (1992): 44-49.

24. Stuart J. Youngner et al., "'Brain Death' and Organ Retrieval: A Cross-Sectional Survey of Knowledge and Concepts among Health Professionals," *JAMA* 261 (1989): 2205-10.

25. Daniel Wikler and Alan J. Weisbard, "Appropriate Confusion over 'Brain Death,'" *JAMA* 261 (1989): 2246.

26. Margareta Sanner, "A Comparison of Public Attitudes toward Autopsy, Organ Donation, and Anatomic Dissection: A Swedish Survey," *JAMA* 271 (1994): 284–88, at 287.

27. Green and Wikler, "Brain Death and Personal Identity."

28. Robert M. Arnold and Stuart Youngner, "The Dead Donor Rule: Should We Stretch It, Bend It, or Abandon It?" *Kennedy Institute of Ethics Journal* 3 (1993): 263-278.

29. Some of the many works defending this view include: Green and Wikler, "Brain Death and Personal Identity"; Gervais, *Redefining Death*; Truog and Fackler, "Rethinking Brain Death"; and Robert M. Veatch, *Death, Dying, and the Biological Revolution* (New Haven: Yale University Press, 1989).

30. The Multi-Society Task Force on PVS, "Medical Aspects of the Persistent Vegetative State," *NEJM* 330 (1994): 1499-1508 and 1572-79; D. Alan Shewmon, "Anencephaly: Selected Medical Aspects," *Hastings Center Report* 18, no. 5 (1988): 11-19.

31. Nancy L. Childs and Walt N. Mercer, "Brief Report: Late Improvement in Consciousness after Post-Traumatic Vegetative State," *NEJM* 334 (1996): 24-25; James L Bernat, "The Boundaries of the Persistent Vegetative State," *Journal of Clinical Ethics* 3 (1992): 176-80.

32. Medical Task Force on Anencephaly, "The Infant with Anencephaly," *NEJM* 322 (1990): 669-74; Shewmon, "Anencephaly: Selected Medical Aspects."

33. Jeffrey R. Botkin and Stephen G. Post, "Confusion in the Determination of Death: Distinguishing Philosophy from Physiology," *Perspectives in Biology and Medicine* 36 (1993): 129-38.

34. The Multi-Society Task Force on PVS, "Medical Aspects of the Persistent Vegetative State."

35. Marcia Angell, "After Quinlan: The Dilemma of the Persistent Vegetative State," *NEJM* 330 (1994): 1524-25.

36. Wikler, "Brain Death: A Durable Consensus?"

37. President's Commission, *Defining Death,* p. 84.

38. Report of the Ad Hoc Committee of the Harvard Medical School to Examine the Definition of Brain Death, "A Definition of Irreversible Coma," *JAMA* 205 (1968): 337-40.

39. "University of Pittsburgh Medical Center Policy and Procedure Manual: Management of Terminally Ill Patients Who May Become Organ Donors after Death," *Kennedy Institute of Ethics Journal* 3 (1993): Al-AI5; Stuart Youngner and Robert Arnold, "Ethical, Psychosocial, and Public Policy Implications of Procuring Organs from Non-Heart-Beating Cadaver Donors," *JAMA* 269 (1993): 2769-74. Of note, the June 1993 issue of the *Kennedy Institute of Ethics Journal* is devoted to this topic in its entirety.

40. Joanne Lynn, "Are the Patients Who Become Organ Donors Under the Pittsburgh Protocol for 'Non-Heart-Beating Donors' Really Dead?" *Kennedy Institute of Ethics Journal* 3 (1993): 167-78.

41. Joyce L. Peabody, Janet R. Emery, and Stephen Ashwal, "Experience with Anencephalic Infants as Prospective Organ Donors," *NEJM* 321 (1989): 344-50.

42. See for example, Norman Fost, "The New Body Snatchers: On Scott's 'The Body as Property,' *American Bar Foundation Research Journal* 3 (1983): 718-32; John A. Robertson, "Relaxing the Death Standard for Organ Donation in Pediatric Situations," *Technology: Ethical, Legal, and Public Policy Issues,* ed. D. Mathieu (Boulder, Col.: Westview Press, 1988), pp. 69-76; Arnold and Youngner, "The Dead Donor Rule."

43. AMA Council on Ethical and Judicial Affairs, "The Use of Anencephalic Neonates as Organ Donors," *JAMA* 273 (1995): 1614-18. After extensive debate among AMA members, the Council retracted this position statement. See Charles W. Plows, "Reconsideration of AMA Opinion on Anencephalic Neonates as Organ Donors," *JAMA* 275 (1996): 443-44.

44. Youngner et al., "'Brain Death' and Organ Retrieval."

45. Jiro Nudeshima, "Obstacles to Brain Death and Organ Transplantation in Japan," *Lancet* 338 (1991): 1063-64.

46. Robert S. Olick, "Brain Death, Religious Freedom, and Public Policy: New Jersey's Landmark Legislative Initiative," *Kennedy Institute of Ethics Journal* 1 (1991): 275-88.

47. Linda L. Emanuel, "Reexamining Death: The Asymptotic Model and a Bounded Zone Definition," *Hastings Center Report* 25, no. 4 (1995): 27-35.

3. Ethical Issues in Living Related Donor Liver Transplantation

R. W. Strong and S. V. Lynch

The quest to save life and stave off death are traditional goals in medicine. The scientific and clinical endeavors in transplantation in the last half of this century have seen these goals come to fruition for many patients. Commensurate with these milestones "a new dimension of urgency and finality"[1] was born. There is little wonder that the law of the land and the ethical issues lag behind the rapid advances and that the pace-setting activities by the few have outstripped comprehension and acceptance by the many.

Over many centuries the Western practice of medicine has been committed to the Hippocratic principle, to act in the patient's best medical interest, irrespective of outside influences. This doctor-patient relationship has been eloquently enunciated by Starzl.[2] "It is doubtful if many doctors who actually care for the sick and the infirm, plan their actions on the basis of the predicted effect upon society. Instead, the dominant tradition is for the physician to provide the best care of which he is capable for those who either seek his services or are assigned to his responsibility; by and large this is done without regard for the conceivably broader issue of whether treatment is justifiable on social grounds. His reasons may include pride, altruism, compassion, curiosity, a spirit of competition, even avarice, or a combination of all these things. The foregoing viewpoint is a narrow one, but there is no reason to believe that it should be abandoned in the face of advancing technocracy. It has shielded the ill from the caprices and moral judgements of other men through centuries of evolving philosophical, religious, and legal doctrines. It has placed the concept of the sanctity of human life on a practical foundation since the respon-

Originally published in *Transplantation Proceedings* 28, no. 4 (August 1966): 2366–69. Reprinted by permission of Appleton & Lange, Inc.

sibility of one person for another could not be more clearly defined than through the doctor-patient relationship, irrespective of the reasons for the contract entered into between the two involved parties."

The Hippocratic tradition is "relentlessly militantly individualistic. It is as if in all the world there was only one physician and one patient."[3] There appears to be an ever-increasing conflict between the desire to represent the patients' interests above all outside influences and the total social benefit where the aggregate good for patients as a whole, is maximized. With the development of modern medicine, the old guidelines of paternalism and individualism are being overtaken by a social ethical goal in which the basic social philosophy of the broader society will ultimately make the choice of the ethical principles employed.[3] However, social conscience is not a guarantee for ethical behavior and it is important that those medical practitioners most closely involved need to participate in these deliberations, as part of a society to which they belong together with their ability to make contributions by virtue of their medical expertise. Medical ethics is a growth industry and it needs the involvement of medical practitioners to add reality.

Since the first successful living related kidney transplant was performed in 1954, there has been a considerable amount of ethical debate. Medical ethics guides medical practitioners by a code of conduct that encompasses the principles of patient autonomy, justice, beneficence, and non-maleficence. The principle of non-maleficence, "above all, do no harm," is obviously at variance with the practice of using living donors for organ transplantation. The procedure to remove an organ from a healthy donor, not to improve the health of the donor but to benefit another, differs from all other surgical procedures. How can one reconcile this predicament? Does a potential donor own his own organs and does autonomy allow removal if he so desires? Nobody owns their organs and the State limits the individual's autonomy over them. You can legally refuse all medical treatment even if this causes great risk to your life and you can prostitute your body for financial gain, but you do not own your organs. In many ways, your personal autonomy is overridden by State paternalism.[4]

Catholic theologians, in considering the earlier precepts of the Church that had forbidden individuals any authority upon parts of their bodies other than when directed to their natural purpose, concluded that "human existence would be impossible if morality were to forbid all actions which could endanger our life, health, or physical integrity. Indeed, one admires the individual who throws himself into the water to save his drowning fellow man, and there is assuredly nothing immoral about the desire to accept a limited risk in order to save a loved one from certain death."[5]

Schreiner, in considering the physical well-being of a kidney donor and the basic principle of autonomy, stated, "if giving a kidney is for his spiritual or psychological good, and this is recognized as part of a total person, the particular mutilation would seem to be permissible under the extension of the physical totality to the totality of a person. But we cannot extend the principle of totality to society in general."[6]

The major role of the transplant surgeon should be to decide whether the process is justifiable on the basis of low risk to the potential donor and a reasonable probability of success for the recipient. In the early period of renal transplantation, it was impossible to predict the result with any degree of certainty in an individual case and discussion revolved around the risk-benefit of the procedure. The donor was required to accept the immediate operative and unknown long-term consequences in order to achieve a potential long-term gain for the recipient. If the result of a kidney transplant was a one-year graft survival of, say less than 25 percent, then surely the risk-benefit was far greater than if the graft survival was more than 80 percent, and it seemed unacceptable to subject the living donor to the procedure. Even forty years after the first living related kidney transplant, it is impossible to elucidate the likelihood of risks that may be incurred by the donor patient (eg, renal trauma, renal tumor, hypertension).

Informed consent is an essential prerequisite. The potential donor must:[7]
1. Understand the procedure and the risks and *imponderables*
2. Not be coerced
3. Provide a voluntary answer
4. Be mentally competent and of legal age

The gradual improvement in results over the years is reflected in five-year graft survival of around 90 percent in major centers, and according to Bonomini, living donor kidney transplantation when performed under strict ethical and medical guidelines is a necessary and acceptable practice with low risk to the donor and high benefit for the recipient.[8] The contrary view has been taken by Michielsen, who believes the risks for the donor are out of proportion to the benefit for the recipient and the only reason for using living donors would be the shortage of cadaver donors.[9] The reality is, of course, that the greatest obstacle to transplantation programs is the shortage of cadaver donor organs, which means that living related organ donation is not obsolete.

In liver transplant programs, the challenge of the shortage of size-matched whole liver grafts for pediatric patients was met by the innovative introduction of reduced-size grafts from adult cadaver donors. As experience increased, the results proved to be equivalent to those achieved with whole liver grafts and even superior when applied to small infants. However, the reduction in waiting list mortality was offset by an increase in the number of adults awaiting transplantation. The redistribution rather than expansion of the resource would be of questionable value, when accompanied by an increase in adult waiting list mortality.

The use of liver partition to produce two grafts—the right hemi-liver for an adult and the left segmental graft for a child—appeared to overcome the obvious disadvantage of discarding a portion of the allograft. The early results were less than satisfactory. Poor donor organ selection and anatomic variation negated the possibility of providing two suitable grafts in many cases and necessitated compromise. The conversion of an elective patient to an urgent retransplantation candidate because of technical failure risked the patient's life and devalued the very reason for performing split-liver transplants: to increase the organ supply. It was considered that the procedure was not justified in elective patients unless the donor anatomy permitted division into two grafts, without compromise.[10] The increasing discrepancy between the supply and demand for donor livers has seen a gradual increase in the use of the method, particularly in Europe, where the results achieved are equivalent to those reported for whole liver and reduced-size grafts by the European Transplant Registry.[11] In Brisbane, experience with 20 split-liver transplants (unpublished data) has yielded equivalent results to those achieved in the total program.

The concept of partial liver transplantation from a living donor evolved from the experience with liver resection for a variety of disease processes, together with the experience in transplantation of reduced-size and split-liver grafts from cadaveric donors. The performance of a safe partial hepatectomy with maintenance of hepatic function and avoidance of injury to both the donor and to the allograft is mandatory. The risk to the donor is that associated with a major operation in the form of perioperative complications and long-term sequelae. The only benefit is a psychological one. The risk for the recipient is comparable to that experienced with the use of a reduced-size graft as obtained from liver partition for split-liver transplantation. The perceived benefits for the recipient, when transplanted electively, are a reduction in pretransplant mortality, avoidance of pretransplant debilitating complications, and deterioration, which severely compromises the chance of success after transplantation and the uniform good quality of the graft.[12] The originally proposed theoretical immunologic advantage has proved to be erroneous.

Should an elective living related liver transplant (LRLT) be performed in preference to a cadaver donor transplant? There is no single answer to this question. Circumstances vary from country to country. The basis of any answer must be that there is some measurable advantage for the recipient or the use of a living donor is not justified. Although the results of LRLT reported so far are excellent, there are no controlled studies comparing one with the other and no data, therefore, to show a measurable advantage. There may be a measurable advantage for liver transplant programs overall. The increased supply of donor organs resulting from the introduction of LRLT not only reduces the waiting list mortality, but allows other patients to receive a cadaver donor organ at an earlier period than they would have otherwise achieved and prior to severe deterioration, with the potential for improved posttransplant survival.

Proposing the argument that LRLT gives an overall benefit to liver transplant programs is ethically unacceptable. The principle of individual totality, physically and spiritually, does not extend to society in general. As stated by Schreiner, "the principle of totality can pertain only to the individual person and not to a group."[6] The voluntary consent of a potential donor must be truly informed consent. It needs to include an assessment of the recipient's potential to receive a cadaver organ and the likely time frame with respect to others on the waiting list. The decision by the potential donor must be in relationship to his or her particular loved one and not to the need to increase the organ supply. There may be a powerful motivation of love and altruism by parents toward their child and this is commendable, but transplant surgeons must not allow them to be inflicted by undue hazards. Although the risk for the donor in LRLT is as yet unknown, there has been one donor death reported[13] and morbidity of 3 percent to 17 percent in reported series.[14] It would be expected that it would be at least commensurate with that experienced in living related kidney transplantation—mortality 0.06 percent and medical morbidity 2 percent to 10 percent. In the early report from Kyoto, 41 percent of donors had complaints such as fatigue, wound pain, gastritis, and duodenal ulcer.[15] The disturbing number of psychosocial problems experienced by families in the early series from Chicago reported by Whitington et al.[12] adds credence to the notion that there are significant risks and concerns for the welfare of the donor and the family.

Is it possible to gain a valid consent? Busuttil in 1991 doubted that it was possible: "How can a parent be expected to make an informed, uncoerced, free choice when asked to consider donating an organ to his/her dying child? In this emotionally charged arena, there is a fine line between asking for the donation, and compelling the parent to donate."[16] In 1995, the same author reported his experience with nine LRLTs and concluded "we believe that living donor liver transplantation has the potential to emerge as the preferred treatment option for paediatric patients in need of liver transplantation for whom it is an option."[17] There was no reference to doubts about obtaining a valid consent, which presumably is now possible.

It would appear from recent publications that there has been an increased use of LRLT procedures in Europe and the United States.[14,17,18] The early reservations, skepticism, and even condemnation appears to have been replaced by cautious optimism and even enthusiasm. Success is a major factor in the acceptance of a new therapeutic endeavor. Recognition of the success of the procedure, coupled with an increased discrepancy between the supply and the demand for liver grafts from brain-dead donors, have been instrumental in the more widespread implementation of the procedure. Human need can cause a change in attitude and values.[19] The ethical issues have not changed; medical acceptance has changed.

The notion that LRLT is necessary because of the relative scarcity of the precious resource (the donor organ) has been questioned by McMaster and Czerniak.[20] They argued that in Europe many cadaver donor livers were not being used because of organizational problems and that the perceived shortage was not as great as had been proposed. For the moment, let us assume that there is a major shortfall in the availability of donor livers to meet the needs of patients awaiting a liver transplant. What about the other side of the equation? Is the expanding transplant activity justified? Here, the bioethical principle of justice needs to expounded. Surely, with a scarce resource, justice demands optimal use for maximal social and patient benefit. The pressures on individual transplant program development and continued viability have resulted in numbers of candidates for transplantation being accepted, where recurrent disease leaves little prospect of survival beyond a limited, finite period. It is a moral imperative that there be an efficient use of the limited resource and justice is very much in question with some of the decision-making processes. Is there a fair selection of candidates, given the scarce resource? To be worthy of trust, we must be honest. It is society that empowers us to act and their scrutiny and judgment of our activities may not be able to be defended. Before an argument can be made to expand LRLT activity, transplant programs must put their houses in order, with justice being done and seen to be done.

Is LRLT an option in an urgent situation? The overwhelming desire of parents to save their child can blind them to the potential dangers, which they may, at that time, consider irrelevant. The element of urgency removes time for reflection and reconsideration, which are basic steps in living donor renal programs. An evaluation of the likely outcome must be made. As gate-keepers, the transplant team must not allow heroic parents to participate in an unworthy enterprise, where the chance of survival of the recipient is poor. "The desperation of illness never justifies the infliction of a hopeless remedy."[21] If there is no alternative and analysis indicates that the prognosis for the recipient's recovery is reasonably good, with likely minimal harm to the donor, it seems reasonable to agree to the parents' strong motivation to participate. The "statistics of probability" is used as an aid in providing a solution to a humanistic problem.[21]

Although there have been more than 500 LRLTs performed worldwide, approximately half have been formed in countries where organ transplantation from brain-dead donors is not practiced or almost nonexistent. With no alternative, the community acceptance living of organ donation is high, and declining to be a donor for loved one in such an environment would be exceptional, bordering on martyrdom. The transplant surgeons in these countries have embraced the concept with prodigious fervor, but it may have been a retrograde step for the progress of transplantation in such communities. Previous concerted efforts to introduce cadaver organ transplantation dissipated somewhat, to the disadvantage of other patients in need, such as potential recipients for heart and most adult liver candidates. Notwithstanding these comments, the rights of individuals to donate or not donate through self-determination, without coercion and armed with all the facts, should be respected.

The obligation of transplant teams who embark on LRLT is to accept the burden of the decision-making process, the advice and the outcome of the procedure. The motivation must not be self-interest but to do what is right and good. Scientific progress has propelled us toward deity before we have had time to become men and it is incumbent on us to maintain integrity and seek the moral high ground. To do less is to abrogate our responsibilities and to denigrate our privileged position.

REFERENCES

1. Cowen Z: *Med J Aust* 2:627, 1968.
2. Starzl TE: *Ann Int Med* 67 suppl 32: 1967.
3. Veatch RM: In Land W, Dossetor JB (eds): *Organ Replacement Therapy: Ethics, Justice, Commerce.* Berlin, Springer-Verlag, p 3, 1990.
4. Dossetor JB: Emerging ethical issues in transplantation. *Proceedings, First Canadian Symposium on Multi-organ Transplantation.* p 131, 1988.
5. Hamburger J, Crosnier J: In Rapaport F, Dausset J (eds): *Human Transplantation.* Orlando, Grune & Stratton, p 37, 1968.
6. Schreiner GE: In Wolstenholme G, O'Connor M (eds): *Law and Ethics in Transplantation.* London, Churchill, p 130, 1968.
7. Diethelm A: *Ann Surg* 211:505, 1990.
8. Bonomini V: In Land W, Dossetor JB (eds): *Organ Replacement Therapy: Ethics, Justice, Commerce.* Berlin, Springer-Verlag, p 25, 1990
9. Michielsen P: In Land W, Dossetor JB (eds): *Organ Replacement Therapy: Ethics, Justice, Commerce.* Berlin, Springer-Verlag, p 32, 1990.
10. Lynch SV, Strong RW, Ong TH, et al: *Transplant Rev* 6:89, 1992.
11. de Ville de Goyet: *J Transplant* 59:137, 1995.
12. Whitington PF, Siegler M, Broelsch CE: In Land W, Dossetor JB (eds): *Organ Replacement Therapy: Ethics, Justice, Commerce.* Berlin, Springer-Verlag, p 117, 1990.
13. Broelsch CE, Burdelski M, Rogiers X, et al: *Hepatology* 20(suppl 1):495, 1994
14. Slooff MJH: *Transplant Int* 8:65, 1995.
15. Marimoto T, Yamaoka Y, Tanaka K, et al: *N Engl J Med* 329:363, 1993.
16. Busuttil RW: *Transplant Proc* 23:43, 1991.
17. Jurim O, Shackelton CR, McDiarmid SV, et al: *Am J Surg* 169:529, 1995
18. Otte JB: *Transplant Int* 8:69, 1995.
19. Hunt R, Arras J: *Ethical Issues in Modem Medicine.* Palo Alto, C.A. Mayfield, p 2, 1977.
20. McMaster P, Czerniak A: In Land W, Dossetor JB (eds): *Organ Replacement Therapy: Ethics, Justice, Commerce.* Berlin, Springer-Verlag, p 130, 1990.
21. Moore FD: *Transplant Proc* 20:1061, 1988.

4. Kidney Transplantation from Unrelated Living Donors: Time to Reclaim a Discarded Opportunity

Andrew S. Levey, Susan Hou, and Harry L. Bush Jr.

Before dialysis therapy was routinely available in the United States, both related and unrelated living donors were accepted for renal transplantation. By 1965, data from the Registry in Human Kidney Transplantation indicated that the success of kidney transplantation from unrelated living donors and from cadaveric donors was similar.[1] With the increasing availability of dialysis, most centers discouraged transplantation from poorly matched living donors on the premise that a cadaveric kidney provides an equal benefit to the recipient, without risk to a living donor. In the past twenty years, the results of transplantation have improved to such an extent that today this therapy is a safe, effective, routine treatment for end-stage renal disease. Nevertheless, living persons who are not related to the recipient are still rejected as potential kidney donors. It is now time to reevaluate the ethical and medical justifications for this policy. For the reasons outlined below, we suggest that transplantation from unrelated living donors is an acceptable practice and that for many patients on dialysis, it may be the preferred treatment.

There has been a spectacular improvement in the outcome of cadaveric kidney transplantation from unrelated donors as a result of advances in immunologic management, including HLA matching, blood transfusions, and immunosuppression with cyclosporine.[2-4] Patient survival after one year is now approximately 90 percent and is equal to or greater than survival in patients on dialysis. First-year graft survival is 75 to 85 percent in many centers, and the quality of life for patients with functioning grafts is superior to the quality of life for patients on dialysis.[5,6] Thus, cadaveric transplantation

Originally published in *The New England Journal of Medicine* 314, no. 14 (April 3, 1986): 914-16. Copyright © 1986 Massachusetts Medical Society. All rights reserved.

TABLE I. DIALYSIS AND TRANSPLANTATION
IN THE UNITED STATES, 1980 TO 1984.*

Year	New Dialysis Patients During Year	Transplantations From Living Related Donors During Year	Cadaveric Transplantations During Year	Patients on Dialysis at Year End	Patients Awaiting Transplants at Year End
1980	19,687	1275	3422	52,364	5072
1981	21,367	1458	3427	58,924	5773
1982	22,797	1677	3681	65,765	6720
1983	24,218	1796	4333	71,961	7137
1984	27,113	1704	5264	78,479	8562

*Source of data is the End-Stage Renal Disease Network Coordinating Council.[7]

should now be considered routinely for most young and middle-aged patients with renal failure.

However, the supply of cadaveric kidneys is not adequate to meet the demand. As shown in Table 1, the rate of kidney transplantation lags far behind the incidence of end-stage renal disease.[7] As the incidence of end-stage renal disease continues to rise, and as the success of transplantation improves, the demand for cadaveric kidneys will also increase. There is no indication that the supply of kidneys will increase to meet this growing demand.[8] The chief obstacles to organ procurement are physician failure to refer potential donors and family refusal to consent to organ donation. The result is that only 15 percent of potential cadaveric donors provide organs for transplantation. Efforts to increase referrals have achieved only limited success, and only about 50 percent of the population is willing to donate.[9,10] It is not known to what extent the recently enacted National Organ Transplant Act (P.L. 98-507) will increase donations. On the other hand, lowering highway speed limits, raising the legal drinking age, enforcing strict drunk-driving laws, and requiring the use of seat belts and child-restraint devices have reduced the number of fatal motor-vehicle accidents and may reduce the potential supply of cadaveric donor organs.[11,12]

In principle, the success of transplantation from living unrelated donors should be equal or superior to the success of cadaveric transplantation, for several reasons. First, the detrimental effects of poor HLA matching occur in both instances.[13,14] Although good matches can sometimes be achieved in cadaveric transplantation, the selection of recipients for cadaveric kidneys on the basis of HLA matching requires a large pool of potential recipients, and it increases the waiting time for transplantation.[15] Even large cooperative organ-sharing programs can find well-matched kidneys for only a minority of patients.[14]

Second, the beneficial effects of blood transfusions from unspecified donors before transplantation should apply equally to transplantations from cadaveric donors and living unrelated donors. However, donor-specific transfusions before transplantation, which improve graft survival dramatically, are possible only when the donors are living.[16]

Third, immunosuppression can be initiated before transplantation from a living unrelated donor, but not until the time of the surgery in transplantation from a cadaveric donor. Laboratory studies have shown that immunosuppressive techniques appear to be more effective when they are begun before transplantation.[17] Moreover, some approaches, such as total-lymphoid irradiation,[18] must be initiated before surgery.

Fourth, complications such as donor hypotension, technical errors during nephrectomy, and renal injury during preservation, which may occur during procurement of cadaveric kidneys, are associated with renal ischemia and compromised graft function. Such complications occur far less frequently in transplantations from living donors.

Fifth, with a living donor, the transplantation can be planned in advance, thus ensuring that the recipient's medical condition is optimal and reducing the possibility of intraoperative and postoperative complications. The advantages of a planned transplantation are particularly important for patients who require bilateral nephrectomies before the procedure.

In summary, the potential advantages of transplantations from living related donors may lead to superior graft function and survival. Indeed, preliminary studies have shown the results of these procedures to be excellent, whether or not donor-specific transfusions are used.[19-22]

The risks of nephrectomy to the donor are minimal. Studies of kidney donors up to twenty years after nephrectomy have defined the consequences of kidney donation.[23-27] Death during the operation is extremely rare; it occurs in only 0.03 percent of procedures—one death in 3,200 operations (Hebert L: personal communication). Major, but temporary, morbidity occurs in 2 to 3 percent of donors. The complications include deep wound infections, pulmonary emboli, and bleeding requiring reoperation. In addition, 10 to 20 percent of patients have superficial wound infections, pulmonary and urinary infections, pneumothorax, or other minor problems. The long-term effects on the renal function of donors have also been studied. Renal failure from "hyperfiltration" in the remaining kidney has not been reported. Generally, serum creatinine levels stabilize at slightly increased values (by 0.1 to 0.3 mg per decaliter), and urinary excretion of protein increases slightly (by 50 to 100 mg per day). The blood pressure is slightly higher than before nephrectomy (by approximately 5 mm Hg), and 10 to 20 percent of donors have mild hypertension that is controlled with medication—a prevalence of hypertension similar to that in the general population. Studies of the effects of nephrectomy on the donor have been criticized for the lack of appropriate control populations for comparison; nonetheless, even the most careful scrutiny reaffirms the long-held belief in the safety of donor nephrectomy.

In fact, the benefits of organ donation to the donor may be considerable. Studies of kidney donors who are related to the recipient have revealed that they experience long-lasting positive feelings about their decision to donate, regardless of the success of the transplantation.[28,29] Many donors report an increased self-esteem and sense of worth. In addition, some report an indirect benefit from the improved health of the recipient.

These considerations suggest that for many patients, kidney transplantation from unrelated living donors may be medically and ethically justifiable. Although the number of potential donors is not known, the number of recipients who might benefit from such transplantations is very large (Table 1). We propose that it is time to take up this debate again, to study carefully the results of the transplantations of this type that have already been performed, and to establish guidelines for this practice. We think that well-informed adults are able to evaluate the risks and benefits of kidney donation and to decide for themselves whether to offer the "gift of life." The current practice of rejecting unrelated living donors seems overprotective and denies important benefits to both the donors and the recipients.

We expect that potential unrelated donors would be spouses or others who have a close personal relationship with the recipient and who would initially be approached by the recipient. Alternatively, for persons who wished to donate to an unknown recipient, a national program could be established to match potential donors and recipients on the basis of objective medical and immunologic criteria. The acceptance of unrelated living donors would raise the specter of persons being coerced to donate. However, two safeguards can protect the welfare of potential donors. First, professional associations of physicians who are involved in transplantations have established firm guidelines that condemn coercion and the offering of financial rewards to obtain organs for transplantation, and that threaten the expulsion of members engaging in such practices.[30,31] Moreover, the National Organ Transplant Act specifically forbids the sale of human organs. Second, individual physicians must exercise heightened vigilance in accepting unrelated donors. Such donors should undergo careful evaluations to assess their motives, their relationship with the potential recipient, their understanding of the risks and benefits of kidney donation, and the voluntary nature of their decision. A donor advocate—someone who is not involved in the care of the recipient—should be appointed, and written informed consent to the donation should be obtained. Currently, these procedures are followed routinely in the evaluation of potential related living donors.

In our view, transplantation from an unrelated living donor is indicated for patients in whom transplantation is recommended but for whom neither a living related donor nor a cadaveric donor is available. This approach may also be considered as an alternative to cadaveric transplantation for selected patients in whom a planned transplant operation would provide an advantage—i.e., those who would benefit from donor-specific transfusions or other pretransplantation immunosuppression, those who require pretransplantation bilateral nephrectomies, and those who choose to avoid the long wait for a cadaveric organ. The results of transplantations from unrelated living donors should be studied carefully to guide future practice. In addition to benefiting the recipient and donor, the acceptance of kidneys from unrelated living donors would reduce the demand for cadaveric kidneys and therefore benefit all those who need kidney transplantations.

REFERENCES

1. Barnes BA. Survival data of renal transplantations in patients. *N Engl J Med* 1965; 272:776-9.

2. Levey AS. The improving prognosis after kidney transplantation: new strategies to overcome immunologic rejection. *Arch Intern Med* 1984; 144:2382-7.

3. Terasaki PI, Perdue ST, Sasaki N, Mickey MR, Whitby L. Improving success rates of kidney transplantation. *JAMA* 1983; 250:1065-8.

4. Strom TB. The improving utility of renal transplantation in the management of end-stage renal disease. *Am J Med* 1982; 73:105-24.

5. Johnson JP, McCauley CR, Copley JB The quality of life of hemodialysis and transplant patients. *Kidney Int* 1982; 22:286-91.

6. Evans RW, Manninen DL, Garrison LP Jr, et al. The quality of life of patients with end-stage renal disease. *N Engl J Med* 1985; 312:553-9.

7. End-Stage Renal Disease Network Coordinating Council. *Program report 1984.* Tampa, Fla.: National Forum of End-Stage Renal Disease Networks, 1985.

8. Bart KJ, Macon EJ, Whittier FC, Baldwin RJ, Blount JH. Cadaveric kidneys for transplantation: a paradox of shortage in the face of plenty. *Transplantation* 1981; 31:379-82.

9. Bart KJ, Macon EJ, Humphries AL Jr, et al. Increasing the supply of cadaveric kidneys for transplantation. *Transplantation* 1981; 31:383-7.

10. Manninen DL, Evans RW. Public attitudes and behavior regarding organ donation. *JAMA* 1985; 253:3111-5.

11. Wearing of seat belts reduces car casualties. *Lancet* 1983; 2:1377.

12. Decker MD, Dewey MJ, Hutcheson RH Jr, Schaffner W. The use and efficacy of child restraint devices: the Tennessee experience, 1982 and 1983. *JAMA* 1984; 252:2571-5.

13. Opelz GE. Correlation of HLA matching with kidney graft survival in patients with or without cyclosporine treatment. *Transplantation* 1985; 40:240-3.

14. Sanfilippo F, Vaughn WK, Spees EK, Light JA, LeFor WM. Benefits of HLA-A and HLA-B matching on graft and patient outcome after cadaveric-donor renal transplantation. *N Engl J Med* 1984; 311:358-64.

15. Pliskin JS. On the probability of finding an HL-A- and ABO-compatible cadaver organ for transplantation: the dependency on time. *Transplantation* 1975; 20:181-5.

16. Salvatierra O. Advantages of continued use of kidney transplantation from living donors. *Transplant Proc* 1985; 17:Suppl 2:18-22.

17. Strom TB, Tilney NL. Renal transplantation: clinical aspects. In: Brenner BM, Rector FJ, eds. *The kidney.* Philadelphia: WB Saunders, 1986, pp. 1941-76.

18. Najarian JS, Sutherland DER, Ferguson RM, et al. Total lymphoid irradiation and kidney transplantation: a clinical experience. *Transplant Proc* 1981; 13:417-24.

19. Sollinger HW, Burlingham WJ, Sparks EMF, Glass NR, Belzer FO. Donor-specific transfusions in unrelated and related HLA-mismatched donor-recipient combinations. *Transplantation* 1984; 38:612-5.

20. Anderson CB, Tyler JD, Sicard GA, Anderman CK, Rodney GE, Etheredge EE. Pretreatment of renal allograft recipients with immunosuppression and donor-specific blood. *Transplantation* 1984; 38:664-8.

21. Hoette M, Razany F, Tavora E, et al. Living non-related kidney donors for transplantation. *Kidney Int* 1986; 29:430 (abstract).

22. Berloco P, Alfani D, Famulari A, et al. Utilization of living donor organs for clinical transplantation. *Transplant Proc* 1985; 17:Suppl 2:13-7.

23. Odgen DA. Consequences of renal donation in man. *Am J Kidney Dis* 1983; 2:501-11.

24. Vincenti F, Amend WJC Jr, Kaysen G, et al. Long-term renal function in kidney donors: sustained compensatory hyperfiltration with no adverse effects. *Transplantation* 1983; 36:626-9.

25. Weiland D, Sutherland DER, Chavers B, Simmons RL, Ascher NL, Najarian JS. Information on 628 living-related kidney donors at a single institution, with long-term follow-up in 472 cases. *Transplant Proc* 1984; 16:5-7,

26. Anderson CF, Velosa JA, Frohnert PP, et al. The risks of unilateral nephrectomy: status of kidney donors 10 to 20 years postoperatively. *Mayo Clinic Proc* 1985; 60:367-74.

27. Miller IJ, Suthanthiran M, Riggio RR, et al. Impact of renal donation: long-term clinical and biochemical follow-up of living donors in a single center. *Am J Med* 1985; 79:201-8.

28. Marshall JR, Fellner CH. Kidney donors revisited. *Am J Psychiatry* 1977; 134:575-6.

29. Simmons RG. Long-term reactions of renal recipients and donors. In Levy NB, ed. *Psychonephrology 2: psychological problems in kidney failure and their treatment.* New York: Plenum Press, 1983, pp. 275-87.

30. Council of the Transplantation Society. Commercialisation in transplantation: the problems and some guidelines for practice. *Lancet* 1985; 2:715-6.

31. Carpenter CB, Ettenger RB, Strom TB. "Free-market" approach to organ donation. *N Engl J Med* 1984; 310:395-6.

5. Rights, Symbolism, and Public Policy in Fetal Tissue Transplants

John A. Robertson

Fetal tissue transplants hold great hope for many patients. Extensive work with animal models has shown that human fetal brain cells transplanted into the substantia nigra of monkeys with exogenously produced Parkinson's disease have restored their function. Physicians expect similar results in humans, to the benefit of thousands of patients.[1] Experimental evidence is also strong that fetal islet cell transplants will restore normal insulin function in diabetics.[2] And fetal thymus and liver transplants may have utility for blood and immune system disorders.

CLARIFYING THE ISSUES

As with many issues in bioethics, careful analysis will help elucidate the normative conflict, showing both areas of agreement and irreducible conflict. An essential distinction in the fetal tissue controversy is between procuring tissue from family planning abortions and procuring tissue from abortions performed expressly to provide tissue for transplant. Although opponents of fetal tissue transplants have often conflated the two, tissue from family planning abortions may be used without implying approval of abortions to produce tissue. Indeed, with ample tissue available from family planning abortions, the latter scenario may never occur.

A second important distinction is that between retrieving tissue for transplant from dead and from live fetuses. Only the use of tissue from dead fetuses is at issue. Researchers are not proposing to maintain nonviable

Originally published in *Hastings Center Report* (December 1988). Reproduced by permission. © The Hastings Center.

fetuses ex utero to procure tissue, or to take tissue from them before they are dead, practices that current regulations and law prohibit.[3]

A third set of issues concern tissue procurement procedures. If fetal tissue transplants do occur, questions about the timing, substance, and process of consent must be addressed, as well as the role of nonprofit and for-profit agencies in retrieving and distributing fetal tissue. As with solid organ transplantation, effective tissue procurement may occur without buying and selling fetal tissue.

At present there are few legal barriers to research or therapeutic use of donated fetal tissue for transplant. The Uniform Anatomical Gift Act (UAGA) in all states treats fetal remains like other cadaveric remains and allows next of kin to donate the tissue, though a few states have laws banning experimental use of aborted fetuses.[4] Federal regulations for fetal research, enacted in 1976 after careful study by the National Commission for the Protection of Human Subjects of Biomedical and Behavioral Research, permit research activities "involving the dead fetus, mascerated fetal material or cells, tissue, or organs excised from a dead fetus . . . in accordance with any applicable state or local laws regarding such activities."[5]

The most immediate public policy question is whether these rules should be changed to prohibit experimental or therapeutic fetal tissue transplants, as the most extreme opponents urge. A second public policy issue is whether federal funding of fetal tissue research should occur. A third set of policy issues concerns the circumstances and procedures by which fetal tissue will be retrieved.

TISSUE FROM FAMILY PLANNING ABORTIONS

Fetal tissue transplant research for Parkinson's disease, diabetes, and other disorders will use tissue retrieved from the one and a half million abortions performed annually in the United States to end unwanted pregnancies. Nearly 80 percent of induced abortions are performed between the sixth and eleventh weeks of gestation, at which time neural and other tissue is sufficiently developed to be retrieved and transplanted.[6] Abortions performed at fourteen to sixteen weeks provide pancreatic tissue used in diabetes research, but it may prove possible to use pancreases retrieved earlier.[7]

No need now or in the foreseeable future exists to have a family member conceive and abort to produce fetal tissue. The neural tissue to be transplanted in Parkinson's disease lacks antigenicity, thus obviating the need for a close match between donor and recipient. Fetal pancreas is more antigenetic, but processing can reduce this, also making family connection less important.

The key question is whether women who abort to end unwanted pregnancies may donate the aborted fetuses for use in medical research or therapy by persons who have no connection with or influence on the decision to terminate the pregnancy. One's views on abortion need not determine one's answer to this question, because the abortion and subsequent transplant use are clearly separated. But some opposed to abortion object that transplanting fetal tissue involves complicity in an immoral act and will legitimate and even encourage abortion. Analysis of these concerns will show that they are insufficient to justify a public policy that bans or refuses to fund research or therapy with fetal tissue from induced abortion.

COMPLICITY IN ABORTION

Even proponents of the complicity argument recognize that not all situations of subsequent benefit make one morally complicitous in a prior evil act. For example, James Burtchaell claims that complicity occurs not merely from partaking of benefit but only when one enters into a "supportive alliance" with the underlying evil that makes the benefit possible. He distinguishes "a neutral or even an opponent and an ally" of the underlying evil by "the way in which one does or does not hold oneself apart from the enterprise and its purposes."[8]

On this analysis, a researcher using fetal tissue from an elective abortion is not necessarily an accomplice with the abortionist and woman choosing abortion. The researcher and recipient have no role in the abortion process. They will not have requested it, and may have no knowledge of who performed the abortion or where it occurred since a third-party intermediary will procure the tissue. They may be morally opposed to abortion, and surely are not compromised because they choose to salvage some good from an abortion that will occur regardless of their research or therapeutic goals.

A useful analogy is transplant of organs and tissue from homicide victims. Families of murder victims are often asked to donate organs and bodies for research, therapy, and education. If they consent, organ procurement agencies retrieve the organs and distribute them to recipients. No one would seriously argue that the surgeon who transplants the victim's kidneys, heart, liver, or corneas, or the recipient of the organs, becomes an accomplice in the homicide that made the organs available, even if aware of the source. Nor is the medical student who uses the cadaver of a murder victim to study anatomy.

If organs from murder victims may be used without complicity in the murder that makes the organs available, then fetal remains could also be used without complicity in the abortion. Burtchaell's approach to the problem of complicity assumes that researchers necessarily applaud the underlying act of abortion. But one may benefit from another's evil act without applauding or approving of that evil. X may disapprove of Y's murder of Z, even though X gains an inheritance or a promotion as a result. Indeed, one might even question Burtchaell's assumption that X becomes an accomplice in Y's prior act if he subsequently applauds it. Applauding Y's murder of Z might be insensitive or callous. But that alone would not make one morally responsible for, complicitous in, the murder that has already occurred. In any event, the willingness to derive benefit from another's wrongful death does not create complicity in that death because the beneficiary played no role in causing it.

The complicity argument against use of aborted fetuses often draws an analogy to a perceived reluctance to use the results of unethical medical research carried out by the Nazis. Burtchaell and others have claimed that it would make us retroactively accomplices in the Nazi horrors to use the results of their lethal research.[9] This ignores, however, the clear separation between the perpetrator and beneficiary of the immoral act that breaks the chain of moral complicity for that act.

Thus one could rely on Nazi-generated data while decrying the horrendous acts of Nazi doctors that produced the data. Nor would it necessarily dishonor those unfortunate victims. Indeed, it could reasonably be viewed as retrospectively honoring them by saving others. The Jewish doctors who made systematic studies of starvation in the Warsaw ghetto to reap some good from the evil being done to their brethren were not accomplices in that evil nor are doctors and patients who now benefit from their studies.[10]

If the complicity claim is doubtful when the underlying immorality of the act is clear, as with Nazi-produced data or transplants from murder victims, it is considerably weakened when the act making the benefit possible is legal and its immorality vigorously debated, as is the case with abortion. Even persons opposed to abortion might agree that perceptions of complicity should not determine public policy on fetal tissue transplants.

Legitimizing, Entrenching, and Encouraging Abortion

A second objection is that salvaging tissue for transplant from aborted fetuses will make abortion less morally offensive and more easily tolerated both by individual pregnant women and by society, and perhaps transform it into a morally positive act. This will encourage abortions that would not otherwise occur, and dilute support for reversing the legal acceptability of abortion, in effect creating complicity in future abortions.[11]

But the feared impact on abortion practices and attitudes is highly speculative, particularly at a time when few fetal transplants have occurred. The main motivation for abortion is the desire to avoid the burdens of an unwanted pregnancy. The fact that fetal remains may be donated for transplant will continue to be of little significance in the total array of factors that lead a woman to abort a pregnancy.

Having decided to abort a woman may feel better if she then donates the fetal remains. But this does not show that tissue donation will lead to a termination decision that would not otherwise have occurred, particularly if the decision to abort is made before the opportunity to donate the remains is offered. Perhaps a few more abortions will occur because of the general knowledge that tissue can be donated for transplant, but it is highly unlikely that donation—as opposed to contraceptive practices and sex education—will contribute significantly to the rate of abortion.[12]

Nor does the use of fetal remains for transplant mean that a public otherwise ready to outlaw abortion would refrain from doing so. Legal acceptance of abortion flows from the wide disagreement that exists over early fetal status. If a majority agreed that fetuses should be respected as persons despite the burdens placed on pregnant women, such possible secondary benefits of induced abortion as fetal tissue transplants would not prevent a change in the legality of abortion.

Indeed, one could make the same argument against organ transplants from homicide, suicide, and accident victims. The willingness to use their organs might be seen to encourage or legitimate such deaths, or at least make it harder to enact lower speed limits, seatbelt, gun control, and drunk driving laws to prevent them. After all, the need to prevent murder, suicide, and fatal accidents becomes less pressing if some good to others might come from use of victims' organs for transplant. In either case, the connection is too tenuous and speculative to ban organ or fetal tissue transplants.

In sum, fetal tissue transplants are practically and morally separate from decisions to end unwanted pregnancy. Given that abortion is legal and occurring on a large scale, the willingness to use resulting tissue for transplant neither creates complicity in past abortions nor appears significantly to encourage more future abortions. Such ethical concerns and speculations are not sufficient, given the possible good to others, to justify banning use of fetal tissue for research or therapy.

ABORTING TO OBTAIN TISSUE FOR TRANSPLANT

Central to the argument for transplanting fetal tissue from family planning abortions has been the assumption that the abortion occurs independently of the need for tissue, and that permitting such transplants does not also entail pregnancy and abortion to produce fetal tissue.

But successful tissue transplants may create the need to abort to produce fetal tissue in two future situations. One situation would arise if histocompatability between the fetus and recipient were necessary for effective fetal transplants. Female relatives, spouses, or even unrelated persons might then seek to conceive to provide properly matched fetal tissue for transplant.

The second situation would arise if fetal transplants were so successful that demand far outstripped supply, such as might occur if the treatment were advantageous to most patients with Parkinson's disease and diabetes, or if the number of surgical family planning abortions decreased. Pressure on supply might also occur if tissue from several aborted fetuses were needed to produce one viable transplant.

The hypothetical possibility of such situations is not a sufficient reason to ban all tissue transplants from family planning abortions. But should such abortions be banned if the imagined situations occurred? Most commentators assume that conception and abortion for tissue procurement is so clearly unethical that the prospect hardly merits discussion.[13] Accordingly, they would ban all tissue transplants from related persons and deny the donor the right to designate the recipient of a fetal tissue transplant.

Analysis will show, however, that the question is more ethically complicated than generally assumed, and should not be the driving force in setting policy for tissue transplants from family planning abortions.

A Hypothetical Situation

Consider first the situation where a woman pregnant with her husband's child learns that tissue from her fetus could cure severe neurologic disease in herself or a close relative, such as her husband, child, parent, father or mother-in-law, sibling, or brother or sister-in-law. May she ethically abort the pregnancy to obtain tissue for transplant to the relative? Or may a woman not yet pregnant, conceive a fetus that she will then abort to provide tissue for transplant to herself or to her relative?

To focus analysis on fetal welfare, assume in each case that no other viable tissue source exists, and that the advanced state of neurologic disease has become a major tragedy for the patient and family. The woman has broached the question of abortion to obtain tissue without any direct pressure or inducements from the family or others. Her husband accepts an abortion for transplant purposes if she is willing, but exerts no pressure on her to abort.

The Woman Is Already Pregnant

If the woman is already pregnant, the question is whether a first trimester fetus that would otherwise have been carried to term may be sacrificed to procure tissue for transplant to the woman herself or to a sick family member. The answer depends on the value placed on early fetuses and on the acceptable reasons for abortion. One may distinguish between fetuses that have developed the neurologic and cognitive capacity for sentience and interests in themselves, and those so neurologically immature that they cannot experience harm.[14] While aborting fetuses at that earlier stage prevents them from achieving their potential it does not harm or wrong them, since they are insufficiently developed to experience harm.[15]

Although aborting the fetus at that early stage does not wrong the fetus, it may impose symbolic costs measurable in terms of the reduced respect for human life generally that a willingness to abort early fetuses connotes. Still, the abortion may be ethically acceptable if the good sought sufficiently outweighs the symbolic devaluation of life that occurs when fetuses that cannot be harmed in their own right are aborted. Many persons find that the burdens of unwanted pregnancy outweigh the symbolic devaluation of human life. Others would require a more compelling reason for abortion, such as protecting the mother's life or health, avoiding the birth of a handicapped child, or avoiding the burdens of a pregnancy due to rape or incest.

By comparison, abortion to obtain tissue to save one's own life or the life of a close relative seems equally, if not more compelling. If abortion in the case of an unwanted pregnancy is deemed permissible, surely abortion to obtain tissue to save another person's life is. Indeed, aborting to obtain tissue would seem as compelling as the most stringent reasons for permitting abortion. In fact, many would find this motive more compelling than the desire to end an unwanted pregnancy.

Of course, aborting a wanted pregnancy to prevent severe neurologic disease in oneself or a close relative will hardly be done joyfully, and will place the mother in an excruciating dilemma. A fetus that could be carried to term will have to be sacrificed to save a parent, spouse, sibling, or child who already exists. Such a tragic choice will induce fear and trembling, and engender loss or grief whatever the decision. Yet one cannot say that the choice to abort is ethically impermissible. There is no sound ethical basis for prohibiting *this* sacrifice of the fetus when its sacrifice to end an unwanted pregnancy or pursue other goals is permitted.

Public attitudes toward a woman aborting an otherwise wanted pregnancy to benefit a family member would most likely reflect attitudes toward abortion generally. Those who are against abortion in all circumstances will object to abortions done to treat severe neurologic disease in the mother or in a family member. Similarly, persons who accept family planning abortions should have no objection to abortion to procure tissue for transplant, since fetal status is no more compelling and the interest of the woman in controlling her body and reproductive capacity is similar.

Since neither group forms a majority, however, persons who object to family planning abortions but accept abortions necessary to protect the mother's health, in cases of rape or incest, or to prevent the birth of a handicapped child will determine whether a majority of people approve.[16] It is conceivable that many persons in this swing group would find abortion to produce tissue for transplant to a family member to be acceptable. The benefit of alleviating severe neurologic disease is arguably as great as the benefits in the cases they accept as justifiable abortion, and more compelling than abortions done for family planning purposes.

Conceiving and Aborting for Transplant Purposes

What is the objection, then, when a woman not yet pregnant seeks to conceive in order to abort and provide tissue for transplant?

In terms of fetal welfare, no greater harm occurs to the fetus conceived expressly to be aborted, as long as the abortion occurs at a stage at which the fetus is insufficiently developed to experience harm, such as during the first trimester. Of course, such deliberate creation may have greater symbolic significance, because it denotes a willingness to use fetuses as a means or object to serve other ends. However, aborting when already pregnant to procure tissue for transplant (or aborting for the more customary reasons) also denotes a willingness to use the fetus as a means to other ends.

As long as abortion of an existing pregnancy for transplant purposes is ethically accepted, conceiving in order to abort and procure tissue for transplant should also be ethically acceptable when necessary to alleviate great suffering in others.[17] People could reasonably find that the additional symbolic devaluation is negligible, or in any case, insufficient to outweigh the substantial gain to transplant recipients that deliberate creation provides.

Many people, no doubt, will resist this conclusion, even if they accept abortion to procure tissue when the woman is already pregnant. Whether rational or not, they assign moral or symbolic significance to deliberate creation, and are less ready to sanction such a practice. Others who accept abortion for tissue procurement when the woman is already pregnant will find an insufficient difference in deliberate creation to outweigh the resulting good. Public acceptability of such a practice thus depends on how the swing group that views abortion only for very stringent reasons views the fact of deliberate creation for the purpose of abortion. If it would accept abortion to produce tissue when the pregnancy is unplanned, it might accept conception to produce fetal tissue as well.

In sum, deliberate creation of fetuses to be aborted for tissue procurement is more ethically complex, and more defensible, than its current widespread dismissal would suggest. Such a practice is, or course, not in itself desirable, but in a specific situation of strong personal or familial need may be more justified than previously thought. In any case, the fear that fetal tissue transplants will lead to abortions performed solely to obtain tissue for transplant should not prevent use of tissue from abortions not performed for that purpose.

RECRUITING UNRELATED FETAL TISSUE DONORS

The strongest case for conception and abortion to produce fetal tissue—if the need arose—is to save oneself or a close relative from death or serious harm. But many patients in need would lack a female relative willing to donate. May unrelated women be recruited for this purpose?

If the hypothetical need arose, a strong case for unrelated fetal tissue donors can be made. If a relative may provide tissue, why not a stranger who chooses to do so altruistically? At this point concerns about fetal status become less important, and the focus shifts toward the welfare of the donor. But the physical effects of pregnancy and abortion to produce fetal tissue are roughly comparable to the effects of kidney or bone marrow donation, though somewhat less since general anesthesia will not be involved. While few unrelated persons now act as kidney donors, there is a national registry for unrelated bone marrow donors. Even if fetal tissue donation were psychologically more complicated, the risks to the woman would appear to within the boundaries of autonomous choice.

Some persons might object that this will turn women into "fetal tissue farms," thus denigrating their inherent worth as persons. This charge could also be made against any living donor, whether of kidney, bone marrow, blood, sperm, or egg. Insofar as persons donate body parts, they may be viewed as mere tissue or organ producers. Indeed, women who bear children are always in danger of being viewed as "breeders." But such views oversimplify the complex emotional reality of organ and tissue donation and of human reproduction. The risk of misperception does not justify barring women from freely choosing to be fetal tissue donors.

Special attention should be given to consent procedures that will protect the woman from being coerced or unduly pressured by prospective recipients and their families just as occurs with living related kidney and marrow donors. Waiting periods, consent advisors and monitors, and other devices to guarantee free, informed consent are clearly justified.[18]

THE WOMAN'S RIGHT TO DISPOSE OF FETAL TISSUE

The UAGA and federal research regulations give the mother the right to make or withhold donations of fetal remains for research or therapy, subject to objection by the father.[19] Yet some ethicists claim that the decision to abort disqualifies the mother from playing any role in disposition of fetal remains.[20] If accepted, this argument would lead either to procuring fetal tissue without parental consent or to a total ban on fetal transplants. But the argument is mistaken on two grounds.

Its major premise is that the person disposing of cadaveric remains acts as a guardian or proxy for the deceased. Since the woman has chosen to kill the fetus by abortion, she is no longer qualified to act as proxy. But this premise is seriously flawed. Deceased persons or fetuses no longer have interests to be protected, as the notion of proxy implies. Control of human remains is assigned to next of kin because of their own interests and feelings about how cadaveric remains are treated, not because they are best situated to implement the deceased's prior wishes concerning disposition of his cadaver. The latter concern is particulariy inappropriate in the case of an aborted fetus, which could have had no specific wishes concerning disposition of its remains.

A second mistake is the assumption that a woman has no interest in what happens to the fetus that she chooses to abort. As a product of her body and potential heir that she has for her own compelling reasons chosen to abort she may care deeply about whether fetal remains are contributed to research or therapy to help others. Given that interest, there is good reason to respect her wishes, as current law does. Indeed, in case of conflict between her and the father over disposition one could argue that her interests control because the fetus was removed from her body.

An alternative policy requiring that fetal remains be used without parental consent or not at all is unacceptable. American public policy has vigorously rejected routine salvage of body parts without family consent as a way to increase the supply of organs for transplant.[21] Even presumed consent, which would take organs unless the family actually objects, has been largely rejected.[22] Depriving the mother (and father who agrees to the abortion) of the power to veto fetal tissue transplants would single out fetal tissue for transplant use without family consent. Such a radical change in tissue procurement practice is not needed to satisfy the demand for fetal tissue. It serves only to punish women who abort.

The alternative would be to ban fetal tissue transplants altogether. But this solution burns the house to roast the pig, in effect banning tissue transplants because the parent is not permitted to consent. As we have seen, however, a ban on all fetal transplants is not justified.

In short, the ethical case for denying the woman who aborts dispositional control of fetal remains is not persuasive. She cannot insist that fetal remains be used for transplant because no donor has the right to require that intended donees accept anatomical gifts, but she should retain the existing legal right to veto use of fetal remains for transplant research or therapy. Her consent to donation of fetal tissue should be routinely sought.

THE CONSENT PROCESS AND ABORTION

If the woman retains the right to determine whether fetal tissue is used for research or therapy, the main ethical concern is to assure that her choice about tissue donation and the abortion is free and informed. A clear separation of the two decisions will assure that tissue donation is not a prerequisite to performance of the abortion. Also, it will prevent the prospect of donating fetal remains from influencing the decision to abort, a preferable policy when sufficient tissue from family planning abortions is available.

To that end, the request to donate fetal tissue should be made only after the woman has consented to the abortion.[23] The alternative of waiting until the abortion has been performed would add little protection and not be practical. In addition, the person requesting consent to tissue donation and performing the abortion should not be the person using the donated tissue in research or therapy, a constraint widely followed in cadaveric organ procurement.

Federal regulations governing fetal research also state that "no procedural changes which may cause greater than minimal risk to the fetus or pregnant woman will be introduced into the procedure for terminating the pregnancy solely in the interest of the activity."[24] While this policy is partially intended to protect fetuses from later or more painful abortions, it also aims to protect women from prolonging pregnancy or undergoing more onerous abortion procedures to obtain tissue.

Some changes in abortion procedures to enhance tissue procurement pose little additional risk and should be permitted. For example, reductions in the amount of suction, use of a larger bore needle, and ultrasound-guided placement of the suction instrument in evacuation abortions would, without increasing risk, facilitate tissue retrieval by preventing masceration of the fetus.

More problematic would be changes such as substitution of prostaglandin-induced labor and delivery or hysterectomy for less risky methods, or postponement of abortion to late in the first trimester or to the second trimester. Apart from her desire to facilitate tissue donation, these changes would not appear to be in the woman's interest.

Asking a woman who is aborting to take on these extra burdens can be ethically justified only if necessary to obtain viable tissue. Because sufficient fetal tissue may now be obtained without increasing the burdens of abortion, the current federal regulations are sound.

A different policy should be considered if changes in timing or method of abortion became necessary to procure viable tissue for transplant. If the need were clearly shown, there is no objection in principle to asking a woman to assume some additional burdens for the sake of tissue procurement. If the woman is already pregnant and determined to have an abortion, the additional risks of postponing the abortion a few weeks or even changing to a prostaglandin abortion would be well within the range of risks that persons may voluntarily choose to benefit others. However, special procedures to protect the woman's autonomy would be in order.

COMMERCIALIZATION OF FETAL TISSUE

In addition to ethical concerns about fetal and maternal welfare, opponents of fetal tissue transplants have raised the specter of fetal tissue procurement leading to a commercial market in abortions and in fetal tissue.

Paying money to women to abort or to donate once they abort is generally perceived as damaging to human dignity, as would be commercial buying and selling of fetal tissue. Such market transactions risk exploiting women and their reproductive capacity and may denigrate the human dignity of aborted fetuses by treating them as market commodities.[25]

Most commentators and advisory bodies that have considered fetal tissue transplants recommend that market transactions in abortions and fetal tissue be prohibited.[26] The National Organ Transplant Act of 1984, which bans the payment of "valuable consideration" for the donation or distribution of solid organs, was amended in 1988 to ban sales of fetal organs and "subparts thereof."[27] Also, several states prohibit the sale of fetal tissue and organs.[28]

At present such policies are easily supported, for they would have little impact on the supply of fetal tissue. There is no reason to think that women who abort unwanted pregnancies would not donate fetal tissue altruistically. Indeed, many women who abort are likely to donate fetal remains in the hope that some additional good might result from the abortion. Paying them to donate—buying their aborted fetuses—is thus unnecessary.

But what if altruistic donations did not produce a sufficient supply of fetal tissue for transplant, or the need for histocompatible tissue required hiring women to be impregnated to produce a sufficient supply of fetal tissue? Would such payments be unethical? Should current legal policy still be maintained? Answering those questions would require balancing the risks of exploiting women and the symbolic costs of perceived commodification against the benefits to needy patients and the rights of women to determine use of their reproductive capacity.

No doubt many people would object to hiring women to become pregnant and abort. However, if pregnancy and abortion to produce fetal tissue is ethically defensible, then money payments in some circumstances may also be defensible, given obligations of beneficence and respect for persons, the lack of alternative tissue sources, and social practices in which some tissue donors are paid.[29] Legal policy might then be reconsidered to permit payments when essential to save the life or protect the health of transplant recipients who lack other alternatives. However, resolution of this difficult issue should await the actual occurrence of the need to pay to obtain fetal tissue for transplant. In the meantime, research and therapy with fetal tissue should proceed without payments to women to abort or to donate fetal tissue.

Current bans on buying and selling fetal tissue do not—and should not— prohibit making reasonable payments to recover the costs of retrieving fetal tissue. The law and ethics of organ procurement allow for payment of costs incurred in the acquisition of organs.[30] Organ donor families, for example, are not asked to pay for the costs of maintaining brain-dead cadavers or for surgically removing the organs that they donate. The same principle should apply to fetal tissue donations. Two related issues concern paying the donor's abortion expenses and paying other tissue retrieval costs.

Paying Abortion Expenses

Paying the cost of the abortion should occur only in those instances in which the abortion is performed solely to obtain tissues for transplant—a mere hypothetical possibility at present. In that case, paying for the abortion is not a fee to donate tissue, but payment of the costs of acquiring the donated tissue, comparable to paying the cost of the nephrectomy that makes a kidney donation possible. Other out-of-pocket costs incurred by the donor could also be reimbursed without violating federal law or ethical constraints.

In contrast, when the abortion is performed for reasons unrelated to tissue procurements, paying abortion expenses amounts to paying the women to donate the tissue. This payment would constitute a sale of fetal tissue and should not be permitted if fetal tissue sales are prohibited.[31] The willingness of most women to donate without a fee should make payment of abortion expenses unnecessary.

Retrieval Costs and For-Profit Agencies

In the past researchers have obtained fetal tissue through informal contacts with physicians doing abortions, often in the same institution. More recently, agencies that retrieve tissue from abortion facilities and distribute it to researchers have developed. In some cases for-profit firms that specialize in processing the tissue for transplant may enter the field.

What role will money payments play in the operation of retrieval agencies? Under existing law tissue procurement agencies will be unable to pay women to donate fetal tissue. However, they should be free to pay the costs of personnel directly involved in retrieval, whether employees of the procurement agency or of the facility performing the abortion. For example, a retrieval agency may reimburse the abortion clinic for using its space and staff to obtain consent for tissue donations and to retrieve tissue from aborted fetuses.[32]

In distributing fetal tissue to researchers and physicians, retrieval agencies should be able to recoup the expenses of procuring the tissue, including overhead and other operating expenses of the agency itself. Such payment is consistent with heart and kidney transplant recipients (or their payors) paying for the analogous costs of organ procurement.

If the retrieval agency is a for-profit research enterprise, some profit margin should also be recognized in the amount it charges the recipient of the tissue. While some persons might argue that allowing any profit amounts to a sale of fetal tissue that risks treating it as a market commodity, those who organize resources and invest capital to provide viable fetal tissue for transplant are performing a useful social activity. Fears about treating donors and fetuses as commodities might justify policies against buying tissue from donors and abortion facilities. But they should not prevent giving for-profit firms the incentives necessary to organize the resources required to obtain fetal tissue altruistically. Such a practice would be consistent with the role of for-profit physicians, hospitals, drug companies and air transport services in organ transplantation.

Federal Funding

While existing federal regulations permit transplant research with tissue from aborted fetuses when state law permits, the question of whether the federal government should fund fetal tissue research nevertheless remains. A special panel was recently convened by the National Institutes of Health to advise the Assistant Secretary for Health on whether intramural and extramural research programs involving fetal tissue transplants should be supported.[33] The panel gave a positive recommendation, with restrictions on tissue procurement comparable to the existing federal regulations, but its approval does not guarantee that federal research funding will occur.[34]

Because funding decisions ordinarily do not infringe constitutional rights, the government is not obligated to fund fetal tissue research (or therapy), no matter how desirable it appears.[35] However, the arguments strongly favor supporting such research. Of overriding importance is the potential benefit to thousands of patients suffering from severe disease. Federal funding will also allow the government to play a more active oversight role than if it leaves the field entirely to private funding, as occurred with in vitro fertilization research.[36]

The arguments against federal research funding come from right-to-life groups that would remove the federal government entirely from any financial support of abortion in the United States. Research funding, however, does not subsidize the abortions making the tissue available. Nor, as we have seen, does it place an imprimatur of legitimacy on abortion, or encourage to any great extent abortions that would not otherwise have occurred.

If the politics of abortion lead to withdrawal of direct government funding of research with tissue from family planning abortions, the government should not penalize institutions that conduct such research with nonfederal funds by denying them other research assistance. The symbolic gains of refusing to fund other medical research in institutions doing nonfederally funded research with aborted fetuses are too few to justify the burden on researchers. Clearly at that point the link to abortion is too attenuated to claim complicity in or encouragement of it.

These same issues will be refought if fetal tissue transplants became a proven therapy for Parkinson's disease, diabetes, or other disorders. While the government is not constitutionally obligated to fund a given therapy, the case for federal funding of treatment is even stronger than for funding of research, because the benefits to patients are clearer. A policy of denying Medicare or Medicaid funding for safe and effective fetal tissue transplants would deprive needy patients of essential therapies simply to avoid speculative concerns about complicity and encouragement of abortion. A more prudent approach would be to fund all therapies that meet the general funding standards for these programs. Alternatively, the government's funding policies should distinguish between therapies dependent on tissue retrieved from family planning abortions and those dependent on tissue from abortions performed to provide tissue for transplant.

LEGAL BANS ON FETAL TISSUE TRANSPLANTS

While the UAGA in every state permits the mother to donate fetal tissue for transplant research and therapy, eight states ban the experimental use of dead aborted fetuses.[37] None of these laws distinguish tissue from family planning abortions and abortions performed solely to obtain fetal tissue. Six of the eight states ban experimental but not nonexperimental use of aborted fetuses. None ban similar uses of other cadaveric tissue, including cadavers that resulted from homicide.[38]

As a policy matter, the case for a legal ban on all research uses of dead fetal tissue is weak. Given that the use of fetal remains from lawful abortions is at issue, such laws are difficult to sustain. They purport to show the state's respect for prenatal life, but they do it in such an irrational way that they are clearly vulnerable to constitutional attack on several grounds, including vagueness, irrationality, and interference with the right to abort and the recipient's right to medical care.[39] A case invalidating the Louisiana law will be a potent precedent in future attacks on these laws.[40]

Even laws that prohibited intrafamilial donations or donor designation of recipients, which aim to prevent women from conceiving and aborting to produce fetal tissue, would be vulnerable if such practices were necessary to provide transplants to sick patients.[41] If the woman is already pregnant, such laws would prevent her from aborting to provide tissue. If not yet pregnant, they would arguably interfere with marital and procreative privacy or the recipient's right to life and medical care. A state's interest in preventing women from becoming "tissue farms," from abusing the reproductive process, or from being pressured to donate would not justify intrusion on such fundamental rights when the patient had no other alternative.[42]

SYMBOLIC AND RIGHTS-BASED CONCERNS

Ethical concerns should not bar research with fetal tissue implants as a therapy for serious illness. Although many persons have ethical reservations about abortion, a wide range of opinion would likely support many research uses of fetal tissue, particularly when the abortions occur for reasons other than tissue procurement.

The use of fetal tissue inevitably implicates the same feelings that abortion engenders. The disparate issues raised, however, can be treated separately, so that ethical concerns and the politics of abortion do not impede the progress of important research. For example, transplants with fetal tissue from family planning abortions do not necessarily entail approval of pregnancy and abortion undertaken to produce tissue for transplant. Nor will recognizing the woman's right to donate fetal tissue cause fetuses to be bought and sold, or women to be paid to abort.

In the final analysis, fetal tissue transplants raise symbolic questions as well as questions of rights. The symbolic issues raised by fetal tissue transplants cut in many directions. Sorting out symbolic and rights-based concerns will help to respect both important ethical values and the need for progress in medical science.

REFERENCES

The author gratefully acknowledges the helpful comments of Richard Markovits, Douglas Laycock, Michael Sharlot, Alan Fine, Albert R. Jonsen, George J. Annas, Arthur L. Caplan, Pat Cain, and Jean Love on a much longer version of this article.

1. Alan Fine, "The Ethics of Fetal Tissue Transplants," *Hastings Center Report* 18:3 June 1988), 5-8.

2. Kevin Lafferty, statement to the Fetal Tissue Transplantation Research Panel, National Institutes of Health, September 15, 1988.

3. 45 CFR 46.209; John A. Robertson, "Relaxing the Death Standard for Pediatric Organ Donations," in *Organ Substitution Technology:* Ethical, Legal, and Public Policy Issues (Boulder, CO: Westview Press, 1988), 69-77.

4. John A. Robertson, "Fetal Tissue Transplants," *Washington University Law Quarterly* 66:3 (November 1988).

5. 45 CFR 46.210.

6. Stanley K. Henshaw *et al.*, "A Portrait of American Women Who Obtain Abortions," *Family Planning Perspectives* 17:2 (1985), 90-96.

7. Lafferty, "Statement."

8. James Burtchaell, "Case Study: University Policy on Experimental Use of Aborted Fetal Tissue," *IRB: A Review of Human Subjects Research* 10:4 (July/August 1988), 7-11.

9. Burtchaell, "Case Study," 10; Phillip Shabecoff, "Head of E.P.A. Bars Nazi Data in Study in Gas," *New York Times*, March 23, 1988, 1.

10. Leonard Tushnet, *The Uses of Adversity: Studies of Starvation in the Warsaw Ghetto* (New York: Thomas Yoseloff, 1966); "Minnesota Scientist Plans to Publish a Nazi Study," *New York Times*, May 12, 1988, 9.

11. Tamar Lewin, "Medical Use of Fetal Tissue Spurs New Abortion Debate," *New York Times*, Aug. 16, 1987, A1.

12. John A. Robertson, "Fetal Tissue Transplants."

13. Mary B. Mahowald, Jerry Silver, and Robert A. Ratcheson, "The Ethical Options in Transplanting Fetal Tissue," *Hastings Law Journal* 39:5 (July 1988), 1079-1107.

14. Cliford Grobstein, *Science and the Unborn* (New York: Basic Books, 1988).

15. John A. Robertson, "Gestational Burdens and Fetal Status: A Defense of *Roe v. Wade*," *American Journal of Law and Medicine* 13:2/3 (1988), 189-212; John Bigelow and Robert Pargetter, "Morality, Potential Persons, and Abortion," *American Philosophical Quarterly* 25 (1988), 173-81.

16. See, for example, "America's Abortion Dilemma," *Newsweek*, January 14, 1985, 22-26.

17. John A. Robertson, "Embryos, Families, and Procreative Liberty: The Legal Structure of the New Reproduction," *Southern California Law Review* (1986), 939-1041.

18. John A. Robertson, "Taking Consent Seriously: IRB Interventions in the Consent Process," *IRB: A Review of Human Subjects Research* 4:5 (May 1982), 1-5.

19. Uniform Anatomical Gift Act, 8A U.L.A. 15-16 (West 1983 and Supp. 1987) (Table of Jurisdictions Wherein Act Has Been Adopted); 45 CFR 46.207(b).

20. Burtchaell, "Case Study," 8; Mary B. Mahowald, "Placing Wedges Along a Slippery Slope: Use of Fetal Neural Tissue for Transplantation," *Clinical Research* 36 (1988), 220-23.

21. John A. Robertson, "Supply and Distribution of Hearts for Transplantation: Legal, Ethical, and Policy Issues," *Circulation* 75 (1987), 77-88.

22. Robertson, "Supply and Distribution"; Department of Health and Human Services, *Organ Transplantation: Issues and Recommendations, Report of the Task Force on Organ Transplantation*, April 1986, 30.

23. 45 CFR 46.206(a).

24. 45 CFR 46.206(a)(4).

25. Margaret Radin, "Market Inalienability," *Harvard Law Review* 100 (1987), 1849-1931; Thomas H. Murray, "Gifts of the Body and the Needs of Strangers," *Hastings Center Report* 17:2 (April 1987), 30-38.

26. Fine, "The Ethics of Fetal Tissue Transplants"; Mahowald, Silver, and Ratcheson, "The Ethical Options."

27. 42 U.S.C.A. No. 247e (West Supp. 1985).

28. Ark. Stat. Ann. §82-439 (Supp. 1985); Ill. Stat. Ann. ch. 38, &81.54(7) (Smith-Hurd 1983); La. Civ. Code Ann. art. 9:122 (Supp. 1987); Ohio Rev. Code Ann. §2919.14 (Page 1985); Okla. Stat. tit. 63 §1-753 (1987); Fla. Stat. Ann. §873.05 (West Supp. 1987); Mass. Gen. Laws Ann. ch. 112, §1593 (19640); Me. Rev. Stat. Ann. tit. 22, §1593 (1964); Mich. Comp. Laws Ann. §333.2690 (West); Minn. Stat. Ann. §145.422 (West Supp. 1986); N.D. Cent. Code §14-02.2-02 (1981); Nev. Rev. Stat. §451.015 (1985); R.I. Gen. Laws §11-54-1(f) (Supp. 1987); Tenn. Code Ann. §39-4-208 (Supp. 1987); Tex. Penal Code Ann. §42.10, 48.02 (Vernon 1974 and Supp.

1988); Wyo. Stat. §35-6-115 (1986); 18 Pa. Cons. Stat. 3216 (Purdon 1983). See also "Note, Regulating the Sale of Human Organs," *Virginia Law Review* 71 (1985), 1015-38.

29. John A. Robertson, "Technology and Motherhood: Legal and Ethical Issues in Human Egg Donation," *Case Western Reserve Law Review* 39:1 (1988).

30. National Organ Transplant Act, 42 U.S.C.A. 274e (West Supp. 1985).

31. National Organ Transplant Act.

32. National Organ Transplant Act.

33. G. Kolata, "Federal Agency Bars Implanting of Fetal Tissue," *New York Times*, April 16, 1988, 1.

34. "Fetal Tissue 'Acceptable' for Research," *Washington Post*, September 17, 1988, 1; Barbara Culliton, "White House wants Fetal Research Ban," *Science* (Sept. 16, 1988), 1423.

35. *McCrae v. Harris*, 448 U.S. 297 (1980); *Beal v. Doe*, 432 U.S. 438 (1977); *Poelker v. Doe*, 432 U.S. 519 (1977) (*per curiam*).

36. John Fletcher and Kenneth Ryan, "Federal Regulations for Fetal Research: A Case for Reform," *Law, Medicine, and Health Care* 15:3 (Fall 1987), 126-28.

37. Ark. Stat. Ann. §82-438 (Supp. 1985); Ariz. Rev. Stat. Ann. §36-2302 (1986); Ind. Code Ann. §35-1-58.5.6 (West 1986); Ill. Ann. Stat. ch. 38, §81-54 (7) (Smith-Hurd 1983); La. Rev. Stat. Ann. §1299.35.13 (West 1986); Ohio Rev. Code Ann. §2919.14 (Page 1985); Okla. Stat. tit. 63, §1-735; N.M. Stat. Ann. §§24-9A-3, 24-9A-3,24-9A-5 (1986).

38. A Missouri law bans use of fetal tissue produced for transplant purposes, but not fetal tissue from family planning abortions. Missouri HB No. 1479 (1988).

39. Robertson, "Fetal Tissue Transplants"; "Note: State Prohibition of Fetal Experimentation and the Fundamental Rights of Privacy," *Columbia Law Review* 88 (1988), 1073-1109.

40. *Margaret S. v. Edwards*, 794 F.2d 944 (5th Cir. 1986).

41. Robertson, "Fetal Tissue Transplants."

42. Danis, "Fetal Tissue Transplants."

6. Are There Really Alternatives to the Use of Fetal Tissue from Elective Abortions in Transplantation Research?

*Daniel J. Garry, Arthur L. Caplan,
Dorothy E. Vawter, and Warren Kearney*

Human fetal tissue has been described as having tremendous plasticity and availability, and as possibly being less prone to rejection than adult tissue. These properties have led many researchers to consider it a possible source of transplantable tissue for patients with incurable debilitating diseases, such as diabetes mellitus and Parkinson's, Alzheimer's, and Huntington's diseases.

The use of human fetal tissue in research involving transplantation in human recipients has become the center of a heated controversy in the United States. In March 1988 the Department of Health and Human Services placed a moratorium on the funding of research involving the transplantation of tissue obtained during induced abortions. Later that year, an advisory panel of the National Institutes of Health (NIH) concluded that the use of such tissue is acceptable public policy under certain conditions.[1] Despite this decision, the moratorium has been extended indefinitely by the secretary of Health and Human Services, Louis W. Sullivan. Congressional efforts to overturn it have been unsuccessful. In vetoing an attempt in 1992 to overturn the moratorium, President Bush and many current and former administration officials argued that alternative sources of human fetal tissue should be used in transplantation research.[2] The assistant secretary of health, James O. Mason, and the NIH director, Bernadine Healy, maintain that ectopic pregnancies and spontaneously aborted fetuses are "feasible" sources of tissue. Consequently, millions of dollars have been budgeted and the NIH has solicited proposals and awarded funding to establish a bank of fetal tissue obtained from ectopic pregnancies and spontaneous abortions that is suitable for transplantation research.

Originally published in *The New England Journal of Medicine* 327, no. 22 (November 26, 1992). Copyright © 1992 Massachusetts Medical Society. All rights reserved.

What is remarkable and disturbing about the current debate is that it remains almost completely devoid of information about alternative sources of fetal tissue. If there are scientific reasons that seriously limit the chances that tissue derived from ectopic pregnancies, spontaneously aborted fetuses, still-born fetuses, or extraembryonic tissue could serve as an alternative to tissue obtained from electively aborted fetuses, then there is very little reason, other than politics, to fund only research using tissue from these sources. Oddly, this is precisely the situation that now exists. None of the alternatives offer a reasonable source of fetal tissue for transplantation research.

ECTOPIC PREGNANCIES

A number of writers have suggested that ectopic pregnancy is a practical and ethically uncontroversial source of human fetal tissue.[2,3] In an ectopic pregnancy, the conceptus is implanted outside the uterus, with the most common sites being the oviduct (in more than 95 percent of cases), the abdominal cavity, and the ovary.[4,5] Such a situation does not result in a successful pregnancy or delivery.

Ectopic pregnancies occur at a rate of 16.8 per 1,000 reported pregnancies.[6] In 1987 there were 88,000 ectopic pregnancies in the United States. Some tubal pregnancies resolve naturally or abort spontaneously. It has been estimated that approximately 60 percent of ectopic pregnancies abort spontaneously early in the first trimester.[7,8] In one study, women with diagnosed ectopic pregnancy were hospitalized for one week to monitor their clinical symptoms and were then discharged and followed as outpatients, with daily clinical examinations and determinations of serum human chorionic gonadotropin levels.[8] The ectopic pregnancy resolved spontaneously in 64 percent; the remaining patients required surgical intervention.[8] Spontaneously aborted ectopic pregnancies rarely produce fetal tissue that is recognizable or viable in culture.[9] Even when they do, the tissue has almost always been ischemic for days before its expulsion.

Ectopic pregnancies that do not abort spontaneously become clinically apparent before the ninth week of gestation. Surgical removal of the ectopic products of conception frequently reveals the absence of any fetal tissue.[9] In one study of sixty-five ectopic pregnancies, thirty-three specimens (51 percent) were morphologically abnormal[10]: eighteen of these specimens had an intact chorionic sac with no recognizable embryo, eight had no recognizable organ differentiation, and seven had systemic abnormalities (i.e., spina bifida, microcephaly, or severe growth retardation).[10] These findings are consistent with a previous report of forty-four specimens from ectopic pregnancies, twenty-eight of which (64 percent) were morphologically abnormal.[11] Yet another recent study of fifty-three proved ectopic pregnancies revealed forty-two specimens (79 percent) to be lacking in fetal tissue or grossly abnormal.[9] In this study, only two of the ectopic pregnancies were viable (i.e., had evidence of myocardial contractility), as observed with ultrasound before the surgical removal of the ectopic conceptus.[9]

Ectopic pregnancy is also linked with a high incidence of hemorrhage, which is associated with probable episodic anoxia to the ectopic fetus. Morphologic examination of 242 ectopic pregnancies revealed that the dilation of the oviduct was due primarily to intratubal hemorrhage. In most cases the growing ectopic fetus had penetrated the wall of the oviduct and assumed an extratubal location.[12] Brenner et al. describe tubal rupture in 297 of 300 ectopic pregnancies, or 99 percent of women who were examined by laparotomy.[13] Tubal rupture casts doubt on the viability and normality of tissues taken from fetuses that develop under such circumstances.

The only circumstance in which tissue from an ectopic pregnancy may be viable occurs when fetal myocardial contractility is observed before surgical removal. Such cases are exceedingly rare and are likely to become more so in the future. Nonsurgical therapy is currently being studied as treatment for ectopic pregnancy in order to preserve fertility. Methotrexate and mifepristone (RU 486), an antiprogestogen, have been administered with some degree of success.[8,14] Pharmacologic advances are likely to reduce or eliminate the already tiny number of ectopic pregnancies that might yield normal, viable fetal tissue.

SPONTANEOUS ABORTIONS

Spontaneously aborted fetuses are another source of tissue often suggested by those who advocate federal funding for tissue banks that do not use fetal tissue from elective abortions. Some authors and government officials claim that such fetuses are both plentiful and ethically appropriate for use in transplantation.[15]

A spontaneous abortion is the unintentional delivery of an embryo or fetus that has died in utero before the twentieth week of gestation. The causes include major chromosomal or other lethal defects in the fetus,[16] infections (e.g., syphilis, rubella, or mycoplasma), and maternal diseases (e.g., diabetes mellitus).[17] Tissue obtained from a fetus that has spontaneously aborted for any of these reasons would hardly be acceptable for transplantation.

Rare causes of spontaneous abortion, such as uterine anomalies (e.g., an incompetent cervix),[18] multiple pregnancy, and intrauterine fetal death as a result of motor vehicle accidents or other trauma (most frequently resulting in fracture of the fetal skull), may produce "normal" fetal tissue.[19] But such tissue is not necessarily viable.

There are few data on the number of spontaneous abortions each year in the United States.[15] Of all recognizable pregnancies, an estimated 15 to 20 percent, or 750,000, end in spontaneous abortion in the first trimester.[7,15,17,20] Chromosomal abnormality is the most frequent cause of such abortions, accounting for 60 percent.[18,21] In general, the earlier the gestational age at the time of spontaneous abortion, the more likely that its cause is a chromosomal abnormality. Trisomies account for 60 percent of all such abnormalities in fetuses aborted spontaneously during the first trimester.[22] Turner's syndrome (in which the fetus has a 45,X karyotype) and polyploidy account for 20 percent each.[22]

Investigators studying the association between certain diseases and chromosomal abnormalities may find spontaneously aborted fetuses the best source of tissue for their purposes. But chromosomally abnormal tissue is not optimal or even acceptable for transplantation, since its growth, development, and function are unreliable.[21]

Most spontaneous abortions occur in the first trimester and are preceded by fetal death in utero.[18] Initially, there is hemorrhage, followed by tissue necrosis and inflammation at or near the site of implantation.[23] The conceptus may then become detached from the uterine wall, and with subsequent uterine contractions the products of conception may be expelled, typically two or three weeks later. Any products that are not expelled must be surgically removed. This long delay in the expulsion of the dead fetus from the body renders the tissue of nearly all spontaneously aborted fetuses unsuitable for transplantation.[23]

Furthermore, most such fetuses are incomplete specimens with no recognizable fetal tissue. One large study recently monitored 1,025 spontaneous abortions over a twelve-month period and found that 77 percent did not contain recognizable fetal tissue.[24] Although 23 percent of the spontaneously aborted pregnancies yielded identifiable fetal tissue, only 3.8 percent produced a recognizable fetus that was not fragmented, stunted, or with some other obvious anomaly.[24]

If 3.8 percent of the approximately 750,000 pregnant women known to abort spontaneously each year in the United States[7,17,19] produce a normal fetus, then the tissue from approximately 28,500 spontaneously aborted fetuses could theoretically be used for transplantation if the fetuses were expelled or surgically removed within hours of fetal death. But even this number is not an accurate indication of the number of fetuses available as a result of spontaneous abortion. Most spontaneously aborted fetuses die in utero two to three weeks before expulsion. In addition, most spontaneous abortions occur outside a health care setting.[21] As a result, the fetal tissue is often contaminated with environmental bacteria and is separated from the appropriate culture medium for many hours. Even in the rare cases in which a spontaneously aborted fetus yields viable fetal tissue, the high rate of major chromosomal anomalies associated with such abortions makes it obligatory to test such tissue for chromosomal abnormalities. Chromosomal analysis requires approximately ten days and would probably necessitate the preservation of the fetal tissue until the test results became available. Thus, the quality of the tissue might be further compromised by the need for lengthy storage while its condition is established. Finally, it is not known how many women would consent to the use of tissue from their spontaneous abortions. But the unexpected and often tragic circumstances surrounding the event make it likely that some would refuse.

In sum, obtaining tissue from a dead fetus after a spontaneous abortion is morally acceptable to most people because the fetal death is perceived as tragic, not immoral. However, the overwhelming number of spontaneous abortions occur outside a medical setting, involve a fetus with chromosomal or other abnormalities, yield an incompletely developed fetus, or yield only nonviable tissue (because of the two-to-three-week period of ischemia before expulsion). And some women will not allow fetal remains to be used for transplantation research. Thus, spontaneously aborted fetuses are not reliable or safe as a source of normal, viable fetal tissue.

STILLBIRTHS

Stillbirth is defined by the National Center for Health Statistics as fetal death in or after the twentieth week of gestation.[25] In 1983 there were approximately 30,280 stillbirths in the United States.[25] In a typical clinical scenario, a woman who has had an uneventful pregnancy might present to the outpatient clinic anxiously reporting that she has been unaware of fetal movement for one or two days.[26] Sonographic examination would reveal fetal death. After the delivery of the stillbirth, postmortem examination often reveals a macerated fetus.[26]

An analysis of 765 consecutive stillbirths showed the identifiable causes of fetal death to be anoxia (in 43 percent), hemorrhage (16 percent), congenital anomalies (10 percent), diabetes mellitus (5 percent), and trauma (2 percent).[27] Other studies report that in approximately half the cases the cause of death is unknown.[26,28]

After a fetus dies in utero, it is usually retained for a time and then delivered spontaneously. A recent review of the literature indicates that at least 75 percent of women go into labor spontaneously within two weeks of fetal death and that the rest deliver within another two weeks.[26] Tissue from these fetuses is not viable. Attempts to culture tissue from stillborn fetuses have rarely succeeded.[28]

Moreover, stillbirths do not yield tissue that is at the stage of development required for most transplants. Neural tissue, for example, must usually be obtained from fetuses of less than twelve weeks' gestational age. The procurement of tissue from stillbirths raises little ethical concern. In fact, in some states the Uniform Anatomical Gift Act explicitly permits the use of tissue from stillbirths in transplantation. In practice, however, getting informed consent from a woman just after a stillbirth is problematic. In sum, the source that raises the least ethical concern is unlikely to provide any tissue suitable for transplantation research.

EXTRAEMBRYONIC TISSUE

Extraembryonic tissue—that is, the placenta and yolk sac—can provide some fetal tissue for transplantation.[3] Such tissue can be obtained from living fetuses early in gestation by diagnostic procedures such as chorionic-villus sampling and amniocentesis. Alternatively, extraembryonic tissue may be available after an abortion.

Fetal tissue from a placenta has unique characteristics. Placental trophoblasts lack major histocompatibility complex Class II antigens and may therefore be less immunogenic than embryonic tissue.[3] Although placental tissue cannot provide fetal islet or neuronal cells, it can be used to develop certain cell lines that might conceivably be engineered genetically to produce insulin or neurotransmitters such as dopamine.

Yolk-sac tissue is a well-recognized source of hematopoietic stem cells. This tissue could be proliferated in vitro, cryopreserved, and later transplanted into recipients with hematologic disorders. Conceivably, yolk-sac tissue may be an alternative to the use of fetal-liver cells in transplantation.

Extraembryonic tissue can be used for transplantation in only a limited number of patients, such as those with hematologic defects. The use of extraembryonic tissue obtained by diagnostic testing of living fetuses raises ethical questions. It is unknown what volume of tissue is safe to remove during such procedures. Nor is there agreement about how consent for the use of this tissue should be obtained. Many would deem it unethical to undertake procedures with the sole intention of removing extraembryonic tissue for research or transplantation.

ALTERNATIVE SOURCES OR POLITICAL DIVERSION?

Ectopic pregnancies, spontaneously aborted fetuses, and stillbirths would at best be rare and unpredictable sources of normal, viable fetal tissue. Since the availability of useful tissue from any of these sources is unpredictable, it is difficult for researchers and transplantation surgeons to make optimal use of it when it becomes available. Moreover, the incidence of abnormality associated with these categories of tissue is extraordinarily high. As a result, the transplantation of tissue obtained from these sources may expose the recipients to higher risks than those associated with other possible sources of fetal tissue, and the use of such tissue may slow or interfere with scientific progress in understanding the efficacy of fetal-tissue transplants. The only advantage to using these types of tissue is that some perceive them as raising less ethical concern with respect to tissue procurement. Even if this were true, the moral advantages perceived by some would not seem to outweigh the disadvantages to scientific progress and the increased risks imposed on human subjects that are entailed in the use of these types of fetal tissue.

REFERENCES

1. Vawter DE, Caplan AL. Strange brew: the politics and ethics of fetal tissue transplant research in the United States. *J Lab Clin Med* 1992;120:30-4.

2. Nolan K. The use of embryo or fetus in transplantation: what there is to lose. *Transplant Proc* 1990;22:1028-9.

3. Fung CHK, Lo JW. Alternatives to using fetal tissue from induced abortions. *JAMA* 1990;264:34.

4. Elias S, LeBeau M, Simpson JL, Martin AO. Chromosome analysis of ectopic human conceptuses. *Am J Obstet Gynecol* 1981;141:698-703.

5. Martin JN Jr, Sessums JK, Martin RW, Pryor JA, Morrison JC. Abdominal pregnancy: current concepts of management. *Obstet Gynecol* 1988;71:549-57.

6. Nederhof KP, Lawson HW, Saftlas AF, Atrash HK, Finch EL. Ectopic pregnancy surveillance, United States, 1970-1987. *MMWR CDC Surveill Summ* 1990;39(SS-4):9-17.

7. Rubin GL, Peterson HB, Dorfman SF, et al. Ectopic pregnancy in the United States: 1970 through 1978. *JAMA* 1983;249:1725-9.

8. Fernandez H, Rainhorn JD, Papiernik E, Bellet D, Frydman R. Spontaneous resolution of ectopic pregnancy. *Obstet Gynecol* 1988;71:171-4.

9. Rochester D, Panella JS, Port RB. Rosenfeld M, Rawal U. Ectopic pregnancy: surgical-pathologic correlation with US. *Radiology* 1987;165:843-6.

10. Poland BJ, Dill FJ, Styblo C. Embryonic development in ectopic human pregnancy. *Teratology* 1976;14:315-21.

11. Stratford BF. Abnormalities of early human development. *Am J Obstet Gynecol* 1970;107:1223-32.

12. Budowick M, Johnson TR Jr, Genadry R, Parmley TH, Woodruff]D. The histopathology of the developing tubal ectopic pregnancy. *Fertil Steril* 1980;34:169-71.

13. Brenner PF, Roy S, Mishell DR Jr. Ectopic pregnancy: a study of 300 consecutive surgically treated cases. *JAMA* 1980;243:673-6.

14. Leach RE, Ory SJ. Modern management of ectopic pregnancy. *J Reprod Mod* 1989;34:324-38.

15. Thorne ED, Michejda M. Fetal tissue from spontaneous abortions: a new alternative for transplantation research? *Fetal Ther* 1989;4:37-42.

16. Leading work-related diseases and injuries—United States. *JAMA* 1985; 254:1891-2.

17. Kalter H. Diabetes and spontaneous abortion: a historical review. *Am J Obstet Gynecol* 1987;156:1243-53.

18. Developmental and genetic abnormalities. In: Huisjes HJ. *Spontaneous abortion.* Vol. 8 of Current reviews in obstetrics & gynaecology. Edinburgh, Scotland: Churchill Livtngstone, 1984:34-61.

19. Stafford PA, Biddinger PW, Zumwalt RE. Lethal intrauterine fetal trauma. *Am Obstet Gynecol* 1988;159:485-9.

20. Edmonds DK, Lindsay KS, Miller JF, Williamson E, Wood PJ. Early embryonic mortality in women. *Fert Steril* 1982;38:447-53.

21. Boue J, Bou A, Lazar P. Retrospective and prospective epidemiological studies of 1500 karyotyped spontaneous human abortions. *Teratology* 1975;12:11-26.

22. Simpson JL, Golbus MS, Martin AO, Sarto GE. *Genetics in obstetrics and gynecology.* New York: Grune & Stratton, 1982:125.

23. Strobino BA, Pantel-Silverman J. First-trimester vaginal bleeding and the loss of chromosomally normal and abnormal conceptions. *Am J Obstet Gynecol* 1987;157:1150-4.

24. Winter PM, Knowles SAS. Bieber FR, Baraitser M. *The malformed fetus and stillbirth: a diagnostic approach.* New York: John Wiley, 1988:14.

25. Infant, maternal, and neonatal mortality rates, and fetal mortality ratios, by race: 1960 to 1983. In: Bureau of the Census. *Statistical abstract of the United States: 1987.* 107th ed. Washington, D.C.: Government Printing Office, 1986:74.

26. Pitkin RM. Fetal death: diagnosis and management. *Am J Obstet Gynecol* 1987;157:583-9.

27. Morrison I, Olsen J. Weight-specific stillbirths and associated causes of death: an analysis of 765 stillbirths. *Am J Obstet Gynecol* 1985;152:975-80.

28. Rayburn W, Sander C, Barr M Jr, Rygiel R. The stillborn fetus: placental histologic examination in determining a cause. *Obstet Gynecol* 1985;65: 637-40.

7. The Use of Anencephalic Neonates as Organ Donors

Council on Ethical and Judicial Affairs,
American Medical Association

Hundreds of children die each year of cardiac, hepatic, or renal failure because there are not enough hearts, livers, or kidneys available for transplantation from other children. Consequently, various measures have been considered over the years to increase the organ supply for pediatric transplantation. One approach that has received particular attention is the possibility of using organs from anencephalic neonates.[1-3] Because anencephalic neonates face a certain and generally imminent death and because they lack any degree of consciousness, many commentators have proposed that organs of anencephalic neonates be used for transplantation, and many parents of such neonates request that their child's organs be given to other children. Permitting such organ donation would allow some good to come from a truly tragic situation, sustaining the lives of other children and providing psychological relief for those parents who wish to give meaning to the short life of the anencephalic neonate. Indeed, two years ago, parents of an anencephalic neonate went before the Florida Supreme Court, seeking permission to donate their anencephalic child's organs.[4] However, under current law, which requires persons to be dead before their life-sustaining organs may be removed for transplantation, it is not possible to use the organs of anencephalic neonates. Accordingly, the Florida court denied the parents' request, and the use of organs from anencephalic neonates remains a matter of debate rather than practice.

In 1988, this Council examined the ethical issues surrounding the use of organs from anencephalic neonates and concluded that it is ethically acceptable to remove organs from anencephalic neonates only after they have died,

Originally published in *JAMA* 273, no. 20 (May 24/31, 1995): 1614-18.

whether the death occurs by cessation of cardiac function or brain function.[5] In June 1994, after more than a year of deliberation, the Council revised its position and issued a new opinion. During its deliberations, the Council considered input from interested persons, including professionals and lay persons, and consulted the published literature on the use of organs from anencephalic neonates. The new opinion states that it is ethically acceptable to transplant the organs of anencephalic neonates even before the neonates die, as long as there is parental consent and certain other safeguards are followed.[6] This opinion is consistent with the majority view among experts in medicine and ethics. In a survey of leading medical experts in anencephaly and leading experts in ethics, two thirds of those surveyed stated that they consider the use of organs from anencephalic infants "intrinsically moral," and more than half stated their support for a change in the law to permit such use.[7(pS834),8(ppS617-S618)]

In this report, the Council presents its rationale for changing its position. The Council recognizes that, even with a change in its position, current law would have to be modified to permit parental donation of organs from an anencephahe neonate before the death of the neonate. In the past, the law has often changed to reflect evolution in ethical thought. Indeed, a report by a committee at Harvard Medical School[9] spurred the modification of the definition of death to mean either the complete cessation of cardiac function or the complete cessation of brain function. The Council presents this report in the hope that it will generate a similar public consensus in favor of permitting parental donation of organs from anencephalic neonates before the neonates die.

SHORTAGE OF ORGANS FOR TRANSPLANTATION IN INFANTS AND YOUNG CHILDREN

For patients of all ages, the demand for organs far outweighs the supply;[3,10] the shortage of organs is particularly acute when the patient needing the transplant is a young child or infant.[10-12] Newborns and other young children usually can benefit from organ transplants only if the organs are taken from children of similar size. However, there is a serious shortage of pediatric organ donors.[12,13] As a result, each year approximately 500 children need heart transplants, another 500 need liver replacements, and approximately 400 to 500 children in the United States need kidney transplants.[3,14] With the scarcity of hearts, livers, and kidneys available for transplantation, 30 to 50 percent of children younger than two years die while waiting for transplants.[15] Overall, 40 to 70 percent of children on the transplant waiting list die while waiting for a suitable organ.[3] These figures are undoubtedly underestimates of the shortage of pediatric organs. With the long waiting lists for the organs, many children in need never make it onto the lists because they would not have high enough priority to receive an organ or because they do not live long enough to have their names entered on the waiting list. Some commentators have therefore proposed that parents be allowed to donate organs from anencephalic neonates for transplantation.

ANECEPHALY

Anencephaly is a developmental abnormality of the central nervous system that results in the "congenital absence of a major portion of the brain, skull, and scalp."[16] Because anencephalic neonates lack functioning cerebral hemispheres, they never experience any degree of consciousness.[16,17(p1575)] They never have thoughts, feelings, sensations, desires, or emotions. There is no purposeful action, social interaction, memory, pain, or suffering. Anencephalic neonates have fully or partially functioning brain stem tissue. Accordingly, they are able to maintain at least some of the body's autonomic function (i.e., unconscious activity), including the functions of the heart, lungs, kidneys, and intestinal tract, as well as certain reflex actions. They may be able to breathe, suck, engage in spontaneous movements of their eyes, arms, and legs, respond to noxious stimuli with crying or avoidance maneuvers, and exhibit facial expressions typical of healthy infants.[16(pp671-672)] While all of this activity gives the appearance that the anencephalic neonate has some degree of consciousness, there is none. Anencephalic neonates are totally unaware of their existence and the environment in which they live.

The life span of an anencephalic neonate is generally very short. Many die within a few hours, less than half survive more than a day,[18] and fewer than 10 percent survive more than a week.[16(p671)] However, because these neonates often do not receive aggressive treatment, their potential life span is probably longer than their actual life span.[16(p671)] Indeed, in a recent court case,[19] an anencephalic child, Stephanie Keene, lived for two and a half years before dying (*Washington Post*, April 7, 1995:B3).

BENEFITS OF PERMITTING PARENTAL DONATION OF ORGANS FROM ANENCEPHALY NEONATES

The argument in favor of parental donation of organs from anencephalic neonates is compelling—many children will be saved from death, and many other children will realize a substantial improvement in their quality of life. As Benjamin Freedman[20] has observed, "organ transplantation is not simply an ethical enterprise but one that is, in its current stage of development, a moral imperative" for society. While society need not require donation of organs or fund all organ transplantations, there is a compelling social interest in permitting the use of organ transplantation as a medical therapy.

Organ transplantation from anencephalic neonates can bring profound benefit not only to the recipients of the organs but also to the parents of the anencephalic neonate. When confronted with the tragedy of bearing a child who can never experience consciousness and who will die in a matter of days, parents may find much of their psychological distress alleviated by the good that results from donating their child's organs and thereby providing lifesaving benefits to other children. Indeed, many parents of anencephalic neonates very much want to donate the organs of their anencephalic offspring to children whose only hope for life is an organ transplant.[3(p923),4(p589),21]

OBJECTIONS TO PARENTAL DONATION OF ORGANS FROM ANENCEPHALIC NEONATES

Several objections are commonly raised against proposals for parental donation of organs from anencephalic neonates: (1) donation violates the prohibition against removal of life-necessary organs from living persons, (2) false diagnosis of anencephaly may result in the death of neonates who could achieve consciousness, (3) permitting donation from anencephalic neonates may open the door to organ removal from patients who are in a persistent vegetative state or in other severely disabling conditions, (4) anencephalic neonates would rarely be a source of organs for transplantation, and (5) allowing donation of organs from anencephalic neonates will undermine public confidence in the organ transplantation system. As discussed herein, however, these concerns do not justify a prohibition on parental donation of organs from anencephalic infants.

1. Prohibition Against Removal from Living Persons

Both law and ethics require that persons be dead before their life-necessary, nonrenewable organs are taken (the "dead donor" rule).[22] This critical principle ensures that one person's life will not be sacrificed for the benefit of another person, even to preserve the life of that other person.[23] While this principle must be vigorously maintained, it must not be applied without regard to whether its application serves its purposes. After consideration of the purposes of the general prohibition against removal of life-necessary organs before death, it is clear that those purposes would not be compromised by permitting parental donation of organs from anencephalic neonates.

Protecting the interests of persons from whom organs are taken.—Ordinarily, the dead donor rule protects the fundamental interest in life of persons from whom organs are taken. However, it does not make sense to speak of an interest of anencephalic neonates in staying alive. Because they have never experienced consciousness and will never experience consciousness, anencephalic neonates cannot have interests of any kind.[24,25(pp127-128)] They cannot experience any pleasure or pain; they have no thoughts, memories, or sensations; and they have no ability to communicate. If their lives are shortened, they lose days of life, but they have no awareness of that loss. If there is a loss, it is a loss for others, whether for their parents or society generally. Similarly, the value in the life of an anencephalic neonate is a value only for others. The neonate feels no better or worse by living longer or by not living at all. Accordingly, prohibiting parental donation of organs from anencephalic neonates cannot be justified in terms of protecting the interests of the neonates themselves.

Providing reassurance to other individuals.—By protecting the interests of persons from whom organs are taken, the dead donor rule provides reassurance to other individuals that, if they choose to become organ donors, their lives will not be shortened by the removal of their organs for the benefit of someone in need of an organ transplant. While this is a critical purpose of the dead donor rule, parental donation of organs from anencephalic neonates will not undermine the rule's reassuring role. People who are contemplating organ donation never can become anencephalic. Accordingly, even if an exception to the dead donor rule is created for anencephalic neonates, people contemplating organ donation will know that they will still always receive the protection of the dead donor rule.

Preserving the value of respect for life.—The dead donor rule, like other prohibitions against killing, reflects the high value that society places on life and emphasizes that all life must be respected and treated with dignity, whatever the quality of life.[26] While respect for life is a value of utmost importance, it is not clear what implications that value has for the treatment of anencephalic neonates. First, it is important to emphasize that respect for the essential worth of life is an absolute value in the sense that it exists irrespective of a person's quality of life. However, it is not an absolute value in the sense of overriding all other values. Rather, it must be balanced with other important social values, including, as in this case, the fundamental social value of saving lives. Thus, for example, when allocating organs for transplantation among different potential recipients, it is permissible to give the organs to the individuals who will derive the most benefit from the organs even though other potential recipients have the same essential worth.

Because the anencephalic neonate is incapable of having an interest in staying alive, respect for the essential worth of the anencephalic neonate does not necessarily entail the preservation of its life. Indeed, it is well accepted that parents of anencephalic neonates always have the option of discontinuing life-sustaining treatment for anencephalic neonates. Society's clear acceptance of parental freedom to discontinue life-sustaining treatment for anencephalic neonates has occurred without evidence that it has diminished society's overall respect for the value of life. When life-sustaining treatment is discontinued, society shows its respect for the anencephalic neonate by treating the neonate as it would other irreversibly and seriously ill patients whose life-sustaining treatment is discontinued. For example, the neonate's corpse may not be desecrated, and the neonate is given a proper burial. Similarly, because the anencephalic infant is incapable of having an interest in staying alive, respect for the essential worth of the infant does not necessarily entail a prohibition on parental donation of the anencephalic neonate's organs before the neonate's death. Instead, society should show its respect for the anencephalic neonate by treating the neonate as it does persons whose organs are removed for transplantation after their death. In short, permitting parental donation of organs from anencephalic neonates is consistent with the social value of respect for life.

Indeed, the primary argument in favor of permitting parental donation is an argument based on the value of respect for life. The whole point of allowing such donation is to ensure that many lives that would otherwise be lost are saved.

2. Accuracy of Diagnosis

There has been concern that allowing parental donation of organs from anencephalic neonates could lead to parental donation of organs from infants with similar, severe conditions but who are not anencephalic.[27] Indeed, when researchers at Loma Linda University Medical Center conducted a protocol involving anencephalic neonates, some physicians referred infants to the protocol who were not in fact anencephalic (*Am Med News*, July 25, 1994:14). Misdiagnoses of infants as anencephalic have been documented in the medical literature and detected by surveillance programs.[16(p670)]

Nevertheless, while the possibility of misdiagnoses cannot be entirely eliminated, it can readily be reduced to an insignificant level with the adoption of appropriate safeguards. The diagnosis of anencephaly is highly reliable. As the Medical Task Force on Anencephaly[16(p670)] observed, "The appearance of the infant with anencephaly is unique, and the diagnosis can be made with virtual certainty when [the four defining] criteria [of anencephaly] are met." A prominent critic of parental donation of organs from anencephalic neonates has written that "[i]n the great majority of cases, the diagnosis of anencephaly is very obvious, and there is little, if any, chance of mistaking it for another condition."[28] With such a high degree of certainty, it is unlikely that anencephaly would be any more difficult (and perhaps even easier) to diagnose than brain death, which is currently accepted as a basis for organ donation from other patients. Problems with diagnosis of anencephaly occur primarily because the diagnosis is being made by a physician with insufficient expertise; as a corollary, there is little risk of misdiagnosis when the diagnosis is made by a physician with sufficient expertise. To ensure that the diagnosis of anencephaly is as accurate as possible, the diagnosis should be confirmed by two physicians with special expertise in diagnosing anencephaly who are not part of the organ transplant team. While this requirement may preclude the use of some organs, since two specialists may not always be readily available, it is an important safeguard. In some cases, even with the involvement of experts, it will not be clear whether the neonate is anencephalic.[16(p670)] In such cases, as others have argued,[29(p389)] parental donation of the organs should be prohibited until the neonate has died.

3. Slippery Slope Concerns

Some commentators oppose parental donation of organs from anencephalic neonates based on their belief that it would open the door to abuses of other persons: creating an exception to the dead donor rule to use organs from anencephalic neonates may result in further exceptions to enable organ removal from other persons with serious disabilities.[23(p8)] For example, many fear that individuals who are in a persistent vegetative state,[27(p1776)] infants with profound neurological injury, and elderly adults with severe dementia[23(p8)] would also be considered acceptable sources of organs.

The problem with this argument, as with other slippery slope arguments, is that any change in policy can be challenged on slippery slope grounds. When patients requested permission to reject life-sustaining treatment, opponents argued that granting such permission would open the way to euthanasia. Permitting the use of contraceptives, particularly those that work after fertilization, opens the way to abortion. It is not enough, therefore, simply to invoke a slippery slope argument. Rather, it must be shown that the slippery slope risk is a serious one in the particular issue under consideration.

There is an important reason why the slippery slope risk is not a serious one if society decides to permit parental donation of organs from anencephalic neonates. Anencephalic neonates are unique among persons because they have no history of consciousness and no possibility of ever being conscious. Infants with other severely disabling conditions have at least some degree of consciousness as do elderly persons with severe dementia. Accordingly, unlike anencephalic neonates, severely disabled infants and adults have interests, including interests in staying alive. While patients who are in a persistent vegetative state no longer are conscious, they once were conscious and have therefore previously established an identity and a set of interests.[25(pp128-129,194)] Society's treatment of living wills or other advance directives that were written by persons who have become permanently unconscious demonstrates society's recognition of the fact that a person retains interests even after becoming permanently unconscious. Under current law, a person's advance directive will be honored even if the person becomes persistently vegetative, and it will be honored because it is in the person's interest to have it honored. Accordingly, even if families disagree with the person's choices in the advance directive, they have no authority to have the directive over-ridden. In short, because anencephalic neonates and other disabled persons differ on the very factor that justifies parental donation of organs from anencephalic neonates, there is little force to the analogy between organ removal from anencephalic neonates and organ removal from other persons with severely disabling conditions.

To be sure, there may be some temporary problems with drawing a distinction between neonates with anencephaly and those with similar but less severe abnormalities. Physicians and parents may be upset if society does not allow use of organs from infants who are less severely affected. However, prohibiting the use of organs from anencephalic infants is not going to solve their concern. It still leaves the physicians and parents with no ability to have organs taken from the less severely affected children. Second, this is likely to be a problem that will disappear over time as people come to understand that organs only from anencephalic infants can be used.

4. Number of Children Who Would Benefit

Critics of parental donation of organs from anencephalic neonates have argued that too few children would benefit from the organs of anencephalic neonates. These critics observe that, while estimates of the number of anencephalic births generally are within the range of 1,000 to 2,000 births per year,[13(p116),16(p671),27(p1774)] most anencephalic neonates are stillborn, and organs from some live-born anencephalic neonates are not suitable for transplantation.[27(p1774)] As a result, the number of children who could benefit from the organs of anencephalic neonates may be considerably smaller than 1,000; indeed, according to one estimate, no more than about twenty infants a year would gain a long-term survival from a heart or liver transplant, and no more than another twenty-five infants would receive a long-term benefit from kidney transplantation.[27(p1775)]

This concern about the number of children who would benefit should not be a barrier to parental donation of organs from anencephalic neonates. First, the estimates are probably much too low. The estimate of only twenty long-term survivals from heart or liver transplants depends on a series of assumptions, most of which are unreliable. According to one assumption, only 40 percent of live-born anencephalic neonates would have birth weights high enough for them to have usable organs. In addition, the estimate assumes that another 15 to 25 percent of hearts and livers will not be usable because of malformations.[27(p1774)] Yet, in a study of twelve live-born anencephalic neonates, researchers found that, on admission of the neonates to the study protocol, the hearts and livers of almost all the neonates were suitable for transplantation.[15(pp346-348)] The estimate also assumes that no more than 25 percent of usable organs would actually be used.[27(p1775)] However, because of advances in organ transplantation technology in the six years since this assumption was made, it is likely that many more organs would be usable. Each anencephalic neonate may be able to provide four lifesaving organs (heart, liver, and kidneys). More importantly, even assuming that there would be only twenty long-term survivals gained each year and that only long-term survivals matter, it is not clear why that should be an objection to parental donation of organs from anencephalic neonates. Among the different goals that health care can achieve, saving lives is of fundamental importance; indeed, it is never insignificant to save twenty lives.

To be sure, there are limits to the price that society can or should pay to save lives, but none of the other arguments against parental donation of organs from anencephalic neonates suggests that such limits would be reached if parental donation were permitted.

5. Public Trust in the Organ Procurement System

Some commentators suggest that creating an exception to the dead donor rule may undermine society's confidence in the organ procurement system and cause a chilling effect on overall organ donations.[13(p1119),27(p1776)] According to this view, even though use of organs from anencephalic neonates might be morally justified when considered in isolation, creating an exception to the dead donor rule will have undesirable effects in the broader social context in which members of the public harbor concerns about physicians removing organs prematurely from dying patients for transplantations. However, the modification of the definition of death to include the complete cessation of ·brain function was a far more fundamental change in social policy than the change proposed here, and the move to brain-based conceptions of death occurred explicitly to facilitate organ procurement.[9] Moreover, that change required an exception to the previously clear rule that people would not be considered dead until there was complete cessation of cardiopulmonary function. Inasmuch as the change in the definition of death has not compromised the effectiveness of the organ procurement system but has led to greater numbers of lives saved by organ transplantation, it is likely that permitting parental donation of organs from anencephalic neonates will also lead to greater numbers of lives saved rather than to compromise of the organ procurement system. In addition, while it is true that existing organ procurement practices should not be changed without due deliberation, change should be possible in response to important, unmet social needs and evolving understanding of the ethical and scientific issues surrounding anencephaly.

Accordingly, rather than prohibiting parental donation of organs from anencephalic neonates, certain safeguards should be used to preserve public trust in the organ procurement system. First, parental donation of organs from anencephalic neonates should occur only if the discussion of donation is initiated by the parents of the neonates, not if it is initiated by members of the health care team. Second, parental donation should not occur without the fully informed consent of the parents of the anencephalic neonate. Third, a pilot program for parental donation of organs from anencephalic neonates should be undertaken to assess its impact before the practice becomes widespread. For example, a single, major medical center could establish a protocol for organ retrieval from anencephalic neonates.

If parents are ever permitted to donate the organs of anencephalic neonates, it is critical that they retain the freedom not to donate. While the Council believes that it is ethically permissible to donate organs of anencephalic neonates, people have very different views about the appropriateness of donation, just as people have very different views about the appropriateness of treating patients in a persistent vegetative state with a ventilator.[31,32] At all times, parents should be permitted to choose among treatment of their anencephalic neonate, withdrawal of treatment, and donation of organs.

Conclusion

For the reasons described herein, the Council has developed the following opinion, which has been revised minimally since its original issuance in June 1994 to clarify the Council's intent (substantive additions are italicized):

2.162 Anencephalic Neonates as Organ Donors. Anencephaly is a congenital absence of a major portion of the brain, skull, and scalp. Neonates with this condition are born without a forebrain and without a cerebrum. While anencephalic neonates are born with a rudimentary functional brain stem, their lack of a functioning cerebrum permanently forecloses the possibility of consciousness.

It is ethically permissible to consider the anencephalic neonate as a potential organ donor, although still alive under the current definition of death, only if: (1) the diagnosis of anencephaly is certain and is confimed by two physicians *with special expertise* who are not part of the organ transplant team; (2) the parents of the neonate *initiate any discussions about organ retrieval and* indicate their desire for retrieval in writing; and (3) there is compliance with the Council's Guidelines for the Transplantation of Organs (see Opinion 2.16, Organ Transplantation Guidelines).

In the alternative, a family wishing to donate the organs of their anencephalic neonate may choose to provide the neonate with ventilator assistance and other medical therapies that might sustain organ perfusion and viability until such time as a determination of death can be made in accordance with current medical standards and relevant law. In this situation, the family should be informed of the possibility that the organs might deteriorate in the process, rendering them unsuitable for transplantation.

It is normally required that a person be legally dead before removal of their life-necessary organs (the "dead donor rule"). The use of the anencephalic neonate as a live donor is a limited exception to the general standard because of the fact that the infant has never experienced, and will never experience, consciousness.

(Although this modified version of Opinion 2.162 will not appear in the published volume of the American Medical Association's *Code of Medical Ethics* until the next issue in 1996, the modified version took effect on its issuance in December 1994. The June 1994 version of this opinion is printed at page 30 of the council on Ethical and Judicial Affairs, *Code of Medical Ethics: Current Opinions With Annotations*, Chicago, Ill: American Medical Association, 1994.)

REFERENCES

1. Fletcher JC, Robertson JA, Harrison MR. Primates and anencephalics as sources for pediatric organ transplants. *Fetal Ther*. 1986;1:150-164.

2. Caplan AL. Ethical issues in the use of anencephalic infants as a source of organs and tissues for transplantation. *Transplant Proc*. 1988;20(4, suppl 5):42-49.

3. Friedman JA. Taking the camel by the nose: the anencephalic as a source for pediatric organ transplants. *Columbia Law Rev*. 1990;90:917-978.

4. *In re TACP*, 609 So 2d 588 (Fla 1992).

5. Council on Ethical and Judicial Affairs. Anencephalic infants as organ donors. In: *Code of Medical Ethics: Reports*. Vol 1. Chicago, Ill: American Medical Association; 1992:49-52.

6. Council on Ethical and Judicial Affairs, American Medical Association. *Code of Medical Ethics: Current Opinions With Annotations*. Chicago, Ill: American Medical Association; 1994:§2.162.

7. Walters JW. Anencephalic infants as organ sources: current attitudes and prospects. *BioLaw*. 1992;III:S834-S837.

8. Walters JW. The question of anencephalic infants as organ sources. *BioLaw*. 1991;II:S613-S624.

9. Report of the Ad Hoc Committee of the Harvard Medical School to Examine the Defmition of Brain Death: a definition of irreversible coma. *JAMA*. 1968;205:337-340.

10. Iglehart J. Transplantation: the problem of limited resources. *N Engl J Med*. 1983;309.123-128.

11. Harrison MR. Organ procurement for children: the anencephalic fetus as donor. *Lancet*. 1986;2:1383-1386.

12. Guttman FM. Organ transplantation in children. *Pediatr Ann*. 1982;11:910-915.

13. Committee on Bioethics, American Academy of Pediatrics. Infants with anencephaly as organ sources: ethical considerations. *Pediatrics*. 1992;89:1116-1119.

14. Brandon B. Anencephalic infants as organ donors: a question of life or death. *Case Western Reserve Law Rev*. 1990;40:781-824.

15. Peabody JL, Emery JR, Ashwal S. Experience with anencephalic infants as prospective organ donors. *N Engl J Med*.1989;321:344-350.

16. Medical Task Force on Anencephaly. The infant with anencephaly. *N Engl J Med.* 1990;322:669-674.

17. Multi-Society Task Force on PVS. Medical aspects of the persistent vegetative state: (second of two parts). *N Engl J Med.* 1994;330:1572-1579.

18. Botkin JR. Anencephalic infants as organ donors. *Pediatrics.* 1988;82:250-256.

19. In *re Baby "K,"* 16 F3d 590 (4th Cir 1994).

20. Freedman B. The anencephalic organ donor: affect, analysis, and ethics. *Transplant Proc.* 1988; 20(4, suppl 5):57-63.

21. Fost N. Organs from anencephalic infants: an idea whose time has not yet come. *Hastings Cent Rep.* 1988;18(5):5-10.

22. Arnold RM, Youngner SJ. The dead donor rule: should we stretch it, bend it, or abandon it? *Kennedy Inst Ethics J.* 1993;2:263-278.

23. Capron AM. Anencephalic donors: separate the dead from the dying. *Hastings Cent Rep.* 1987;17 (1): 5-9.

24. Robertson JA. Policy issues in a non-heart-beating donor protocol. *Kennedy Inst Ethics J.* 1993;3:241-250.

25. Buchanan AE, Brock DW. *Deciding for Others: The Ethics of Surrogate Decision Making.* Cambridge, England: Cambridge University Press; 1989.

26. Orentlicher D. Physician-assisted dying: the conflict with fundamental principles of American law. In: Blank RH, Bonnicksen AL, eds. *Medicine Unbound: The Human Body and the Limits of Medical Intervention.* New York, NY: Columbia University Press; 1994, pp. 257-268.

27. Shewmon DA, Capron AM, Peacock WJ, Schulman BL. The use of anencephalic infants as organ donors: a critique. *JAMA.* 1989;261:1773-1781.

28. Shewmon DA. Anencephaly: selected medical aspects. *Hastings Cent Rep.* 1988;18(5):11-19.

29. Truog RD, Fletcher JC. Anencephalic enewborns: can organs be transplanted before brain death? *N Engl J Med.* 1989;321:388-390.

30. Childress JF. Reasons not to use anencephalics' organs for transplantation prior to death. *BioLaw.* 1992;III:S845-S847.

31. Angell M. The case of Helga Wanglie: a new kind of 'right to die' case. *N Engl J Med.* 1991;325: 511-512.

32. Miles SH. Informed demand for 'non-beneficial' medical treatment. *N Engl J Med.* 1991;325:512-515.

8. The Use of Anencephalic Infants as Organ Sources: A Critique

D. Alan Shewmon, Alexander M. Capron,
Warwick J. Peacock, and
Barbara L. Schulman

In July 1988, Loma Linda (California) University Medical Center suspended the controversial protocol under which it had been the only center in the United States with an active program for harvesting organs from anencephalic infants for transplantation (*Los Angeles Times*, August 19, 1988:[pt I]3; *Los Angeles Times*, August 24, 1988:[pt I]25).[1] In reaching this decision (following thirteen failed attempts to obtain organs from such babies during the preceding seven months), the protocol's principal author acknowledged that critics had been justified in worrying about such issues as the consequences for the anencephalic infant and the expansion of the category of potential donors to infants with less severe defects. The experience of the Loma Linda program clearly indicates that substantial ethical as well as practical issues remain to be resolved before any further effort is made to employ anencephalic infants as organ "donors."

The attempt to harvest organs from anencephalics itself reflects the difficulties physicians have faced in responding to the growing demand for suitable donors generated by recent progress in pediatric organ transplantation. The first difficulty is that death in organ donors is usually diagnosed through the use of brain-based criteria (typically referred to as "brain death").[2,3] Yet, the sorts of injuries (such as highway accidents) that can destroy the brain, while leaving the other organs intact for transplantation, are much rarer in infants than in adults and older children. Aside from use of contrast angiography, diagnostic criteria for infant brain death have not been validated, and certainty of diagnosis is much less easily attained than in older patients,[4,5] recent guidelines[6-8] notwithstanding.

The difficulties in obtaining adequate numbers of infant cadavers with arti-

Originally published in *JAMA* 261, no. 12 (March 24/31, 1989): 1773-80.

ficially supported vital functions have led some physicians to search for alternative sources of organs, such as other animal species, human fetuses, and even dying—but still living—human infants. Anencephalic infants are the main group so far proposed. Objections to using them as organ sources before death has been diagnosed and declared, which we discuss, led to the Loma Linda protocol under which organs were to be harvested only after death had been declared in infants receiving ventilatory support. In this article, we also discuss the issues raised by this now-suspended approach to obtaining infant organs.

HISTORICAL REVIEW

During the past twenty-five years, there have been a number of reports of heart[9-11] and kidney[12-28] transplants using anencephalic donors, with varying results. In most of the U.S. cases of kidney transplants, the donors were declared dead prior to removal of organs; although the basis for determining death was not always stated, when reported it was the cessation of heart beat and respiration. In the few cases of heart transplants, death was putatively declared on the basis of neurological criteria.

These previous reports of the use of anencephalic infants raise several serious issues, the first of which is the physicians' lack of clarity about the status of these patients. For example, Lawson et al.,[17] describing kidney harvesting from an infant of thirty-seven weeks' gestation, stated that "the anencephalic fetus was delivered by cesarean section and was kept on a sterile field while the nephrectomies were performed. No attempt was made to resuscitate the fetus during the nephrectomies." Plainly, the source of the kidneys was a live-born infant, no longer a fetus; had the infant been stillborn, the kidneys would have been unusable.

Second, without announcing that a less demanding standard was employed, in some cases determinations of death appear to have been made that would have been unacceptable in nonanencephalic patients. For example, Iitaka and colleagues[21] regarded the anencephalic as a cadaver "once assisted ventilation is required," apparently not because this is the usual criterion for death but because "thereafter the condition of the donor deteriorates rapidly." The deviation from usual standards was particularly notable in two anencephalic heart transplant cases in the late 1960s.[9,10] It seems dubious that the cited criteria of a flat electroencephalogram and absence of all neurological functions would have applied to the anencephalic infants, because it is unclear how even to perform an electroencephalogram on these patients and because there is no reason for the neural tissue of an anencephalic to cease functioning prior to somatic death. Instead, the timing of the cardiac excision appears to have been based on the moment when the heart stopped beating spontaneously, albeit not irreversibly. That the cessation of heart beat in one case[9] happened to take place conveniently in the operating room after heparinization and cooling to −2.8°C in preparation for the transplant raises further questions as to whether the "donor's" death was entirely spontaneous.

CURRENT DEVELOPMENTS

The problems that lay below the surface in these earlier attempts to transplant organs from anencephalic infants are receiving attention again because of the increased interest in obtaining neonatal organs. Several new arguments have been advanced for the use of these infants as organ sources. First, some have suggested that the inevitability of the rapid demise of anencephalics justifies their use ante mortem.[29,30] This was the rationale for bill 3367 introduced in New Jersey in October 1986 by Assemblyman Walter Kern, Jr, which would have amended the Uniform Anatomical Gift Act (UAGA) to permit parents of an anencephalic infant to donate its organs before death. Second, it has been argued that anencephalics are "brain absent" and therefore should be regarded as equivalent to being "brain dead."[28-30] On this basis, California Senator Milton Marks in 1986 promoted SB 2018, which, as originally formulated, would have expanded the Uniform Deterimination of Death Act (UDDA) to include anencephaly as a basis for diagnosing death, in addition to irreversible cessation of circulatory and respiratory functions or irreversible cessation of all functions of the entire brain.[31] Various groups, including the California Medical Association, opposed the use of live anencephalic infants as organ sources and these bills failed to be adopted. Subsequently, other professional groups, such as the California Nurses Association[32] and the United Network for Organ Sharing,[33] have expressed similar opposition to the application of special standards to anencephalic infants.

Alternatively, some physicians believe that organs can be harvested from these infants without having to change medical and legal standards. Loma Linda University Medical Center, for example, adopted a protocol in December 1987 under which anencephalic infants would receive ventilatory support at birth and then be monitored for up to seven days or until all brain functions had ceased.[1] Hoping to increase the likelihood that brain death would occur within the seven-day limit, Loma Linda modified the protocol in April 1988 to delay ventilatory support until the infant began to manifest major respiratory or circulatory difficulties. The program was finally discontinued in July 1988 because few of these infants actually became brain dead under such circumstances (*Los Angeles Times*, August 19, 1988:(pt I]3).[1] In light of the heavy reliance on apnea as the major criterion in determining death in this approach, Ohio State Representative Tom Watkins proposed Substitute HB 718 to establish a special legal category of "respiratory brain death," under which anencephalic infants could be declared dead based only on apnea.

These various approaches, which have also been seriously considered at several other medical centers across the country though not implemented,[1,34] raise several important issues. First, should anencephalics be carried to term and then used as organ donors while still alive though dying? Second, can death be reliably determined in artificially supported anencephalic infants, and if so, should they be so maintained to enhance their utility as organ sources? An affirmative response to one or both questions is given by those who favor allowing parents of anencephalics to "salvage something positive" out of the tragedy by donating their child's organs to save the life of another child. Plainly, this argument has a great deal of appeal, and multiple popular accounts of these situations, as well as the experience of donor referral centers, make it apparent that this wish is strongly felt by some of the parents of anencephalics (*San Francisco Chronicle*, May 5, 1986:1; *New York Times*, September 9, 1986:Cl). From a utilitarian standpoint, providing legal sanction for the harvesting of organs from anencephalics might seem a way to maximize net utility for society as a whole. Such a conclusion may be short-sighted, however, because either legalizing organ removal from live anencephalics or applying unvalidated criteria for death might undermine the very goal of promoting infant organ transplantation and endanger society in the process, while actually producing surprisingly few usable organs.

MEDICAL UTILITY

It is possible to calculate the approximate number of patients who would benefit from anencephalic organs if no ethical or legal barriers to their retrieval existed. (A fuller explanation of these figures and a more complete set of references are provided in a recent article by one of us [D.A.S.].[35]) The prevalence rate of anencephaly has been declining steadily over the past several decades almost everywhere in the world.[36-42] In the United States in the late 1980s, a conservative estimate is around 0.3 per 1,000 total births.[35] Given a national birth rate of 3.75 million per year,[43] this yields an estimate of 1,125 anencephalic infants potentially born each year in this country. Probably around 20 percent of pregnancies nationwide are screened for neural tube defects during the second trimester by means of either ultrasound or maternal serum alpha-fetoprotein testing and 95 percent of the detected anencephalic fetuses are electively aborted (Linda Dobbs, RN, Southern California regional coordinator for the alpha-fetoprotein screening program, UCLA Medical Center, Los Angeles, Calif, oral communication, July 1988), making the number of anencephalic births per year around 911. Some two-thirds of anencephalics are stillborn,[39(pp68,75-76,84,109),41,44] reducing the annual number of live-born anencephalics to 304.

Slightly more than half of anencephalic births are premature (less than thirty-seven weeks' gestation)[39(pp55-56),45] and some 50 to 80 percent have birth weights less than 2500 g.[45,46] Taking 60 percent as the proportion of anencephalics too small to provide transplantable organs, the annual number of useful anencephalics is 122. If as many as two-thirds of the parents of these infants would be willing to donate their child's organs while still living, the number of donated, useful anencephalics decreases to eighty-one.

But not all transplantable organs are actually used. In particular, the experience with grafting infant kidneys has been disappointing relative to the success rate with older donors; moreover, the technique of chronic peritoneal dialysis in infancy has improved enough that pediatric nephrologists generally prefer to treat infants with renal failure by means of dialysis until they reach several years of age, when the likelihood of a successful transplant is much higher.[47,48] For this reason, the kidneys from infant liver or heart donors are typically not salvaged. Around 15 percent of anencephalic hearts will be unusable on account of associated malformation or excessive hypoplasia.[49-53] Size-matching between donor and recipient organs is much more important for liver transplants than for hearts[48,54] and an estimated 25 percent of the livers will be unusable on the basis of malformation or hypoplasia.[50,51(pp79-80),52,53] Thus, the estimated annual number of usable anencephalic kidneys, hearts, and livers reduces to zero, sixty-nine, and sixty-one, respectively.

For various reasons, around 25 percent of referrals of vital organs (all ages combined) are found acceptable by established organ-sharing networks, and the figure for hearts is even less. Some reasons for the nonuse of organs are the desirability of blood-type compatibility for hearts and livers, the need for temporal coincidence of potential donors and compatible potential recipients, and difficulties in transporting organs or sick patients across great distances. Infants with biliary atresia almost always receive first a Kasai procedure and then are placed on the national transplant waiting list at four or five months of age, by which time many are no longer size-compatible with a newborn donor.[55]

Such problems are illustrated by the experience to date at Loma Linda University Medical Center. By the time of discontinuation of their protocol (and including the first case, referred from Canada prior to formal initiation of the protocol), fourteen anencephalic infants had been referred for possible organ donation; three of those were declared brain dead within the specified seven-day limit, yet only a single vital organ, a heart, ended up being transplanted (*Los Angeles Times*, August 19, 1988:[pt I]3).[1]

It would seem that protocols respecting existing standards of brain death are simply not going to yield a sufficient number of usable organs to be worthwhile. Even if laws were relaxed so as to allow the harvesting of organs from live anencephalics soon after birth, it is doubtful that any more than 25 percent and 15 percent of otherwise suitable hearts and livers, respectively, would actually be used, bringing the yearly number of transplanted anencephalic kidneys, hearts, and livers to zero, seventeen, and nine, respectively, at most.

Finally, the net benefit to the infant recipients of these organs is unclear, as the experience with transplantation at this age is still so limited. A long-term survival rate of 50 percent and 20 percent for hearts and livers, respectively, is reasonable, given the current state of the art, reducing the yearly number of children nationwide who would actually benefit from anencephalic kidneys, hearts, and livers to zero, nine, and two, respectively. These figures will undoubtedly increase as transplantation techniques improve. On the other hand, the magnitude of that increase will be offset by the decrease in the natural prevalence of anencephaly and the increase in prenatal screening. An optimistic projection of the annual number of patients benefiting from anencephalic kidneys, hearts, and livers nationwide ten years from now is twenty-five, twelve, and seven, respectively.[35]

When enthusiasts begin to realize that the number of usable organs from anencephalics will fall far short of the demand, even if present laws requiring donor death were to be relaxed, various steps might be taken to increase the supply, even though current proponents would not endorse such extensions of their proposals. The number of donors could be increased, for example, by encouraging the parents of prenatally diagnosed anencephalics not to abort. Although proponents typically advise against allowing financial incentives in this area,[28] the power of human ingenuity to circumvent formal restrictions on economic transactions is well known.

It is even possible that an unlimited supply of anencephalics could be purposefully created by means of in vitro fertilization under the influence of an appropriate teratogen, with hired surrogate mothers to carry the organ sources to term. This may seem farfetched at present, but it is a logical development in the evolving trend of increasing interest in fetuses as "organ farms"[56-59] and an increasing desire to dominate human reproduction technologically.[60] Recently, some women have seriously proposed conceiving in order to abort for the sake of fetal tissue for transplantation, either for themselves or for a relative (*Seattle Times*, March 7, 1988:F1). Although their wishes were not carried out, the mere proposal of such a thing would have been unthinkable only a few years ago. If the present direction of evolution of societal attitudes continues, the day can be foreseen in which "anencephalic factories" are a standard source of transplantable organs, yet it requires little imagination to see that the good of the surviving organ recipients would hardly offset the global harm to society of an approving attitude toward such crass manipulation of human life.

ETHICOLEGAL CONSIDERATIONS

The natural cause of death in anencephaly is ultimately hypoventilation, which renders the vital organs unsuitable for transplantation by the time death could be declared. To make it legal to harvest these organs while still usable would thus require either (1) a revision of the UAGA to allow removal of vital organs from live patients (as proposed in New Jersey), (2) a legal definition of anencephalics as non-human beings or nonpersons or lacking any "interests" (as is frequently stated in the literature) and therefore outside the scope of laws protecting innocent human life, (3) an expansion of the UDDA to include anencephaly as a variant of "brain death" (as proposed in California), or (4) an attempt to accommodate such transplantations to existing laws by giving the anencephalic infant ventilatory support and waiting for traditional brain death to occur (as was attempted at Loma Linda).

Revision of the UAGA to Include Live Anencephalics as Acceptable Donors

The first alternative opens up possibilities for abuse that are only too obvious. The principle behind excepting some human organ donors from being dead ultimately reduces to one of the following: either homicide should be lawful if it is motivated by saving the life of another whose life is not threatened by the person killed, or homicide should be lawful if the victim is about to die anyway. But if these are valid principles for anencephalics, then they are also valid for a whole host of other patients, when, in fact, the law makes no such exceptions. This logical inconsistency might then be used to justify subsequent expansion of the exceptions to include incompetent patients in the final stages of a terminal illness or even prisoners on death row, whose organs would be much more suitable for transplantation than those of anencephalics and whose execution could be timed according to the availability of an optimally matched recipient.

Specifically, using this kind of logic, half of all the infants who die of congenital kidney, heart, and liver disease would better be used as organ sources to preserve the lives of the other half, rather than letting them all die along with their transplantable organs. Even though this sounds preposterous, the experience at transplantation referral centers indicates that the enthusiasm for using anencephalics does indeed quickly extend to other categories of dying infants. As a result of the national interest in Loma Linda's protocol, for example, that institution received from "good" physicians several referrals of infants with less severe anomalies for organ donation, such as "babies born with an abnormal amount of fluid around the brain or those born without kidneys but with a normal brain." Moreover, the referring physicians " 'couldn't understand the difference' between such newborns and anencephalics." Joyce Peabody, MD, chief of neonatology there and primary drafter of the protocol, deserves much credit for her courageously candid statement: "I have become educated by the experience. . . . The slippery slope is real" (*Los Angeles Times*, August 19, 1988:[pt I]3).

Legal Definition of Anencephalics as Nonpersons

The second approach would be based on the philosophical tenet that anencephalics are not human beings, or at least not "persons," thereby eliminating the main ethical problem in killing them. This could be argued on the basis of either their age or their neurological lesion. There are indeed ethicists who maintain that even neurologically normal human infants are not persons, that they therefore have no right to life, and that their killing would not be murder.[61,62] Such philosophers differ on the age at which they believe that postnatal infants become persons, ranging from a few days to several months. Clearly, if one's goal is to increase public enthusiasm for infant organ donation, this is not the best principle to invoke.

A greater number of philosophers, however, maintain that severe neurological impairment is incompatible with personhood. For example, Joseph Fletcher[63] has argued that:

> Any individual of the species *homo sapiens* who falls below the I.Q. 40-mark in a standard Stanford-Binet test, amplified if you like by other tests, is questionably a person; below the 20-mark, not a person. . . . This has bearing, obviously, on decision making in gynecology, obstetrics and pediatrics, as well as in general surgery and medicine.

Singer[64] maintains that:

> If we compare a severely defective human infant with a nonhuman animal, a dog or a pig, for example, we will often find the nonhuman to have superior capacities, both actual and potential, for rationality, self-consciousness, communication, and anything else that can plausibly be considered morally significant. Only the fact that the defective infant is a member of the species *homo sapiens* leads it to be treated differently from the dog or pig. Species membership alone, however, is not morally relevant.

The potential for diagnostic confusion that can invade attempts to draw lines of "personhood" based on neurological deficit is illustrated in the use of the unqualified term hydrocephalic by Lachs[65] in an argument that these children are not persons and that in comparison "pigeons have more personality [and] the indigo bunting more intellect." The fact that anencephaly is one of the few conditions that has been argued as an indication for even third-trimester abortions (partly on the basis of "total or virtual absence of cognitive function")[66] is often cited as a rationale for the legitimacy of killing the same beings a few weeks later, postnatally, for their organs.[67]

Even if it were possible in theory to know with certainty that a particular degree of neurological deficit was incompatible with personhood, it is extremely doubtful that in practice very many would be capable of applying such knowledge to individual cases without risk of error. And even if they, in good conscience, believed they were killing nonpersons for the sake of persons, the majority of the rest of the world—in their inevitable unsophistication—would fail to perceive any distinction between that and murder justified by utilitarian principles, and the general impression that the latter had become legitimate would have disastrous consequences for society.[68] Moreover, it would be presumptuous for anyone to maintain that he or she was certain enough that an anencephalic infant was not a person to be willing to risk committing murder by killing it for its organs, given that a large number of equally intelligent people do regard it as a person, albeit with a severe disability.

Were it conceded, for the sake of argument, that some categories of congenital brain malformations are so extreme as to be clearly incompatible with personhood, there is the obvious problem of knowing where to draw the line along the continuum of severity. In addition to the difficulties in defining anencephaly precisely (see below), infants with other severe congenital neurological anomalies and older children and adults in a persistent vegetative state are functionally similar to anencephalics (insofar as they operate on a brain stem alone) and would also fail to qualify as persons on the same basis. It would be inconsistent to legitimize the removal of organs from anencephalics on the basis that they are nonpersons, while proscribing the use of hydranencephalic, atelencephalic, lissencephalic, and persistently vegetative patients, those with end-stage degenerative brain diseases, and so forth.[69] All of these patients would equally fail to qualify as persons, and their organs would actually be both more usable and more plentiful than those of anencephalics. The impossibility of defining a logically consistent neurological boundary between persons and nonpersons is why even people who ascribe privately to the nonpersonhood theory mostly do not advocate its practical application in law.

Differentiating Anencephalic Infants by Lack of Consciousness

Short of labeling anencephalics nonpersons, many commentators have suggested that these infants can be treated differently from others because they are incapable of experiencing consciousness or pain, and therefore have no interests and cannot be harmed. Although this is undoubtedly true for those with complete craniorachischisis, such infants are of little interest vis-à- vis their organs, because they are almost invariably stillborn. Whether those with relatively intact brain stems have any subjective awareness associated with their responsiveness to the environment is inherently unverifiable, but what is known about the functional capabilities of the brain stem, particularly in newborns, suggests at least keeping an open mind.

In experimental animals, brain stem structures have been shown to mediate complex behaviors, sometimes traditionally assumed to be cortical, including binocular depth perception,[70] habituation, learning, and discriminative conditioning.[71-75] Similarly, decerebrate (anencephalic or hydranen-cephalic) human newborns with relatively intact brain stems can manifest a surprising repertory of complex behaviors, including distinguishing their mothers from others, consolability, conditioning, and associative learning,[76-80] although irritability and decreased ability to habituate are also common.[76,81] Lorber[82] described a remarkable case of a boy with hydranencephaly, diagnosed by pneumoencephalography, who had developed normally as of twenty-one months of age. Although the author suspected the existence of a cerebral cortex somewhere in the head, he was unable to find even a thin mantle between the injected air and the inner table of the skull. Even in normal human newborns, the cerebral cortex, though grossly present, is much less developed microscopically than the brain stem[83(pp56-64,297-98)] and is relatively nonfunctional, as revealed by positron emission tomography.[84] Thus, it is possible, for example that parents of hydranencephalic infants often fail to realize during the first month or two that anything is wrong with their baby.

Without question, decerebrate infants are neurologically much more similar to normal infants than they are to decerebrate adults, and it simply begs the question to apply adult-derived neurophysiological principles to this age group in support of the claim that a functioning cortex is necessary for consciousness or pain perception in newborns. Moreover, the phenomenon of developmental neuroplasticity could, in principle, allow brain-stem structures in the congenital absence of cerebral hemispheres to assume somewhat more complex integrative activity than would ordinarily be the case, as has been suggested in some animal studies.[85-87] Thus, it neither logically nor physiologically follows that anencephalic infants "by definition . . . can neither feel nor experience pain."[88] The main difference between decerebrate and normal newborns lies not so much in their actual functional abilities as in their potential for future cognitive development. Therefore, both prudence and logical consistency demand that we attribute to anencephalic infants at least as much consciousness and capacity for suffering as we attribute to laboratory animals with even smaller brains, which everyone seems to feel obliged to treat "humanely."

Revision of the UDDA to Define Anencephalics as Dead

Suggestions to include anencephaly within the definition of "death" pose many problems, including further expansion to other categories of patients with severe neurological impairments, damage to public confidence in death determinations (and thus a decline in the total number of organs offered for transplantation), and adverse impact on families that do not wish to regard their anencephalic child as dead.

At the heart of the proposals to amend the UDDA or comparable statutes is the assumption that there is no possibility of misdiagnosis or entry into a "slippery slope" of expanding exceptions.[28-30] Nevertheless, serious misdiagnosis is possible; for example, in an epidemiologic study, Baird and Sadovnick[89] came across a case of amniotic band syndrome that was mistaken for anencephaly. Elsewhere, amniotic band syndrome has been reported as an actual *cause* of anencephaly, obviously implying a wide spectrum of severity compatible with that diagnosis.[90,91] Some cases of anencephaly are associated with the facial features of holoprosencephaly, introducing another direction for possible diagnostic confusion.[51(p62),92,93]

More fundamentally, the contention that "brain absence can be clearly defined"[30] and "cannot be expanded to include individuals with less severe anomalies or injuries"[29] is not confirmed by those most experienced in fetal neuropathology. Literally, *anencephaly* means absence of the brain, but the term has been and continues to be used to describe a developmental anomaly in which only the cerebral hemispheres are missing or extremely rudimentary, while the brain stem and varying portions of the diencephalon are present. A major textbook on anencephaly[51(p5)] states: "An almost incomprehensible array of synonyms and classifications of anencephaly exists in the literature; many include entities now considered to be pathogenetically unrelated to the anencephaly spectrum." Another expert on congenital malformations has written: "[Anencephaly] exemplifies the problems and difficulties of teratologic research in man. The terminology is confusing. . . ."[94(p189)] Current usage also implies partial or complete absence of the cranial vault, but one anatomist has stated that "the [calvarial] defect is so widely variable that a rigid classification is almost impossible."[95] (See, for example, the relatively small skull and scalp defect in specimen AN-61 in Figs 1a and 1b of Siebert et al.[93] and in Fig 4-12 of Lemire et al.[83(p62)])

Indeed, anencephaly is not an all-or-none phenomenon, but constitutes an imprecisely defined range of conditions toward one end of a spectrum of congenital malformations related to failure or closure of the neural tube or to its later reopening.[51,96-98] The supratentorial brain tissue in preterm anencephalic fetuses, prior to involution in utero, may surprisingly resemble cerebral hemispheres with a midline fissure present.[93] Clearly, variability in both gestational age and degree of involution for age will result in variability in the amount of supratentorial tissue encountered in "anencephaly" and the consequent impossibility of providing an unequivocal operational definition of the condition based on degree of brain absence. For example, while most anencephalic brains weigh less than 60 g or so, one case of Metnick and Myrianthopoulos[50] (case 1-66) had a normal term brain weight of 391 g. Careful study of the cerebrovasculosa in third-trimester anencephalic fetuses led Bell and Green[99] to conclude that "in many anencephalics parts of both the forebrain and hindbrain are present, although incompletely developed," and to reject "the widely accepted view that the area cerebrovasculosa is totally disorganized, and that anencephaly is characterized by absence of the forebrain." They stressed the variability in degree of neural differentiation in the wall of the forebrain from one case to the next. Others[100,101] have also pointed out that some, even most, anencephalics have rudimentary cerebral hemispheres.

More importantly, the least severe cases of meroanencephaly (meroacrania), in which the forebrain and overlying tissues are only partially absent, are indistinguishable from the most severe cases of microcephaly with encephalocele. The literature is replete with both photographs and descriptions exemplifying the potential for confusion surrounding these two diagnoses.[35] One case in Dallas was diagnosed at the time of birth by the obstetrician as having microcephaly with encephalocele, but was later rediagnosed by a pediatric neurologist and a geneticist as having anencephaly. The parents were told that the infant would die within a few hours, but they eventually took her home and she lived for fourteen months (Joni Burchett, Garland, Texas, oral communication, June 1988).[102] Judging from the published photographs, the "anencephalic" infants reported by Brackbill[81] and by Nielsen and Sedgwick[103] would probably have been diagnosed by many as having microcephaly with encephalocele. That amniotic bands can cause both anencephaly[90,91] and encephalocele[104] highlights the vagueness of the boundary between these two conditions. Because microcephaly with encephalocele constitutes a spectrum of its own, at the other end of which are quite functional individuals, the danger of misapplication of a revised UDDA to living, nonvoluntary organ sources other than anencephalics is far from hypothetical.

Definitional problems aside, the rationales for expanding the statutory definition of death to include "anencephaly" are broad enough to define other categories of dying, neurologically impaired patients as equally "dead," and subsequent expansions of the law would be likely once it became apparent that there are too few usable anencephalic organs to meet transplantation demands. Although present proponents caution against such a development, there is no reason to believe, in the context of today's rapidly changing bioethical mores, that inclusion of anencephaly would be the final such legislative revision.

Indeed, confusion about differences between dying, comatose patients on the one hand and dead bodies on the other emerges repeatedly in the writings of those who would proclaim anencephalics dead. For example, Harrison[29] labels anencephalics as "brain absent" to emphasize their supposed equivalence with "brain-dead" bodies. Yet his language—that one should "not detract from the dignity of [their] dying or abridge [their] right to die"— along with his injunction that the removal of organs should be carried out "in a way that would not conceivably cause suffering" reveal an implicit realization that the anencephalic infant is not dead.

Furthermore, atelencephaly,[105,106] hydranencephaly,[83(p251-255)] and extreme postnatal forebrain destruction resulting in a persistent vegetative state all involve just as much "brain absence" as anencephaly, underneath an intact scalp and skull. Proposals have in fact been made to define patients in a persistent vegetative state as legally dead,[107,108] and the removal of organs from persistently vegetative patients is starting to receive serious discussion in the medical literature.[109] In a recent radio talk show ("Point-Counterpoint." February 20,1988 [KABC, 790 AM, Los Angeles, Calif]) about organ harvesting from anencephalic infants, the mother of a 12-year-old vegetative child called in to say that she would have no qualms about offering her child's organs to benefit another child, if only it were legal. Cranford[110,111] has also stressed the logical connection between the use of anencephalic and persistently vegetative patients as organ donors, forecasting that present trends will soon bring society to the point of considering both as equally legitimate. A physician in France was recently censured for using persistently vegetative patients for nonvoluntary, nonbeneficial, and potentially harmful medical experimentation (*Le Figaro*, February 25, 1988:40). Although such activity horrifies most people today, it will cease to elicit that reaction in a society that has become accustomed to defining patients without a cerebral cortex as "dead" in order to use their bodies for the benefit of others. Revisions in the law that would allow the use of anencephalics, on the basis of their absence of potential for future cognitive functioning, could thereby render novels such as Robin Cook's *Coma* more prophetic than fictional.

Another rationale frequently offered for amending the UDDA to include anencephalics along with other "brain-dead" patients is the supposedly uniform imminence of their death. First of all, this is factually incorrect. In one series,[89] 5 percent lived between one and two weeks. Another study found that, of those with a birth weight greater than 2500 g (and therefore of greatest interest vis-à-vis organs), 8 percent survived between one week and one month and 1 percent lived up to three months.[46,112] In addition, there are documented cases of anencephalic infants surviving sixteen days,[94(p199)] "several weeks,"[83(p62)] thirty-two days,[113] fifty-one days,[80] two months (*Los Angeles Times*, August 19, 1988:[pt I]3), eighty-five days,[103] five and a half months,[81] seven months (personal experience of one of us [W.J.P.]), and fourteen months.[102]

More importantly, the appeal to this logical contradiction—that an anencephalic should be considered legally "dead" on the basis of being about to die—reveals an underlying belief that other "brain-dead" patients are also not *really* dead, but merely near death, and that this somehow renders organ removal appropriate. This position treats brain death as a legal fiction by which to procure organs from still-living patients.

Plainly, reasoning of this or the previous sort erects no barriers to later expansions of the definition of death to other patients near death and/or without neocortical functions, whenever demand for transplantable organs increases. In our desire to increase the number of organ donations, however, it is crucial to keep completely separate the issue of defining death from that of transplantation needs. Manipulating the definition of death—by including anencephalic infants, whose spontaneous breathing, sucking, crying, and the like separate them from the dead bodies that society is usually willing to label cadavers and bury—may undermine the public's already tenuous confidence in brain-based determinations of death. The predictable result will be a decline in the donation of organs from all categories of potential donors, as occurred in England following a highly publicized television program that called into doubt the accuracy of brain-death diagnoses.[114] Interestingly, organ-procurement organizations nationwide noticed a drop-off in referrals as of the beginning of 1988, which happened to correspond to the widespread publicity of Loma Linda's anencephalic protocol, although the extent of causal connection between the two cannot be determined. If the UDDA were revised and the general public therefore concluded that statutory definitions of death were being invented based not on objective biologic properties of the "corpses" but on other patients' need for organs, any temporary increase in the number of organs for tiny infants would have been purchased at the cost of great harm to transplantation generally, which is just now—twenty-one years after the first human-to-human heart transplant—beginning to build a solid base of public acceptance.

Expanding the statutory definition of death to include anencephalics would also cause problems for the parents of such infants who wish to sustain them with nutrition and comfort during the dying process. For the law to proclaim that anencephalics are "dead" would not only contradict the manifest reality of the families' efforts to care for them but might well pose financial barriers for the payment of days (or perhaps weeks) of medical or nursing services for the alleged corpses.

Providing Intensive Care While Awaiting Brain Death

In the hope of obtaining organs from anencephalic infants within the framework of existing statutory definitions of death and requirements that donors of vital organs be dead, some have advocated providing the infant with ventilatory assistance and intensive care while awaiting the occurrence of brain death. This approach is based on three assumptions: (1) that brain death is likely to occur under these circumstances, (2) that brain death in anencephalics can be diagnosed as reliably as in other potential organ donors, and (3) that the provision of intensive care, in the interests not of the infant in question but of someone else, is ethically appropriate.

Concerning the first assumption, the precise cause of death of these infants has never been systematically studied. As the condition involves a spectrum of maldevelopment of brain-stem structures, it is likely that those anencephalic infants who die within the first few hours after birth succumb to hypoventilation due to dysplasia of the respiratory control centers in the lower brain stem. Pressure on and mechanical distortion of the exposed brain stem during the birth process could also result in fatal, though potentially transient, respiratory dysfunction. The minority with better formed brain stems would be susceptible to dying after several days or weeks from multiple endocrine abnormalities, particularly pituitary and adrenal failure,[50,51(pp66-73),115-119] which could render them much less able to withstand the physiological stresses of birth. Hypoventilation would still appear to be the proximate cause of death if a fatal cardiac arrhythmia did not supervene. The small minority of long-surviving anencephalic infants probably die of aspiration or sepsis.

The important point is that there is known progressive destruction of the nervous system, as in the vicious cycle of brain ischemia and swelling within a rigid skull that leads to brain death in patients who, for example, have but suffered head trauma. A squamous epithelial membrane typically covers the exposed neural tissue (as also occurs with spina bifida),[94(p.192),99] protecting it from both infection and exposure to air. Neither does the in utero involution of the cerebrovasculosa, which has no neurological function anyway, affect any other brain structures, particularly the relatively well-formed brain stem.[94(pp191-195),98,99,120] Thus, there is no basis for positing an intrinsic neurological cause of death, and the only anticipated effect of providing mechanical ventilation and intensive care would be to maintain the viability of the brain stem as effectively as that of the other organs, thereby merely postponing an essentially nonneurological death. A fortiori, cooling of the newly delivered anencephalic, as proposed by some,[88] far from hastening brain death, would only serve to protect the integrity of the brain even more, in addition to invalidating the clinical testing for brain death.

The scanty experience to date with intensive care of anencephalic infants supports this theoretical prediction. The infant with the longest survival (fourteen days) in Baird and Sadovnick's[89] series was given life support.[121] Ten out of the twelve live-born anencephalic infants entered into Loma Linda's protocol did not meet that institutional criteria for brain death within the specified seven-day limit, at which point the infants were disconected from the ventilator and allowed to die.[1] Even modifying the protocol, so that resuscitation and ventilatory assistance not be provided until the infant was near death, did not improve the yield over the original procedure of intubation and ventilation immediately after birth. One of those babies survived at home for two months following discharge (*Los Angeles Times*, August 19, 1988:[pt I]3).

But the diagnosis of brain death is problematic even in those few anencephalics who do cease to manifest spontaneous respirations and brain-stem reflexes while receiving assisted ventilation. In nonanencephalic patients, the UDDA requires certainty of both the irreversibility and the totality of brain nonfunction. Certainty of the former ordinarily derives either from a knowledge of the pathophysiological process responsible for the nonfunction or from a demonstration of absence of intracranial blood flow. But the likely causes of death in anencephaly are nonneurological and are therefore in principle potentially reversible. Hypoventilaion and apnea could be caused by electrolyte or endocrine disturbances or by transient edema due to birth trauma to the exposed brain stem, none of which imply intrinsic irreversibility. Moreover, if a vertebral angiogram were performed, there would be no reason to expect it to show absent blood flow to the brain stem.

Establishment of the totality of brain nonfunction is both easier and more difficult in anencephalics. It is easier insofar as the absence of cortical function is self-evident. It is more difficult insofar as there are more peripheral factors that can create a false impression of brain-stem nonfunction. Associated malformations of the retina and optic nerves are common,[51(pp52-53),94(p192),122] so that pupillary nonreactivity should not be interpreted as supportive of a diagnosis of brain death. Similarly, maldevelopment of the middle and/or inner ears[123] could result in absence of reactivity to sound and absence of oculovestibular and perhaps oculocephalic reflexes, invalidating these, too, as evidence for brain death. Some protocols call for meperidine (Demerol) hydrochloride to be administered if the intubated infant shows signs of discomfort and for naloxone hydrochloride (Narcan) to be given at the time of neurological examinations. Even if it is assumed that the naloxone completely cancels the respiratory and general depressant effects of the meperidine, its duration of action is only ten or fifteen minutes, so that neurologically valid observation of the infant would be possible only during around 1 percent of the entire day. If spontaneous aspiration or responsiveness to noxious stimuli were present intermittently, it could easily go unrecognized under these circumstances.

For all these reasons, diagnosing brain death in an anencephalic infant at the moment of loss of a small set of clinically testable brain-stem functions, or even after some arbitrary observation period, would not conform to existing diagnostic standards. Some might say that this is being too punctilious in the case of an infant who is about to die soon anyway. On the other hand, inevability of somatic death is also the case with many nonanencephalic patients who are almost, but not quite, brain dead, yet that does not justify diagnostic corner cutting or proceeding with organ harvesting before actual death in those patients.

Obviously, inaccuracies in the declaration of brain death make no difference whatsoever from the point of view of dying, comatose patients themselves. The importance lies rather with the larger impact on society of establishing a tolerance toward sloppiness in either the conceptualization or implementation of standards for determining death, particularly when this is motivated both by pressure to obtain organs and by an implicit depreciation of a being whose humanity is at least possible, if not probable.

The medical profession and society have always demanded high standards in the diagnosis of death of donors of vital organs, and rightly so. The following are just a few examples of the extreme importance given to the issue of certainty of death, when physicians were trying to formulate reliable diagnostic guidelines for brain death in adults and older children during the 1970s and early 1980s:

"A hopeless prognosis may be an adequate criterion for termination of artificial resuscitation, but the bioethical issue involved is one of 'passive' euthanasia and not brain death. A hopeless prognosis without a pronouncement of death itself would seem inadequate grounds to remove viable organs for transplantation."[124]

"The criteria that physicians use in determining that death has occurred should: (1) Eliminate errors in classifying a living individual as dead, (2) Allow as few errors as possible in classifying a dead body as alive."[3(p161)] (Note the contrast in degree of certainty required against the two types of error.)

"It is particularly important that the most up-to-date and precise assessment of the dying patient's state be made, even if this means that organs must be sacrificed because the techniques for an absolute diagnosis of death are not available."[125]

"A diagnosis of brain death must never be confused with concerns about the quality of residual life in vegetative states. Moreover, a shortage of transplant organs should not be met by changing criteria for diagnosing death, or by the adoption of more lenient or flexible standards."[126]

Even if a particular anencephalic protocol does not purport to go against present laws, a selective lowering of diagnostic standards amounts to the same thing, even if it were to remain hidden from the general public and much of the nonneurological medical profession. It is simply disingenuous to present such approaches as perfectly consistent with existing diagnostic standards. It would be wiser in the long run for advocates to argue straightforwardly for the use of live anencephalics than to force this practice into appearing compatible with existing legal structures by loosening both the concept and the diagnostic standards of death.

Finally, even if some anencephalic infants receiving ventilatory assistance could reliably be determined to be dead by neurological criteria, the difficult ethical issue remains of subjecting one person to invasive, potentially burdensome treatments and prolongation of the dying process, solely for the benefit of another. Although a pure utilitarian calculus might favor just that, current ethical standards still regard respect for the inherent dignity and inviolability of persons as a moral good that outweighs the material evil of someone else's death due to natural causes. In the Loma Linda protocol, the precedents of resuscitation and intensive care solely for the sake of transplantation that were cited as ethical justification all involved already dead bodies, and hence are inapposite for the nonvoluntary prolongation of a dying process for the sake of another. It is certainly true that the care of potential donors near the moment of death may be influenced by plans for transplantation—but this follows concerted efforts aimed at saving the donor's own life, in stark contrast to the conflict of interest inherent from the outset in providing life-prolonging treatment to anencephalic infants. Walters and Ashwal[1] and Fost[127] offer a few arguably acceptable precedents for the nonvoluntary imposition of a burdensome procedure on a minor child for the sake of someone else. The practice of sibling-to-sibling bone marrow transplantation might be cited as a more generally sanctioned example. The main difference between this and the provision of intensive care to anencephalic infants, however, lies in the greater obligation toward the recipient by virtue of the family tie as well as the greater probability of benefit to the recipient, which in the case of awaiting brain death of an anencephalic receiving mechanical ventilation is very low indeed. In particular, it seems that the vast majority of anencephalics receiving ventilatory support will survive the experience, only to have their lives needlessly prolonged without actually benefiting any other child.

PARENTAL COUNSELING

How should one counsel the parents of an anencephalic infant who want to donate their child's organs in order to experience some sense of fulfillment? We do not understand why the proponents of legislative revision consider this to be a major psychiatric problem. Up until the time that certain legislators and surgeons began to promote the idea that organ donation from live anencephalics ought to be an option, the thought never arose more than in passing; parents coped with their grieving process in just the same way that all other parents of terminally ill children do, and health care professionals comforted them just as they comfort all other parents of terminally ill children.

To encourage parents to donate organs from their still-living infant would do nothing more for most parents than to cause them agony over a decision between two options, only one of which is both presently realistic and also wise for society to permit in the future. Although some parents around the time of birth of their anencephalic infant desperately want to add "meaning" to their infant's life and death by giving life to another child, it should be remembered that this noble desire will most often end in further disappointment due to nonuse of the organs. And, if laws were revised to permit organ harvesting from live anencephalics, in the relatively few cases in which "the gift of life" would actually be realized, no one knows the degree to which the donating parents, once over their acute grieving process, might begin to suffer from doubts about the legitimacy of their authorizing what was, in the final analysis, the killing of their own child—a situation potentially analogous to the parental guilt syndrome that can occur years following an elective abortion.[128,129]

On the other hand, parents can be offered the opportunity to donate their child's nonvital organs, such as corneas and heart valves, for transplantation after death and otherwise to cooperate with postmortem investigations aimed at learning more about this condition and its prevention. This may seem to many like a negligible compensation at the moment, but in the long run it may be that what is emotionally better for the parents coincides with what is also better for society.

CONCLUSION

Although the proposal for donation of organs from anencephalics is well intended, it is shortsighted. Attempts to operate within existing laws by waiting for brain death simply do not work, and even if the laws were revised to permit organ harvesting from live anencephalics, the number of children who die each year from congenital kidney, heart, and liver disease would still be insignificantly reduced. Moreover, such radical revisions in the law would ironically undermine the very goal of promoting organ transplantation, and the moral confusion unwittingly introduced into society would constitute a far greater evil than the good done to the relatively few surviving recipients of these organs.

REFERENCES

1. Walters JW, Ashwal S. Organ prolongation in anencephalic infants: ethical and medical issues. *Hastings Cent Rep.* October/November 1988;18: 19-27.

2. Task Force on Organ Transplantation. *Organ Transplantation: Issues and Recommendations.* Rockville, Md: US Dept of Health and Human Services; 1986:27-37.

3. *Defining Death: Medical, Legal and Ethical Issues in the Determination of Death.* Washington, DC: President's Commission for the Study of Ethical Problems in Medicine and Biomedical and Behavioral Research; 1981.

4. Shewmon DA. Caution in the definition and diagnosis of infant brain death. In: Thomasma DC, Monagle JF, eds. *Medical Ethics: A Guide for Health Professionals.* Rockville, Md: Aspen Systems Corp; 1987:38-57.

5. Coulter DL. Neurologic uncertainty in newborn intensive care. *N Engl J Med;* 1987;316:840-844.

6. Task Force for the Determination of Brain Death in Children. Guidelines for the determination of brain death in children. *Ann Neurol.* 1987;21:616-617. (See also *Arch Neurol.* 1987; 44:587-588; *Neurology.* 1987;37:1077-1078; *Pediatrics.* 1987;80:298-300; and *Pediatr Neurol.* 1987; 3:242-243.)

7. Shewmon DA. Commentary on guidelines for the determination of brain death in children. *Ann Neurol.* 1988;24:789-791.

8. Volpe JJ. Brain death determination in the newborn. *Pediatrics.* 1987;80:293-297.

9. Kantrowitz A, Haller JD, Joos H, Cerruti MM, Carstensen HE. Transplantation of the heart in an infant and an adult. *Am J Cardiol.* 1968;22:782-790.

10. Cooley DA, Hallman GL, Bloodwell RD, Nora JJ, Leachman RD. Human heart transplantation: experience with twelve cases. *Am J Cardiol.* 1968;22:804-810.

11. Annas GJ. From Canada with love: anencephalic newborns as organ donors? *Hastings Cent Rep.* December 1987;17:36-38.

12. Goodwin WE, Kaufman JJ, Mims MM, et al. Human renal transplantation, I: clinical experiences with six cases of renal homotransplantation. *J Urol.* 1963;89:13-24.

13. Martin LW, Gonzales LL, West CD, Swartz RA, Sutorius DJ. Homotransplantation of both kidneys from an anencephalic monster to a 17 pound boy with Eagle-Barrett syndrome. *Surgery.* 1969;66:603-607.

14. Fine RN, Korsch BM, Stiles Q, et al. Renal homotransplantation in children. *J Pediatr.* 1970;76:347-357.

15. LaPlante MP, Kaufman JJ, Goldman R, Gonick HC, Martin DC, Goodwin WE. Kidney transplantation in children. *Pediatrics.* 1970;46:665-667.

16. King LR, Gerbie AG, Idriss FS, et al. Human renal transplantation with kidney grafts from the newborn. *Invest Urol.* 1971;8:622-628.

17. Lawson RK, Bennett WM, Campbell RA, Pirofsky B, Hodges CV. Hyperacute renal allograft rejection in the human neonate. *Invest Urol.* 1973;10:444-449.

18. Salvatierra O Jr, Belzer FO. Pediatric cadaver kidneys: their use in renal transplantation. *Arch Surg.* 1975;110:181-183.

19. Dreikorn K, Röhl L, Horsch R. The use of double renal transplants from paediatric cadaver donors. *Br J Urol.* 1977;49:361-364.

20. Kwun YA, Butt KMH, Kim KH, Kountz SL, Moel DI. Successful renal transplantation in a 3-month-old infant. *J Pediatr.* 1978;92:426-429.

21. Iitaka K, Martin LW, Cox JA, McEnery PT, West CD. Transplantation of cadaver kidneys from anencephalic donors. *J Pediatr.* 1978;93:216-220.

22. Martin LW, McEnery PT, Rosenkrantz JG, Cox JA, West CD, LeCoultre C. Renal homotransplantation in children. *J Pediatr Surg.* 1979; 14:571-576.

23. Moel DI, Butt KMH. Renal transplantation in children less than 2 years of age. *J Pediatr.* 1981;99:535-539.

24. Kinnaert P, Vereerstraeten P, Van Asperen de Boer F, et al. Transplantation of both kidneys of an anencephalic to a 23-year-old patient. *Urol.* 1981;7:373-375.

25. Kinnaert P, Persijn G, Cohen B, Van Geertruyden J. Transplantation of kidneys from anencephalic donors. *Transplant Proc.* 1984;16:71-72.

26. Ohshima S, Ono Y, Kinukawa T, Matsuura O, Tsuzuki K, Itoh S. Kidney transplantation from an anencephalic baby: a case report. *J Urol.* 1964;132:546-547.

27. Gutierrez Calzada JL, Martinez JL, Baena V, et al. En bloc kidney and bladder transplartation from an anencephalic donor into an adult recipient., *J Urol.* 1987;138:125-126.

28. Holzgreve W, Beller FK, Buchholz B, Hansmann M, Köhler K. Kidney transplantation from anencephalic donors. *N Engl J Med.* 1987;316:1069-1070.

29. Harrison MR. The anencephalic newborn as organ donor. *Hastings Cent Rep.* April 1986;16:21-22.

30. Harrison MR. Organ procurement for children: the anencephalic fetus as donor. *Lancet.* 1986;2:1383-1386.

31. Capron AM. Anencephalic donors: separate the dead from the dying. *Hastings Cent Rep.* 1987;17:5-9.

32. *Position Statement on Anencephalic Infants as Organ Donors.* San Francisco: California Nurses Association; 1988.

33. *Report of the Ethics Committee* (approved by the Board of Directors). Richmond, Va: United Network for Organ Sharing; February 1989.

34. Ethics and Social Impact Committee, Transplant Policy Center. Anencephalic infants as sources of transplantable organs. *Hastings Cen Rep.* October/November 1988;18:28-30.

35. Shewmon DA. Anencephaly: selected medical aspects. *Hastings Cent Rep.* October/November 1988;18:11-19.

36. Radic A, Dolk H, De Wals R. Declining rate of neural tube defects in three eastern counties of Ireland: 1979-1984. *Irish Med J.* 1987;80:226-228.

37. Romijn JA, Treffers PE. Anencephaly in the Netherlands: a remarkable decline. *Lancet*. 1983; 1:64-65.

38. Leck I. Spina bifida and anencephaly: fewer patients, more problems. *Br Med J*. 1983;286:1679-1680.

39. Elwood JM, Elwood JH. *Epidemiology of Anencephalus and Spina Bifida*. Oxford (England) University Press; 1980:87-90, 107-119.

40. Stein SC, Feldman JG, Friedlander M, Klein RJ. Is myelameningocele a disappearing disease? *Pediatrics*. 1982;69:511-514.

41. Windham GC, Edmonds LD. Current trends in the incidence of neural tube defects. *Pediatrics*. 1982;70:333-337.

42. Borman GB, Howard JK, Chapman CJ. Secular trends in anencephalus prevalence in New Zealand. *NZ Med J*. 1986;99:183-185.

43. *Statistical Abstract of the United States: 1988*. 108th ed. Washington, DC: US Bureau of the Census; 1987:59-60 (Tables 81 and 83).

44. Jorde LB, Fineman RM, Martin RA. Epidemiology of neural tube defects in Utah, 1940-1979. *Am J Epidemiol*. 1984;119:487-495.

45. Cassady G. Anencephaly: a 6 year study of 367 cases. *Am J Obstet Gynecol*. 1969;103:1154-1159.

46. Pomerance JJ, Morrison A, Schifrin BS, Williams RL. Anencephalic infants: life expectancy and organ donation. *J Perinatol*. 1989;9:33-37.

47. Ettenger RE, Fine RN. Renal transplantation. In: Holliday MA, Barratt TM, Vernier L, eds. *Pediatric Nephrology*. 2nd ed. Baltimore,Md: Williams & Wilkins; 1987:828-846.

48. Lum CT, Wassner SJ, Martin DE. Current thinking in transplantation in infants and children. *Pediatr Clin North Am*. 1985;32:1203-1230.

49. Cabasson J, Blanc WA, Joos HA. The anencephalic infant as a possible donor for cardiac transplantation. *Clin Pediatr*. 1969;2:86-89.

50. Melnick M, Myrianthopoulos NC. Studies in neural tube defects, II.: pathologic findings in a prospectively collected series of anencephalics. *J Med Genet*. 1987;26:797-810.

51. Lemire RJ, Beckwith JB, Warkany J. *Anencephaly*. New York. NY: Raven Press; 1978:73-74.

52. David TJ, Nixon A. Congenital malformations associated with anencephaly and iniencephaly. *J Med Genet*. 1976:13:263-265.

53. Naeye RL, Blanc WA. Organ and body growth in anencephaly: a quantitative, morphological study. *Arch Pathol*. 1971;91:140-147.

54. Esquivel CO, Koneru B, Karrer F, et al. Liver transplantation before 1 year of age. *J Pediatr*. 987;110:545-548.

55. Lilly JR, Hall RJ, Altman RP. Liver transplantation and Kasai operation in the first year of life: therapeutic dilemma in biliary atresia. *J Pediatr*. 1987;110:561-562.

56. Mahowald MB, Silver J, Ratcheson RA. The ethical options in transplanting fetal tissue. *Hastings Cent Rep*. February 1987;17:9-15.

57. Warren MA. Can the fetus be an organ farm? *Hastings Cent Rep*. October 1978;8:23-24.

58. Brahams D. Fetal spare parts. *Lancet*. 1988; 1:424.

59. Caplan AL. Should foetuses or infants be utilized as organ donors? *Bioethics*. 1987; 1:119-140.

60. Chargaff E. Engineering a molecular nightmare. *Nature*. 1987;327:199-200.

61. Warren MA. Postscript on infanticide. In: Nasserstrom RA, ed. *Today's Moral Problems*. New York, NY: Macmillan Publishing Co Inc; 1975, pp. 135-136.

62. Tooley M. Abortion and infanticide. In: Gorofitz A, Jameton AL, Macklin R, et al, eds. *Moral Problems in Medicine*. Englewood Cliffs, NJ: Prentice-Hall International Inc; 1976, pp. 297-317.

63. Fletcher J. Indicators of humanhood: a tentative profile of man. *Hastings Cent Rep.* November 1972;2:1-4.

64. Singer P. Sanctity of life or quality of life? *Pediatrics.* 1983;72:128-129.

65. Laches J. Humane treatment and the treatment of humans. *N Engl J Med.* 1976;294:838-840.

66. Chervenak FA, Farley MA, Walters L, Hobbins JC, Mahoney MJ. When is termination of pregnancy during the third trimester morally justifiable? *N Engl J Med.* 1984;310:501-504.

67. Gianelli DM. Pediatric surgeon back in spotlight-with controversial new donor. *Am Med News.* November 6, 1987:48.

68. Coulter DL. Beyond Baby Doe: does infant transplantation justify euthanasia? *J Assoc Persons With Severe Handicaps.* 1988;13:71-75.

69. Arras JD, Shinnar S. Anencephalic newborns as organ donors: a critique. *JAMA.* 1988;259:2284-2285.

70. Feeney DM, Hovda DA. Reinstatement of binocular depth perception by amphetamine and visual experience after visual cortex ablation. *Brain Res.* 1985;342:352-356.

71. Bromiley RB. Conditioned responses in a dog after removal of neocortex. *J Comp Physiol Psychol.* 1948;41:102-110.

72. Travis AM, Woolsey CN. Motor performance of monkeys after bilateral partial and total cerebral decortications. *Am J Phys Med.* 1956;35:273-310.

73. Finger S, Stein DG. Brain Damage and Recovery: Research and Clinical Perspectives. New York, NY: *Academic Press Inc*; 1982, pp. 245-250.

74. Huston JP, Borbély AA. The thalamic rat: general behavior, operant learning with rewarding hypothalamic stimulation, and effects of amphetamine. *Physiol Behav.* 1974; 12:433-448.

75. Norman RJ, Buchwaid JS, Villablanca JR. Classical conditioning with auditory discrimination of the eye blink in decerebrate cats. *Science.* 1977;196:551-553.

76. Francis PL, Self PA, McCaffree MA. Behavioral assessment of a hydranencephalic neonate. *Child Dev.* 1984;55:262-266. (Judging from the author's description, this infant probably suffered from maximal hydrocephalus rather than hydranencephaly.)

77. Aylward GP, Lazzara A, Meyer J. Behavioral and neurological characteristics of a hydranencephalic infant. *Dev Med Child Neurol.* 1978;20:211-277.

78. Berntson GG, Micco DJ. Organization of brain-stem behavioral systems. *Brain Res Bull.* 1976; 1:471-483.

79. Berntson GG, Tuber DS, Ronca AE, Bachman DS. The decerebrate human: associative learning. *Exp Neurol.* 1983;81:77-88.

80. Graham FK, Leavitt LA, Strock BD, Brown JW. Precocious cardiac orienting in a human anencephalic infant. *Science.* 1978; 199:322-324.

81. Brackbill Y. The role of the cortex in orienting: orienting reflex in an anencephalic human infant. *Dev Psych.* 1971;5:195-201.

82. Lorber J. Hydranencephaly with normal development. *Dev Med Child Neurol.* 1965;7:628-633.

83. Lemire RJ, Loeser JD, Leech RW, Alvord EC Jr. *Normal and Abnormal Development of the Human Nervous System.* Hagerstown, Md: Harper & Row Publishers Inc; 1975.

84. Chugani HT, Phelps ME, Mazziotta JC. Positron emission tomography study of human brain functional development. *Ann Neurol.* 1987;22:487-497.

85. Bjursten L-M, Norrsell K, Norrsell U. Behavioural repertory of cats without cerebral cortex from infancy. *Exp Brain Res.* 1976;25:115-130.

86. Hovda DA, Villablanca JR, Shook BL. Sparing of the visual field is associated with less metabolic depression in the superior colliculus of neonatal versus adult hemisphereectomied cats. *Soc Neurosci Abstr.* 1987; 13:1692.

87. Goldman PS, Galkin TW. Prenatal removal of frontal association cortex in the fetal rhesus monkey: anatomical and functional consequences in postnatal life. *Brain Res*. 1978;152:451-458.

88. Fletcher JC, Robertson JA, Harrison MR. Primates and anencephalics as sources for pediatric organ transplants: medical, legal, and ethical issues. *Fetal Ther*. 1986; 1: 150-164.

89. Baird PA, Sadovnick AD. Survival in infants with anencephaly. *Clin Pediatr*. 1984;23:268-271.

90. Harmon JB, Miller CA, Turkel SB. The cerebral malformation of the amniotic band syndrome. *Bull Los Angeles Neurol Soc*. 1978;43:87-90.

91. Urich H, Herrick MK. The amniotic band syndrome as a cause of anencephaly—report of a case. *Acta Neuropathol (Berl)*. 1985;67:190-194.

92. Lemire RJ, Cohen MM Jr, Beckwith JB, Kokich VG, Siebert JR. The facial features of holoprosencephaly in anencephalic human specimens, I: historical review and associated malformations. *Teratology*. 1981;23:297-303.

93. Siebert JR, Kokich VG, Beckwith.TB, Cohen MM Jr, Lemire RJ. The facial features of holoprosencephaly in anencephalic human specimens, II: craniofacial anatomy. *Teratology*. 1981;23:305-315.

94. Warkany J. *Congenital Malformations*. Chicago, Ill: Year Book Medical Publishers Inc, 1971.

95. Chaurasia BD. Calvarial defect in human anencephaly. *Teratology*. 1984;29:165-172.

96. Lemire RJ. Neural tube defects. *JAMA*. 1988;259:558-562.

97. Gardner WJ. Klippel-Feil syndrome, iniencephalus, anencephalus, hindbrain hernia and mirror movements: overdistention of the neural tube. *Child's Brain*. 1979;5:361-379.

98. Wood LR, Smith MT. Generation of anencephaly: 1. aberrant neurulation and 2. conversion of exencephaly to anencephaly. *J Neuropathol Exp Neurol*. 1984;43:620-633.

99. Bell JE, Green RJL. Studies on the area cerebrovasculosa of anencephalic fetuses. *J Pathol*. 1982;137:315-328.

100. Chaurasia BD. Forebrain in human anencephaly. *Anat Anz*. 1977;142:471-478.

101. Terao T, Kawashima Y, Noto H, et al. Neurological control of fetal heart rate in 20 cases of anencephalic fetuses. *Am J Obstet Gynecol*. 1984;149:201-208.

102. Gianelli DM. Anencephalic heart donor creates new ethics debate. *Am Med News*. November 6, 1987:3,47-49.

103. Nielsen JM, Sedgwick RP. Instincts and emotions in an anencephalic monster. *J Nerv Ment Dis*. 1949;110:387-394.

104. Keller H, Neuhauser G, Durkin-Stamm MV, Kaveggia EG, Schaaff A, Sitzmann F. 'ADAM complex' (amniotic deformity, adhesions, mutilations): a pattern of craniofacial and limb defects. *Am J Med Genet*. 1978;2:81-98.

105. Shewmon DA, Sherman MP, Danner R. Atelencephalic microcephaly. *Clin Pediatr*. 1984;23:649-651.

106. Siebert JR, Kokich VG, Warkany J, Lemire R.J. Atelencephalic microcephaly: craniofacial anatomy and morphologic comparisons with holoprosencephaly and anencephaly. *Teratology*. 1987; 36:279-285.

107. Veatch RM. The whole-brain oriented concept of death: an outmoded philosophical formulation. *J Thanatol*. 1975;3:13-30.

108. Youngner SJ, Bartlett ET. Human death and high technology: the failure of the whole-brain formulations. *Ann Intern Med*. 1983;99:252-258.

109. Oski FA, Fost NC, Freeman JM, Seidel HM, Joffe A. Ethical dilemma should organs be taken from this patient? *Contemp Pediatr*. 1987;4:110-117.

110. Cranford RE, Roberts JC. Use of anencephalic infants as organ donors: crossing a threshold. In: Kaufman HH, ed. *Pediatric Brain Death and Organ Retrieval*. New York: Plenum Medical Book Co., 1989.

111. Cranford RE. Anencephalic organ donation raises broader ethical issues. *Hennepin County Med Cent Q*. November 1987;3:2-5, 8.

112. Pomerance JJ, Schifrin BS. Anencephaly and the 'Baby Doe' regulations. *Pediatr Res*. 1987;21(4, pt 2):373A. Abstract.

113. De Morsier G, Bamatter F. Anencéphalie (télencéphaloschizis total) et rhomboschizis avec hétérotopies cérebélleuses médianes: survie de 32 jours. *Arch Psicol Neurol Psichiatr*. 1952;13:2-3.

114. Potts SG. Headaches in Britain over brain death criteria. *Hastings Cent Rep*. April 1987;17:2-3.

115. Carr BR, Parker CR Jr, PorterJC, MacDonald PC, Simpson ER. Regulation of steroid secretion by adrenal tissue of a human anencephalic fetus. *J Clin Endocrinol Metab*. 1980;50:870-873.

116. Cavallo L, Altomare M, Palmieri P, Licci D, Carnimeo F, Mastro F. Endocrine function in four anencephalic infants. *Hormone Res*. 1981;15:159-166.

117. Cawood ML, Heys RF, Oakey RE. Corticosteroid production by the human foetus: evidence from analysis of urine from women pregnant with a normal or anencephalic foetus. *J Endocrinol*. 1976;70:117-126.

118. McGrath P. Aspects of the human pharyngeal hypophysis in normal and anencephalic fetuses and neonates and their possible significance in the mechanism of its control. *J Anat*. 1978;127:65-81.

119. Pajor L, Németh Á, Illés T. Functional morphology of the adrenal cortex in newborns, I: morphometric study. *Acta Morphol Hung*. 1986;34:31-37.

120. Papp A, Csécsei K, Tóth Z, Polgár K, Szeifert GT. Exencephaly in human fetuses. *Clin Genet*. 1986;30:440-444.

121. Baird PA, Sadovnick AD. Survival in liveborn infants with anencephaly. *Ann J Med Genet*. 1987;28:1019-1021.

122. Boniuk V, Ho PK. Ocular findings in anencephaly. *Am J Ophthalmol*. 1979;88:613-617.

123. Friedmann I, Wright JLW, Phelps PD. Temporal bone studies in anencephaly. *J Laryngol Otol*. 1980;94:929-944.

124. Molinari GF. Review of clinical criteria of brain death. *Ann NY Acad Sci*. 1978;315:62-69.

125. Walker AE. *Cerebral Death*. 2nd ed. Baltimore, Md: Urban & Schwarzenberg; 1981:175.

126. Lamb D. *Death, Brain Death and Ethics*. Albany, NY: State University of New York Press; 1985:8.

127. Fost N. Organs from anencephalic infants: an idea whose time has not yet come. *Hastings Cent Rep*. October/November 1988;18:5-10.

128. Rue VM, Speckhard A, Rogers JL, Franz W. *The Psychological Aftermath of Abortion: A White Paper*. Rockville, Md: Office of the Surgeon General; 1987.

129. David H, Rasmussen N, Holst E. Postpartum and postabortion psychotic reactions. *Fam Plan Perspect*. 1981;13:88-91.

9. Should Organs from Patients in Permanent Vegetative State Be Used for Transplantation?

R. Hoffenberg, M. Lock, N. Tilney,
C. Casabona, A. S. Daar, R. D. Guttmann,
I. Kennedy, S. Nundy, J. Radcliffe-Richards,
and R. A. Sells

A shortage of donor organs limits most transplant programs: some patients die of otherwise untreatable end-organ failure, others, in chronic renal failure, are obliged to continue with costly and distressing dialysis procedures. We discuss whether organs taken from patients in a permanent vegetative state (PVS) could be used for transplantation once a decision has been taken to withdraw treatment and allow the patient to die. In the USA, there are an estimated 10,000–25,000 adult patients and 4,000–10,000 children in PVS;[1] figures for the UK are likely to be substantially less pro rata, perhaps 1,000 in all. The UK figure applies to all those who have been vegetative for longer than three months, many of whom die within the first year, so no decision would be taken to withdraw treatment in their lifetimes and they would not be regarded as potential organ donors. As yet, few court decisions have given consent to withdraw treatment from such long-standing cases, but the numbers may increase as the process becomes more widely accepted. There would be obvious benefits if this potential source of organs were to be made available for transplantation, but some arguments have been adduced against this proposition.

First, there is continuing uncertainty and controversy about the definition and diagnosis of PVS, higher brain death, and the recognition of residual consciousness. Errors in diagnosis could result in faulty prognosis.[2,3] Therefore, no decisions should be taken to end the life of patients thought to be in PVS. However, Andrews and colleagues[2] affirm that an accurate diagnosis of PVS can be made if the patient is assessed over a period of time by an experienced team, and that the fear of misdiagnosis should not constitute an argu-

Originally published in *The Lancet* 1997; 350:1320-21. Reprinted by permission.

ment against ending the life of a patient. Second, the ruling of the UK's House of Lords in the case of Tony Bland[4] allowed all treatment including food and water to be withdrawn from patients who had been in PVS for longer than one year without evidence of recovering cerebral function, on the grounds that later restoration of function would be highly improbable. This ruling has been challenged by reports of exceptional individuals who first evinced such recovery after this time.[2] For example, Andrews[5] commented on a recently reported case of a man who first showed signs of recovery of function more than five years after the original injury, but emphasised that this case was "the exception which shouldn't make the rule."

These arguments apply to the general decision to withdraw treatment from patients in PVS; this decision has received legal sanction in the UK and is permitted without overt legal agreement in many other jurisdictions. We are aware of the difficulty involved in making a correct diagnosis of PVS, and, particularly, of distinguishing the locked-in syndrome. However, in this paper we discuss the possible use of organs taken from those patients in whom a decision has already been taken to withdraw treatment and allow them to die. The actual cause of their unresponsive condition is not in this sense relevant.

Once the decision has been taken to withdraw treatment and allow a patient in PVS to die, what are the arguments against the use of their organs for transplantation? First, the law distinguishes between passively allowing to die and actively accelerating death. The former may be permissible, the latter is not. Thus, it would be unlawful to cause the death of a patient by the act of organ removal. Patients with whole-brain or brain-stem death are deemed in law to be dead. When cardiopulmonary support is withdrawn, spontaneous function of the heart and lungs rapidly ceases, the circulation stops, and immediate organ retrieval is allowed. By contrast, patients in PVS are not regarded as dead; they have higher brain death, but retain brain-stem function and are not, therefore, recognised as dead by the US (whole brain) or UK (brain stem) criteria. In the case of PVS, life-support is the provision of nutrition and fluids. When this support is withdrawn, the heart and lungs continue to function until they fail ten to twelve days later because of inanition, electrolyte imbalance, or dehydration. By this time, the organs are no longer in optimum condition and a poor outcome of transplantation is to be expected. To obtain viable transplantable organs, death would have to be accelerated, which is unlawful. If you wait for patients in PVS to die after withdrawal of treatment, the organs are unusable; if you accelerate death, you are acting illegally. So the argument goes that patients in PVS cannot be suitable organ providers. In addition, health-care workers with experience of seeking consent from relatives for the use of organs from patients with whole-brain or brain-stem death anticipate objections if requests are made about patients in PVS. Similarly, opposition among the general public to this practice might damage the overall program for organ donation.

In the possible use of organs of patients in PVS one may ask three separate, but linked, questions. First, should patients in PVS be maintained by supportive treatment until they die "naturally," which could take many years; or might it be morally or legally permissible to accelerate their death? In the UK, the House of Lords accepted that Tony Bland was alive after three years in PVS, but argued that continued treatment was futile because there was no hope of recovery. Since he was regarded as non-sentient, non-cognitive, and wholly unaware of his predicament, he could not be said to have any interest in being kept alive, or, for that matter, in being allowed to die. An American Multi-Society Task Force review of PVS supported the view that "a persistent PVS can be judged to be permanent twelve months after a traumatic injury in adults and children; recovery after this time is exceedingly rare and almost always involves severe disability."[1] For non-traumatic causes, the twelve-month period is reduced to three months. The choice of twelve months as a reasonable time to consider withdrawal of treatment is supported by the British Medical Association[6] and the American Neurological Association.[7] In favor of withdrawal are the lengthy distress of the patient's family and the medical staff who care for a patient whose condition will never improve, and the large amount of skill, effort, and money devoted to the care of such patients. The overall annual cost of keeping patients in PVS alive in the USA has been estimated at between one and seven billion dollars.[1] It is not a responsibility of doctors to preserve life at all costs, especially if treatment would be inordinately painful, damaging, or futile. In such circumstances, a doctor's duty of care to a patient may cease and be directed instead to the interests of the family, carers, or society. It is morally, and now in the UK legally, acceptable to accelerate the death of the patient by withdrawal of treatment.

Second, once the decision has been taken to end the life of a patient in PVS, how should it be done? Should life be allowed to drain away slowly after withdrawal of solid and liquid sustenance, or could a case be made for a more speedy termination of life? Since patients in PVS are presumed to be non-sentient, it is unlikely that they experience distressing thirst or hunger when food and fluids are withdrawn. Such distress would be a strong argument in favour of a more expeditious mode of death, for example, administration of a lethal drug. Indeed, if patients in PVS are thought to be sentient or capable of experiencing pain, discomfort, or distress either before or after a decision has been taken to withdraw food and fluids, a strong case could be made on humane grounds for routine administration of palliative analgesic or psychotropic therapy. A more speedy end to life may also reduce, the misery imposed by a long drawn-out death on family, nursing staff, and others. At present, UK and US law accepts that in some circumstances patients in PVS may be permitted to die slowly through omission of therapy, but no active steps may be taken to accelerate the process.

Third, is it legally, morally, or practically possible to procure organs from patients in PVS for transplantation? The fact that these patients are legally deemed to be alive is a major obstacle to the use of their organs for any purpose. If one has to wait until death, as it is defined in law, then organs will be unsuitable for transplantation. An earlier act of retrieval would kill the patient and is illegal. As the law stands, there is no way out of this dilemma, and it is not possible to use the organs of patients in PVS for transplantation. From a moral point of view, the critical decision is whether or not to terminate life. Although we recognise that there are intuitive psychological distinctions between killing a person and allowing them to die, we believe that, though the means by which death is attained has legal implications, there is no clear moral distinction between allowing to die by omission of treatment and more actively ending life, for instance, by injection of a fatal substance. The outcome is the same.

In the judgment by the House of Lords, Lord Mustill expressed his own uneasy feeling that "however much the terminologies may differ the ethical status of the two courses of action is for all relevant purposes indistinguishable"—what the law refers to as a distinction without a difference. If the legal definition of death were to be changed to include comprehensive irreversible loss of higher brain function, it would be possible to take the life of a patient (or more accurately to stop the heart, since the patient would be defined as dead) by a "lethal" injection, and then to remove the organs needed for transplantation, subject to the usual criteria for consent. Another approach would be not to declare such individuals legally dead, but rather to exempt them from the normal legal prohibitions against "killing" in the way that was considered for anencephalic infants.[7] Arguments in favour of one of these steps would be humanitarian, to obviate the futile use of resources needed to keep alive an individual with no hope of recovery, and to make available organs suitable for transplantation. If such a step were legally permissible, it would be essential to separate the decision to let the patient die from the steps taken to procure organs. In other words, the medical team that decides, in consultation with the family, that no further benefit would come from continued treatment, must be separate and independent from those who request organ donation and from the team that secures the organs.

The recent debate about anencephalic neonates as potential organ donors[7] is relevant to our discussion of patients in PVS, since they are in many ways analogous. The Council on Ethical and Judicial Affairs of the American Medical Association stated in 1995 that it is ethically permissible for an anencephalic neonate to be an organ donor, although still legally alive by virtue of the current definition of death.[7] A survey of leading medical experts in anencephaly and in ethics showed that two-thirds of physicians regarded this decision as "intrinsically moral."[7] If changes in public thinking and the law were to make possible the use of organs from patients in PVS, it would be necessary, as in the case of abortion, to include a conscience clause allowing doctors and nurses the right to refuse to take part in the procedure. For religious, cultural, and other traditional reasons, it is likely that the proposal would be rejected, nevertheless, the arguments in favour are sufficiently compelling to justify serious debate.

REFERENCES

1. Multi-Society Task Force on PVS. Medical aspects of the persistent vegetative state. *N Engl J Med* 1994; 330: 1499-1508 (part 1) and 1572–79 (part 2).

2. Andrews K, Murphy L, Munday R, Littlewood C. Misdiagnosis of the vegetative state: retrospective study in a rehabilitation unit. *BMJ* 1996; 313: 13–16.

3. Crawford R. Misdiagnosing the persistent vegetative state. *BMJ* 1996; 313: 5–6.

4. House of Lords. *Report of the Select Committee on Medical Ethics*. Session 1993-94. London: HM Stationery Office, 1994.

5. Andrews K, cited by Dyer C. Hillsborough survivor emerges from permanent vegetative state. *BMJ* 1997; 314: 996.

6. British Medical Association Ethics Committee. Discussion paper on treatment of patients in PVS. London: *BMA*, 1992.

7. American Neurological Committee on Ethical Affairs Report on PVS. *Ann Neurol* 1993; 33: 386-390.

10. Is Xenografting Morally Wrong?

Arthur L. Caplan

It is tempting to think that a decision about whether or not it is immoral to use animals as sources for transplantable organs and tissues hinges only upon the question of whether or not it is ethical to kill them. But the ethics of xenografting involves more than an analysis of that question. And even the assessment of the morality of killing animals to obtain their parts to use in human beings is more complicated than it might at first glance appear to be.

To decide whether it is ethical to kill animals, a variety of subsidiary questions must be considered. Is it ethical to kill animals to obtain organs and tissues to save human lives or alleviate severe disability when it might not be ethical to kill them for food or sport?[1] Why are animals being considered as sources of organs and tissues—do alternative methods for obtaining replacement parts for human beings exist? What sorts of animals would have to be killed, how would they be killed, and how would they be stored, handled, and treated prior to their deaths?

If it is possible to defend the killing of animals for xenografting then questions as to the morality of subjecting human beings to the risks, both physical and psychological, associated with xenografting must also be weighed. In undertaking a xenograft on a human subject the focus of moral concern ought not to be solely on the animal that will be killed.

Even for those who eat meat or hunt, it might well seem immoral to kill animals for their parts if alternative sources of replacement parts were or might soon be available. The moral acceptability of xenografting will for many, including the prospective recipients of animal parts, be contingent on

Originally published in *Transplantation Proceedings* 24, no. 2 (April 1992): 722-27. Reprinted by permission of Appleton & Lange, Inc.

the presumption that there is no other plausible alternative source of transplantable organs and tissues. Unfortunately, the scarcity that is behind the current interest in xenografting is all too real.

WHY PURSUE XENOGRAFTING?

The supply of organs and tissues available from human cadaveric sources for transplantation in the United States and other nations is entirely inadequate. Many children and adults die or remain disabled due to the shortage of transplantable organs and tissues. Unless some solution is found to the problem of scarcity, the plight of those in need of organs and tissues will only grow worse and the numbers who die solely for want of an organ will continue to grow.

More than one-third of those now awaiting liver transplants die for want of a donor organ. Well over one-half of all children born with fatal congenital deformities of the heart or liver die without a transplant due to the shortage of organs. The percentage of those who die while waiting would actually be higher if all potential candidates were on waiting lists.[2]

Some Americans are not referred for transplants because they cannot afford them. If those with organ failure from economically underdeveloped nations were wait-listed at North American and European transplant centers, the percentage of those who die while awaiting a transplant would be much larger.[3]

More than 150,000 Americans with kidney failure are kept alive by renal dialysis. The cost for this treatment exceeded five billion dollars in 1988. It would be far cheaper and, from the patient perspective as to the quality of life, far more desirable to treat kidney failure by means of transplants. But, there are simply not enough cadaveric kidneys for all who desire and could benefit from a transplant.

The supply of cadaveric organs for pancreas, small intestine, lung, heart-lung transplants for those dying of a wide variety of diseases affecting these organs is not adequate. The same story holds for bone, ligament, dural matter, heart valves, and skin. Moreover, demand for the limited supply of organs and tissues is increasing as more and more medical centers become capable of offering this form of surgery, and as techniques for managing rejection and infection improve.[4]

The shortage of organs and tissues for transplantation has led researchers to pursue a variety of alternatives in order to bridge the gap between supply and demand. Some suggest changing existing public policies governing cadaveric procurement. Others focus on locating alternatives to human cadaveric organs.

Efforts could be made to modify public policy to encourage more persons to serve as organ and tissue donors. Legislation mandating that the option of organ and tissue donation be presented whenever a person dies in a hospital setting has been enacted in the United States but, while leading to increases in both tissue and organ availability, has not been adequately implemented.[5,6] Organs and tissues are still lost because families are not approached about donation. Hospital compliance is not what it should be and the training of those who must identify potential donors and approach families is woefully lacking. Refusal rates to requests to donate are high and there exists a significant degree of mistrust and misunderstanding about donation on the part of the public.[6] Public policies could and should be changed to rectify these problems.

Other proposals to change public policy involve changing laws to permit payment to those who agree to donate or whose families consent to cadaveric donation[7,8] or to move toward a presumed consent system in which the burden of proof is placed on those who do not wish to donate to carry cards or other evidence of their nondonor status. However, cultural and religious attitudes in large segments of American society and in other societies will not support either the creation of markets, bounties, or property status for body parts[9] or the extension of state authority to the seizure of cadaveric organs and tissues.

Allowing markets may lead to criminal activities.[10] Selling irreplaceable body parts is an especially repugnant way to ask a person to earn income or benefits.[11] There is much reluctance on the part of the general public to swap the presumption of individual control over the body, either in life or death, for a policy that might benefit the common good by risking the loss of personal autonomy.[4,11] Nor has the actual experience with presumed consent laws in European nations been such as to justify enthusiasm for the likely results of a shift away from individualism and personal autonomy with respect to the control of cadavers.[12]

Even if drastic changes were made in existing public policies, other factors are working against the prospects for large increases in the human cadaveric organ supply. Improvements in emergency room access and care, the onset of the acquired immunodeficiency syndrome (AIDS) epidemic, ambivalence about cadaveric donation on the part of the public, plus laudable advances in public health measures, such as mandatory seatbelt use, raising the age for legally purchasing liquor, and tougher laws against drunk driving mean that a tremendous increase in the supply of cadaveric organs is unlikely to occur no matter what public policies are adopted.

Most importantly with respect to the moral defensibility of exploring xenografting as an alternative source of organs, even if all human cadaveric organs were somehow made available for transplant, the supply would still not meet the potential demand. The hidden pool of potential transplant recipients would quickly become visible were these organs and tissues to become available.[3,6] The search for alternatives to the use of human cadaveric organs rests on the recognition that scarcity is an insurmountable obstacle.

In recent years surgeons have tried to solve the problem of shortage by using kidneys. and segments of liver, lung, and pancreas from living donors. Transplant teams in a few nations have been testing the feasibility of transplanting lobes of livers between biologically related individuals.[13,14] Teams at Stanford University and the University of Minnesota have used parents as lung donors for their child. Minnesota and some other centers have been experimenting for many years with transplants of the kidney and pancreas from related and unrelated living donors.[15] Many centers around the world have performed bone marrow transplants between biologically unrelated persons.

There are serious problems with and limits to the use of living donors as alternative sources of organs and tissues. The most inviolate limit is that unmatched vital organs, such as the heart, cannot be used. Using living donors for other organs requires subjecting the donors to life-threatening risks, some pain and disfigurement, and some risk of disability. The legitimacy of consent on the part of living donors, especially among family members, is hard to assess. And, since it is not well known whether transplanting lobes or segments of organs or unrelated bone marrow is efficacious, it is not certain that this strategy for getting more organs and tissue is a realistic option much less whether it will prove attractive to a sufficient number of actual donors.

Another alternative to human cadaveric organ transplantation is the development of mechanical or artificial organ and tissue substitutes. Kidney dialysis is one such substitute. The widely publicized efforts to create a total artificial heart, first at the University of Utah and then later at Humana Audubon Hospital in Louisville, Kentucky, represent another, albeit failed effort to create an alternative to transplantation using cadaveric hearts. New generations of mechanical hearts are in the research pipeline as are artificial insulin pumps, artificial lungs, and various types of artificial livers. But, safe, effective, and reliable artificial organs and tissues appear to still be decades away. Ironically, the immediate impact of the available forms of artificial organs is to increase the problem of allocation in the face of scarcity since these devices permit temporary "bridging" of children and adults in need of transplants, thereby increasing the pool of prospective recipients.

It is the plight of those dying of end-stage diseases for want of donor organs from both living and cadaveric human sources that has led a number of research groups to explore the option of using animals as the source of transplantable organs and tissues. Transplant researchers at Loma Linda, the University of Pittsburgh, Stanford, Columbia, and Minnesota as well as in England, China, Belgium, Sweden, Japan, and France, among other countries, are conducting research on xenografting organs and tissues. Some are exploring the feasibility of primate to human transplants. Others are pursuing lines of research that would allow them to utilize animals other than primates as sources.

It is scarcity that grounds the moral case for thinking about animals as sources of organs and tissues. In light of current and potential demand, no other options exist for alleviating the scarcity in the supply of replacement parts. If, however, society were to decide not to perform transplants or to perform only a limited number of them, then the case for xenografting would be considerably weakened. While transplant surgeons and those on waiting lists may find strategies for finding more organs or tissues attractive, another possible response to scarcity is to simply live with it. Those who advocate this response could do so on the grounds that it is not morally necessary to transplant all persons who are in need especially if doing so requires the systematic killing of animals for human purposes.[1,16,17]

IS THE PROBLEM OF SCARCITY RESOLVABLE BY SOME OTHER STRATEGY?

Instead of pursuing the option of xenografting it is possible to argue that the answer to the problem of scarcity is that medicine should simply stop doing transplants entirely or only do as many as can be done with whatever human cadaveric organs and tissues are available. This moral stance might rest on the claim that transplants are simply too expensive and do not work well enough to justify a hunt for alternative sources to human organs. Or someone might view xenografting as unnecessary and immoral on the grounds that prevention makes far more sense than salvage and rescue in dealing with end-stage organ failure. Some forms of transplantation are notoriously expensive. A critic of the xenografting option might argue that it is not wise to spend hundreds of thousands of dollars on heart, liver, or nonrelated bone marrow transplants when the number of people requiring these treatments could be drastically reduced by decreasing the incidence of smoking, alcohol consumption, and the exposure to toxic substances in the workplace and the environment.

The arguments in favor of the "live within your means" position are not persuasive. While prevention of organ and tissue failure is surely to be preferred to rescue by means of transplants, large numbers of persons suffer organ and tissue failure for reasons that are poorly understood and, thus, not amenable to prevention. While individuals should certainly be encouraged to adopt more healthful lifestyles (including the consumption of less animal fat!) there are no proven techniques available for ensuring that people will behave wisely or prudently. Moreover, those who will need transplants in the next few decades are persons for whom prevention is too late. So, while prevention is desirable, the demand for transplants will not diminish for a significant period of time regardless of the efforts undertaken to improve public health.

Transplants are expensive, but many types of transplantation, especially for children and young adults, are very effective in providing a good quality of life for many, many years. The wisdom of doing any medical procedure cannot simply be equated with its overall cost. A more reasonable measure would be to see what is purchased for the price that is charged. If the moral value of spending money for health services is not total price but, cost per year of life saved or, cost relative to the likelihood of saving a life, then there are many other areas of health care that ought to be restricted or abandoned long before accepted forms of transplantation such as heart, liver, and kidney are deemed too expensive or not cost worthy.

ETHICAL PROBLEMS WITH THE XENOGRAFT OPTION

If it is true that the case for pursuing xenografting is a persuasive one then the question of whether xenografting is morally wrong shifts to an analysis of which animals will be used, how they will be kept and killed, and the risks and dangers involved for potential human recipients. Xenografting is still evolving so the ethical issues must be considered under two broad headings; issues associated with basic and clinical experimentation and, if this proves successful, those that would then be associated with the widespread use of xenografts as therapies.

Ethical Issues Raised by
Basic and Clinical Research

In thinking about the ethics of research on xenografting a couple of assumptions can safely be made. The number and type of animals used will be very much a function of cost, prior knowledge of the species, inbred characteristics, ease in handling, and availability. Gorillas are not going to be used in research simply because there are too few of them and they are unlikely to make compliant subjects. Rats and mice will dominate the early stages of research (as they already do) because they are relatively well understood, special-purpose bred, and cheap to acquire and maintain. Few primates will be used for basic or clinical research simply because they are too scarce, too expensive, and too complex to permit controlled study for most experimental purposes.

Even if the number of animals to be used is relatively small, the question still must be faced as to whether it is ethical to use animal models involving species such as rats, chickens, sheep, pigs, monkeys, baboons, and chimps in order to study the feasibility of cross-species xenografting? In part, the answer to this question pivots on whether or not there are plausible alternative models to the use of animals for exploring the two critical steps required for successful xenografting—overcoming immunologic rejection and achieving long-term physiologic function in an organ or tissue.

To some extent, immunologic problems can be examined without killing primates or higher animals by using lower animals or cellular models. But there would not appear to be any viable alternatives or nonhuman substitutes available for understanding the processes involved in rejection. At best it may be possible to utilize animals that have fewer cognitive and intellectual capacities for most forms of basic research with respect to understanding the immunology of xenografting.

When research gets closer to the clinical stage especially when it becomes possible to examine the extent to which xenografted organs and tissues can function posttransplant, it will be necessary to use some animals as donors and recipients that are closely related to human beings. If, in light of the scarcity of human organs, it is ethical to pursue the option of xenografting, then, it would be unethical to subject human beings to any form of xenografting that has not undergone a prior demonstration of both immunologic and physiologic feasibility in animals closely analogous to humans.

The use of animals analogous to humans for basic research on xenografting means that some form of primates must be used both as donors and as recipients. Is it ethical to kill primates, even if only a small number, to demonstrate the feasibility of xenografting in human beings? If primate and humans have the same moral status then it is hard to see how the use of primates could be justified.[1,16,18] Are humans and ape moral equivalents?

At this point, those who want to deny the validity of moral equivalence begin to look for morally significant properties uniquely present in human beings but not in primates. Strong candidates for the property that might make a moral difference sufficient to allow the killing of primates to advance human interests are language, tool-use, rationality, intentionality, consciousness, conscience, and/or empathy. The debate about the morality of killing a primate of some sort to advance human interests by saving human lives then hinges on empirical facts about what particular species of primates can or cannot do in comparison to what humans are capable of doing.[19]

It is indisputable that there are some differences in the capacities and abilities of humans and primates. Chimps can sign but humans have much more to say. Gorillas seem to reason but humans have calculus, novels, and quantum theory. Humans are capable of a much broader range of behavior and intellectual functioning then are any specific primate species.

Many who would protest the use of primates in xenografting research are keen to illustrate that primates possess many of the properties and abilities that are found to contribute moral standing to humans. The fact that one species or another of primate is capable of some degree of intellectual or behavioral ability that seems worthy of moral respect when manifest by humans does not mean that human beings are the moral equivalents of primates. It is one thing to argue that primates ought to have moral standing. It is a very different matter to argue that humans and primates are morally equivalent. One can grant that primates deserve moral consideration without conceding that, on average, the death of a human being is of greater moral significance then is the death of a baboon, a green monkey, or a chimpanzee.

Xenografting involving primates can be morally justified on the grounds that, in general. human beings possess capacities and abilities that confer more moral value upon them than do primates. This is not "speciesism"[1,20] but, rather, a claim of comparative worth that is based on important empirical differences between two classes or sets of creatures.

Perhaps there are empirical reasons to support the claim that it is worth killing primates for humans on the grounds that as groups humans have properties that confer greater moral worth and standing upon them then do other animal species. Human beings are after all moral agents while, at most, animals, even primates, are moral subjects.

Even conceding this point, there is still a problem when it comes time to kill a baboon and a chimp to see if xenografting between them is possible. Critics might ask whether scientists would be willing to kill a retarded child or an adult in a permanent vegetative state in the service of the same scientific goal? It is indisputable that human beings have on average more capacities and abilities than do animals. But there are some individual animals, many of them primates, that have more capacities and abilities than certain individual human beings who lack them due to congenital disorders or as the result of disease or injury. If it is argued that we ought to use animals instead of humans to assess the feasibility of xenografting because humans are more highly developed in terms of intellectual and emotional capacities, capacities that make a moral difference in that they are the basis for moral agency, then why should we not use a severely retarded child instead of a bright chimp or gorilla[20] as subjects in basic or clinical research? Unless those who are doing or wish to engage in basic research on xenografting can answer this question they will be open to the charge of immorality even if they kill primates or other "higher" animals in order to benefit humans who are, as a species, of more moral worth than are animals.

One line of response is to simply say that we are powerful and the primates are less. Therefore they must yield to human purposes if we choose to experiment upon them rather than retarded children. This line of response sounds rather far removed from the kinds of arguments we expect to be mustered in the name of morality. A more promising line of attack on the view that humans and primates or other animals are morally equivalent is to examine a bit more closely why it is that we would not want to use a retarded child instead of a chimp in basic research.

Two reasons might be given for picking a chimp instead of a human being with limited or damaged capacities. We might decide not to use a human being who has lost his or her capacities and abilities out of respect for their former existence. If the person makes a conscious decision to allow his or her body to be used for scientific research prior to having become comatose or brain dead then perhaps those wishes should be honored. If no such advance notice has been given then we ought not to presume anything about what they would have wanted and should forego any involvement in medical research generally and xenografting in particular on the grounds that this is what is demanded out of respect for the persons they once were.

However, severely retarded children or those born with devastating conditions such as anencephaly have never had the capacities and abilities that confer a greater moral standing on humans as compared with animals. Should they be used as the first donors and recipients in xenografting research instead of primates?

The reason they should not has nothing to do with the properties, capacities, and abilities of children or infants who lack and have always lacked significant degrees of intellectual and cognitive function. The reason they should not be used is because of the impact using them would have upon other human beings, especially their parents and relatives. A severely retarded child can still be the object of much love, attention, and devotion from his or her parents. These feelings and the abilities and capacities that generate them are deserving of moral respect. I do not believe animals including primates are capable of such feelings.

If a human mother were to learn that her severely retarded son had been used in lethal xenografting research she would mourn this fact for the rest of her days. A baboon, monkey, orangutan would not. The difference counts in terms of whether it is a monkey or a retarded human being who is selected as a subject in xenografting research.

It may be that parents would want to volunteer their child's organ or tissue for research or they might wish to have their baby with anencephaly serve as the first recipient of an animal organ or tissue. It may be necessary to honor such a choice. Whatever public policies are created to govern our actions toward severely retarded children or babies born with most of their brain missing, these are policies that are meant to be respectful of the sensibilities and interests of other human beings.[21] They do not find their source in some inherent property of the anencephalic infant. It is in the relationships with others, both family and strangers, that the moral worth and standing of these children are grounded.

The case for using animals, even primates, before using a human being with severely limited abilities and capacities is based on the relationships that exist among human beings, which do not have parallels in the animal kingdom. These relationships, such as love, loyalty, empathy, sympathy, family-feeling, protectiveness, shame, community-mindedness, a sense of history, and a sense of responsibility, which ground many moral duties and set the backdrop for distinguishing virtuous conduct and character, do not, despite the sociality of some species, appear to exist among animals.

If animals are to be used then what sorts of guidelines should animal care and use committees or other review bodies follow in reviewing basic research proposals? These committees must ensure that basic research is designed in such a fashion as to minimize the need for animal subjects while maximizing the opportunity to obtain generalizable knowledge. They must also ensure that the animals used are kept in optimal conditions and are handled humanely and killed without pain. These steps will be necessary in order to both respect the moral standing of the animals and to maximize the chance for generating useful knowledge from the use of these animals in research.

Perhaps the most difficult question arising when sufficient data have been obtained to make clinical trials plausible is who ought to be the first subjects in clinical xenografting trials. The baby Fae xenograft case involved an infant because the researchers felt that the scarcity of organs for infants born with congenital defects was so great that morality demanded that infants be the initial subjects selected. Many argued that this choice was mistaken since at the level of initial clinical trials it is morally wrong to use infants, children, or other human beings incapable of giving informed consent to their participation.[17]

If it is true that clinical trials involving xenografting should avoid the initial use of infants, children, and adults who lack the capacity for consent then who ought to go first? Perhaps adults who would not be otherwise eligible for transplants under existing exclusion criteria, the imminently dying, terminally ill volunteers who agree to serve, those who are brain dead, or those needing a second or third transplant when scarcity and prognosis would make it most unlikely they would receive another human organ or tissue.

Similarly, for clinical trials the question arises as to which type of organ or tissue ought be the subject of initial research efforts? Those for which the scarcity of human organs and tissues is greatest or those for which alternatives to animal organs seem the least promising? A strong case can be made that the selection of an organ or tissue to xenograft should be guided by the scarcity of human organs and tissues as well as the results achieved in animal to animal xenografting during basic research.

When clinical trials are designed for human subjects, those undertaking the research must have the qualifications and the background to make it likely that they will generate reliable and replicable results that are quickly made available in the literature. While the use of primates and human beings in research may be morally justified, their use can only be justified when research is designed and conducted in circumstances most likely to maximize the chances of creating knowledge.

Those who will be recruited for clinical trials have the right to know the risks and benefits of the research that can best be inferred from animal and any other relevant studies. They should also know how many subjects will be used before the end-point of this phase of research is reached. The measures taken for coping with any psychological issues raised by the use of animal organs for subjects must be presented. Subjects should also be told about the steps that have been taken to ensure their privacy and confidentiality to the extent they wish these preserved. It is of special importance given the high odds of failure in the initial phase of xenografting on human subjects that procedures be in place for ending the experiment if the subject wishes to withdraw from the research.

Ethical Issues Raised by Therapy

Perhaps the most obvious moral problem that would arise if xenografting proved to be a viable source of organs and tissue for transplantation is whether prospective recipients would be able to accept animal parts when in need of transplants. Some might feel that it is unnatural to do so. But, naturalness is very much a function of familiarity. One hundred years ago surgery and anesthesia were viewed by many as unnatural. People may require support and counseling when faced with the option of xenografting but, facing death, most will probably accept a transplant and decide to deal with the naturalness issue later.

What about systematically breeding, raising, and killing animals for their parts on a large scale? Is it moral to systematically farm and kill animals for spare parts for humans? Would it be right to systematically farm and kill animals for spare parts for other animals, say companion animals?

One response to the issue of breeding and raising animals in order to have a regular supply of organs for xenografting is to argue that this practice does not raise any new or special moral issues since huge numbers of animals are currently bred, raised, and killed solely for consumption. However, animals raised for food are often raised under inhumane and brutal conditions. Nor is there much consideration given to the techniques involved in their slaughter.[1] Animals that are to be used to generate a constant source of organs and tissues for transplant must be raised under conditions that would ensure the healthiest possible animals. The moral obligation to potential recipients would seem to require that systematic farming of animals only be permitted under the most humane circumstances.

Interestingly the issue of whether it is morally permissible to systematically breed, raise, and kill animals to obtain their parts does not raise the same issues of moral equivalence between animals and humans that arise with respect to basic and clinical research. It would obviously be immoral to breed, raise, and kill humans for their parts. The availability of animal organs for transplant on a therapeutic basis is likely to become a matter of economics. The economics of this sort of animal breeding must take into account the costs of creating the healthiest possible animals and the most painless modes of killing. However, should xenografting evolve to the point of therapy, those who perform xenografts must also strive to ensure that access to transplants is equitable.

CONCLUSION

The morality of using animals as sources of organs is contingent on the need to turn to animals as sources. The scarcity of organs and tissues from human sources is real, growing, and unlikely to be solved by any other alternative policies or approaches in the foreseeable future. If xenografting must be explored as an option then the moral justification for doing basic and clinical research involving animals is that it would not be possible to learn about the feasibility of overcoming immunologic and physiologic problems without using animals, and that animals are to be used instead of human subjects whenever possible since human beings have more moral worth than do animals. If xenografting evolves into a therapy then provisions must be made for ensuring the welfare and health of the animals that would be bred, raised, and killed to supply organs and tissues to human beings.

REFERENCES

1. Singer P: *Animal Liberation.* New York: Random House, 1975.
2. Baum B, Bernstein D, Starnes VA, et al.: *Pediatrics* 88:203, 1991.
3. Caplan A: *Transplant Proc* 21:3381, 1989.
4. Caplan A, Siminoff L, Arnold B, et al.: *Surgeon General's Workshop on Organ Donation.* Washington, DC: HRSA, (in press).
5. Caplan A, Virnig B: *Crit Care Clin* 6:1007, 1990.
6. Caplan A: *J Transplant Coordination* 1:78, 1991.
7. Peters TG: *JAMA* 265:1302, 1991.
8. Wight JP: *Br Med J* 303:110, 1991.
9. John Paul II: *Statement on Organ Transplantation.* International Congress of the Society for Organ Sharing, Rome, Italy, June 20, 1991.
10. *New Scientist*: July 13, p 1991.
11. Tufts A: *Lancet* 337:1403, 1991.
12. Eurotransplant Foundation: *Eurotransplant Newsletter* 87:1, 1991.
13. Raia S, Nery JR, Mies S: *Lancet* 26:497, 1989.
14. Strong RW, Lynch SV, Ong TH, et al.: *N Engl J Med* 322:1505, 1990.
15. Elick BA, Der Sutherland K, Gillingham JS, et al: *Transplant Proc* 1990.
16. Regan T, Singer P: *Animal Rights and Human Obligations.* Englewood Cliffs, NJ: Prentice-Hall, 1976.
17. Caplan A: *JAMA* 254:3339,. 1985.
18. Regan T, VanDeVeer D: *And Justice for All.* Totowa: Rowman and Littlefield, 1982.
19. Jasper JM, Nelkin D: *The Animal Rights Crusade.* New York: The Free Press, 1992.
20. Singer P: *Transplant Proc* (this volume).
21. Caplan A: *Bioethics* 1:119, 1987.

11. Transplantation Through a Glass Darkly

James Lindemann Nelson

Bioethical problems take many different forms, and fascinate many different kinds of people. Physicians and philosophers, lawyers and theologians, policy analysts and talk show hosts are all drawn by the blend of practical urgency and moral complexity that characterize these issues.

But there seem to be only two kinds of bioethical problems that typically pull into their orbits not only theorists and practitioners, but pickets and protesters as well. When it comes to the treatment of fetuses and animals, people take to the streets. On the same day that demonstrators on both sides of the abortion issue lamented the Supreme Court's decision in *Casey,* representatives of PETA (People for the Ethical Treatment of Animals) gathered at the University of Pittsburgh to protest the implantation of a baboon's liver in a thirty-five-year-old man—the father of two children—whose own liver had been destroyed by hepatitis B virus.

There is, of course, a big difference in the way the disputes are perceived: abortion's bona fides as a central ethical issue are well established, but despite an upsurge of interest among ethicists over the past decade and a half, concern about animals still seems a bit quirky, too exclusively the domain of zealots who maintain the moral equality of all species, and thereby mark themselves as fundamentally out of sympathy with our basic ethical traditions. Here I try to pull moral consideration of nonhumans closer to the ethical center, arguing that thinking about the fate of nonhumans at our hands shares with abortion—indeed, with many of our culture's most difficult moral issues—a fundamental problem: we don't really know what we are

---

Originally published in *Hastings Center Report* 22, no. 5 (1992): 6-8. Reprinted by permission.

talking about. More concretely, we're at a loss to say what it is about baboons that makes their livers fair game, when we wouldn't dare take vital organs from those of our own species whose abilities to live rich, full lives are no greater than those of the nonhumans we seem so willing to prey upon. Unless we're able to isolate and defend the relevant moral distinction, we should reject the seductive image of solving the problem of organ shortage by maintaining colonies of animals at the ready for transplantation on demand.

MORAL OUTLIERS

Public protest about abortion is not galvanized by concern about the quality of informed consent, or its impact on the doctor-patient relationship. What *does* lie at the center of the dispute is an absolutely crucial kind of ignorance. As a society, we don't know what fetuses are, and, in an important sense, we don't know what pregnant women are either. Are fetuses babies or tissue? Are pregnant women mothers bound by special duties to their unborn children, or independent adults exercising their right to make important self-regarding decisions under the protection of a mantle of privacy? Because we don't know these things, and they matter so much, we have a hard time imagining what responsible compromise might really be like.

And what gets people out into the streets in response to a daring attempt to rescue from certain death a young father of two? What, for that matter, causes medical research advocacy organizations to spend large amounts of money, not on research, but on full-page ads in the *New York Times* defending what scientists do? Is it concerns about justice in the allocation of medical resources? Doubts about the "courage to fail" ethos? Misgivings centered around the independence of IRB review? Surely not. The ground of protest and counterprotest is a similar kind of ignorance about the fundamental terms of the relevant moral discourse: we don't know what animals are, either. We treat them as if they were morally protean; we mold them into anything from much-loved companions and symbols of virtue to mere machines for making food and instruments for scientific research.

Our ignorance as a society about these dark corners of our moral commitments, our lack of consensus about where outliers really fit, is extremely divisive when coupled with individual assurance that there is in fact available knowledge about these matters, that the answers are of surpassing importance, and that there is something suspicious, if not downright evil, about the people who don't get it. While such conclusions cripple civility, and should of course be resisted, our history should be making us nervous. We have so often gotten matters of who counts morally just flatly wrong, and have exacted horrible prices from those shuffled unjustly to the margins of our moral concern.

What fetuses are has at least received a thorough airing in bioethics literature. Gravid women we still find quite puzzling apparently, as witness current concerns about "forced cesareans" and "maternal-fetal conflict," but at least there is an awareness that getting clear about the moral character of pregnancy is a key to understanding the morality of pregnancy terminations. But despite their ubiquity in medical research and practice, determining what animals are is not thought of as a paradigmatic bioethics issue. Yet seeing animals clearly is likely to be at least as difficult as the analogous tasks for fetuses and pregnant women. After all, we have a strong stake in the presumption that nonhumans are things whose moral status is at our discretion: the looser we can keep the moral constraints, the freer we are to do as we like with these extremely useful creatures. Further, there is a sense in which animals really are protean. Human beings are animals; so are protozoa. Drawing some moral distinctions is inescapable when facing such a range, and if there's to be a bright line between entities that really matter and those that don't, the human species may very well seem a reasonable place to draw it.

Choosing this line may appear suspiciously self-serving. Yet, at least at first glance, it looks as though there really could be something ethically serious to be said for us. We don't have to rely on the brute fact that we've got all the power; this is a comfort, as "might makes right" has a dubious history as a basis for moral distinctions. Nor do we have to resort to the bare fact of our common species membership—again, all to the good, as such purely biological bases for moral categorization also have a simply horrifying pedigree. Further, we can avoid invoking the soul as a sort of special moral talisman whose possession elevates us above all others: purely metaphysical entities aren't much use when we're trying to do ethics with an eye to public policy in a pluralistic society. Besides, imagine what we would do if someone were to argue that the subjugation of women was justified on the grounds that all and only men possess "schmouls," an empirically undetectable entity that inexplicably gives them extra moral worth.

The distinction we wish to draw between humans and the rest of creation seems much more respectable than overlapping differences, that will end distinctions based on might, on species, or on sectarian metaphysics. One could say that the appeal to such things as the range and power of the human intellect, the complexity and depth of our interpersonal relationships, our passions, both personal and aesthetic, our sense of morality, and of tragedy makes good sense. If these abilities and vulnerabilities don't matter morally, it's hard to imagine what would.

But if these are the characteristics that matter morally, it is not only baboons who lack them; not all of us humans have them either. Many humans have lost, or will never have, powerful intellects, deep relationships, rich passions, or the intimations of mortality. Think of the profoundly mentally ill, the comatose, and those who have sustained severe brain injuries. While such humans are themselves instances of tragedy, they have no sense of what tragedy is.

Despite this sad fact, our convictions about the importance of simply being human are so strong that we hesitate to use organs from newborns with anencephaly, a condition incompatible with either sensation or life. Given this hesitation, one can imagine the response if a leading transplant surgeon were to call for the maintenance of colonies of mentally handicapped orphans, to be well-cared for until needed, but whose organs would then be "humanely" harvested for use in dying but otherwise "normal" people—infants with hypoplastic left heart syndrome, young fathers with HVB. Yet this scenario—with baboons and other primates substituting for handicapped orphans—is precisely what some transplant surgeons have been advocating since at least the 1960s, and is quite explicitly part of the agenda underlying the recent effort in Pittsburgh. If we are morally repulsed by a call to use handicapped orphans, but are eager to see whether colonies of baboons mightn't become a solution to our endemic lack of transplantable organs, it surely behooves us to have a good answer to the question, "What's so different about the two kinds of creature?"

Perhaps there is a good answer to that question—a difference, or set of overlapping differences, that will end up ethically supporting our practice. Perhaps we could, without arbitrary prejudice, keep all mentally handicapped humans, no matter how damaged or how alone in the world they might be, in the ethical family, so to speak. Perhaps it's appropriate to see all nonhumans, no matter how intelligent or complex their lives might be, as largely discretionary items, to be cast into the outer darkness if anything approaching a serious purpose seems to demand it. Or perhaps the real moral of the story here is that it is not baboons we should respect more, but humans who are their emotional and intellectual peers we should respect less; consider the research and therapeutic bonanza *that* would yield! But defending either of these conclusions would take a powerful argument, and there's very little evidence that any of the people most enthusiastically thumping the tub for more and better xenotransplantation have come up with reasons of the kind that are needed. Typically, their strategy is simply to point to the human cost of not pushing the xenograft agenda—the "three people who die every day waiting for a necessary organ" argument—without any serious attempt to balance that cost against the debit incurred to the victims of those grafts. Nor do we see much effort to set the xenograft strategy against the costs and benefits incurred by trying to enforce the required request laws that are already on the books, or to enact "presumed consent" or "routine retrieval" policies for organ procurement.

DISCERNMENT IN THE DARK

This, of course, returns us to our original problem: we don't even know how to begin that balancing act, and it seems that we aren't very keen on learning.

A simple reliance on our moral intuitions isn't enough. As the history of medical research in the nineteenth and even twentieth century reveals, we have been more than willing to subject those who were "clearly less valuable" to the rigors of research—only then, the ones who were obviously less valuable were Jewish, or people of color. Our gut instincts simply aren't good enough as reliable moral guides when we're dealing with those whom we've pushed to the margin of moral discourse. The question is not whether we're generally able to move deftly within our ordinary understanding of morality, but whether, when it comes to the moral outliers, that ordinary understanding itself is adequate.

Cross-species transplantation crystallizes a certain kind of moral conflict between humans and other animals—perhaps too sharply. Pitting the life of the father of two against that of a baboon is sure to strike most of us as no contest. The glare of the contrast distracts us from such realities as the fact that, at the point of decisionmaking, the animal's death buys only a chance, not a guarantee, or that the outcome of acting is not always better than the outcome of refraining, even when death is inevitable if we stay our hand. If we reflect about our moral duties and liberties more broadly, it may strike us that we are apparently quite comfortable allowing many tragic deaths to occur daily, when what it would take to stop them is not the life of an intelligent animal, but merely the cost of drinks after work.

On the other hand, if we do refuse to take the baboon's life in an effort to save the human's out of a sense that the moral parity between baboons and mentally handicapped humans leaves us no other option, then we need to ask what else that sense of parity implies. The animal who provided the liver in the Pittsburgh case was at least killed in an effort to save the life of an identifiable person. But most of what we do with the lives of animals is—at best—only distantly related to the lives and health of people in general. If it is wrong to kill a baboon to try to save a man's life, is it wrong to kill a pig because sausages taste so good? To kill a kid to make elegant gloves? Critics of xenograft whose main concern is with the "sacrificed" animal may find it relatively easy to adopt vegan diets and eschew wearing leather. But do they really advocate that ill people begin a wholesale boycott of a medical system in which the training and research leading up to its quite standard offerings are, as it were, drenched in the blood of nonhumans?

The implications of all this for the development of xenograft and the creation of "donor" colonies are comparatively clear. There are numerous ways in which we might strive to save and enhance lives, including many that are more efficient than killing animals who resemble us in no small degree— ways that do not burden us by reinforcing our commitment to moral positions we do not fully understand, and may not be able to maintain. If we feel morally constrained to continue organ transplantation as an important way of saving and enhancing human lives, we ought not to try to respond to that moral challenge with the technological fix of a better antirejection drug that will allow us to use nonhumans as organ sources, but rather by figuring out better ways to engage the altruism of the human community, until at last it strikes us all as mighty peculiar that anyone would want to hang on to her organs after death, when she has no use for them.

We ought to drop xenograft research and therapy, investing the resources of human effort, ingenuity, and money it consumes elsewhere. We don't now know what the judgment of history will be, but there's no reason to be sanguine about it. What this uncertainty says for our overall relationship with animals may still be a matter for debate, but there's no compelling need to make matters any worse.

PART TWO
Policy

The huge demand for transplantable organs and tissues may not be solved by expanding the donor pool by adding whole new populations. Part One demonstrated how the quest to alleviate organ shortages has resulted in proposals to use persons as donors that, many argue, fail to make either practical or ethical sense. As a result some in the transplant field and in public policy have turned away from the search for new donor populations. Instead they are seeking ways to maximize the efficiency of the procurement system itself.

The steps involved in organ procurement have not changed drastically during the past few decades. Throughout much of the 1970s and 1980s, procurement policy attempted to address the organ shortage problem in two ways. First, extensive public education programs were launched to increase altruistic organ donation. Second, great efforts were made to increase the administrative efficiency of the existing procurement system. While these efforts did help, it became clear that the future of American organ procurement needed to take a whole new direction.

The fundamental failure of the system prior to 1986 was that the supply of transplantable organs depended solely upon "voluntarism"—altruistic donation which depended on the prospective donor's filling out a donor card. While such a policy made perfect ethical sense in terms of respecting individual autonomy, the huge gap between supply and demand for organs plus the perception that many potential donors were being missed prompted ethicists and policy makers alike to search for more effective laws and policies to increase the supply of organs and tissues.

Instrumental to that policy change were the writings of Arthur Caplan. He asserted that organ donation is a right either of the individual or the

139

family if the individual did not object prior to death. Most importantly he insisted that medical institutions have an obligation to facilitate the opportunity to make a decision to donate. Caplan noted that many potential organ and tissue donors were being missed, not because requests to donate were being refused but because no one had asked for a donation. He argued that the key to increasing the supply of organs and tissues was to insure that families of potential organ and tissue donors were approached about donation whenever a death occurred. Such a policy would not only preserve altruism and choice but would guarantee the opportunity to exercise them.

Discussion of required request in the 1980s led to the passage of "required request" laws at both the state and federal levels. By 1995, forty-three states had enacted laws mandating that requests be made. Hospitals as a condition of their accreditation were required to have policies in place for identifying organ donors and insuring that requests were made. Required request policies made significant strides towards alleviating tissue and cornea shortages. However, the shift in policy has had limited impact on the supply of organs partly because many families refused requests and partly because those making the requests initially received little training in how to do so.

The continuing and worsening gap between supply and demand with respect to organs has led some to argue that those in need of transplants would be better served if the long-standing ethical commitment to altruism and voluntary choice were abandoned. One such proposed system of procurement has come to be known as Mandated Choice: a policy that requires competent adults to decide prospectively whether or not they wish to be organ donors when they die. Aaron Spital believes that the best way to obtain consent where organ donation is concerned is for each adult to decide for themselves what they wish to do. It is the individual not the family who should control consent. In the current system decisions are most frequently made by the family postmortem rather than by the individual prospectively. People simply do not fill out donor cards, or leave any written or oral record of their wishes about donation. Spital asserts that if mandated choice was to become law, if people were forced to choose to be donors or not, most adults would consent to donation and thereby increase the pool of desperately needed organs. Ann Klassen and David Klassen disagree with Spital's conclusions and assert that the moral, societal, and financial costs of mandated choice are simply too high. They suggest that the organ shortages would be better alleviated by finding out why people refuse to donate, rather than mandating more requests.

Presumed Consent, a system by which individuals are considered potential donors upon death unless they specifically note otherwise, has been in place in some European countries such as France, Austria, Spain, Italy, and Belgium for many years. It is not clear that putting the onus on those who want to "opt out" of donation instead of those who wish to "opt in" by carrying a donor card will increase the supply of organs and tissues. Belgium and Spain have seen increases in the supply of organs post the passage of a presumed consent law but France has not. Whether this kind of policy would work in the United States is a source of much controversy.

Presumed Consent breaks completely from the values underlying current policy which presumes that the deceased would not have willed their organs or tissues for donation. L. G. Futterman believes that presumed consent is the most effective way to realize autonomy and achieve a fairer and more protective system of organ procurement. Such a policy, he states, would give the individual ample opportunity to "opt out" of the system, and thus shifting the burden of decision-making under the highly stressful circumstances of what is often an unexpected death from the family and physicians.

In contrast to the Futterman article, Veatch and Pitt believe that Presumed Consent is based on the erroneous assumption that people would donate if asked—an assumption not backed by empirical data. Furthermore, they cite various polls that indicate public apprehension about a policy of presumed consent. They worry that the desire of the majority to get more organs may stifle the ability of religious minorities or other groups who find organ and tissue donation morally problematic.

Other plans to increase the number of organ donors propose using incentives as a method to alleviate demand. For example, Rupert Jarvis advocates a policy wherein admission to future transplant lists be conditional on registration as a potential organ donor. Economic incentives as a way to increase the supply of organs have been fervently debated in the literature since the beginnings of transplantation. The pros and cons of economic incentives appear in Part Three.

Existing policy to increase public awareness about donation has failed to alleviate our nation's organ shortages. The source of resistance to requests for donation remains poorly understood. Furthermore, it is not clear whether consensus exists about any drastic shift away from prevailing public policy governing organ donation. Thus, the debate will and should continue about the advantages and disadvantages of procurement policies based on values other than altruism, individual autonomy, and voluntarism.

Arthur L. Caplan
Daniel H. Coelho

12. Ethical and Policy Issues in the Procurement of Cadaver Organs for Transplantation

Arthur L. Caplan

In the past few years there has been a dramatic rise in the demand for organs for transplantation. Advances in surgical techniques, tissue typing, and the development of powerful immunosuppressive drugs, such as cyclosporine, have made it possible to transplant both a larger number and an increasing variety of organs. Among organs and tissues currently being transplanted from cadavers are kidneys, hearts, lungs, livers, bone marrow, skin, corneas, and pancreases.

Although some of these procedures are still experimental, graft and recipient survival rates for transplantations have shown steady improvement during the past decade.[1,2] Many centers report five-year-graft survival rates of 60 percent among patients who have received kidneys from cadavers. More then 95 percent of those who receive corneas from cadavers have their sight restored. Moreover, recent survival rates for heart transplantation are approaching 50 percent at five years.

This remarkable progress in the field of organ transplantation raises numerous moral and policy problems for the medical profession and the general public. Who ought to pay the high costs associated with these procedures? What rate of survival justifies the labeling of a procedure as therapeutic, and who should be responsible for making such determinations? When the number of organs is insufficient to meet the demand, what policies should be instituted to help increase the availability of these precious tissues?

It is the last question that, in many ways, is the most disturbing of all. The large gap that exists between the available supply and the demand for

Originally published in *The New England Journal of Medicine* 311, no. 15 (October 11, 1984): 981-83. Copyright © 1984 Massachusetts Medical Society. All rights reserved.

organs for transplantation has been well documented. The Centers for Disease Control has estimated that no more than 15 percent of the 20,000 persons who might serve as organ donors actually do so.[3]

The gap between supply and demand with respect to organ transplantation is not only large but growing in proportion to the rapid advances being made in this area. Nationwide, between 6,000 and 10,000 people are being maintained on either hemodialysis or peritoneal dialysis while awaiting a kidney transplant[3]; nearly 4,000 are estimated to be in need of corneal transplants. Indeed, the public has grown all too familiar with televised pleas for a liver, heart, or other tissue to save the life of a relative or friend.

The potential demand for organs is much greater than present levels may indicate. For example, the majority of liver transplantations are performed in children with congenital defects. However, if liver transplantation should prove to be an effective therapeutic option for adults with cirrhosis of the liver, then tens of thousands of persons might be potential recipients. Similar projections can be made for transplantations involving the heart, lungs, and pancreas.[24]

Given the current and potential future demand for cadaver organs, there may be no way to avoid the problem of rationing for many forms of transplantation. Nonetheless, it would appear to be both ethically and medically sensible to examine current public policy with respect to the procurement of organs for transplantation, to determine whether legal or regulatory changes might be effected that would help maximize the supply of tissues available to those in need.

For the past fifteen years this country has been committed to a policy of what might best be termed "voluntarism" in the procurement of tissues for transplantation.[5] As transplantation of certain tissues between genetically related family members became possible during the early 1960s, it soon became evident that physicians required both legal and moral guidance in developing procedures to procure tissue for this purpose.

Since many of the organs used for transplantation during this period were procured from living donors, legal authorities and the courts tended to stress the importance of voluntary consent in the procurement process. There was an understandable concern that family members, particularly those who were minors or had diminished mental capacities, were at some risk of being coerced to make donations against their will. Various court cases recognized the legal right of a person to give consent to the transplantation of tissue as long as he or she was both free from coercion and well informed about the risks and benefits of the procedure. Courts even gave children and the retarded the right to donate, in the belief that they might suffer greatly from the loss of a sibling or other family member.

When the prospects for the transplantation of tissues from cadaver donors improved during the 1960s, public policy was modified in order to encourage this form of donation. In 1968 the Uniform Anatomical Gift Act was enacted, which recognized the legal status of donor cards and "living wills," as well as the authority of the next of kin to make a donation in a situation in which the deceased had not indicated any opposition to donation.

Free choice and voluntarism played key parts in the moral and legal arguments that surrounded the passage of this legislation. Proponents of donor cards, donor statements on driver's licenses, and other forms of living wills argued that a system of cadaver organ procurement built on voluntarism would promote socially desirable virtues, such as altruism, and at the same time, protect the rights of persons who might, for various reasons, oppose the procurement of tissues from cadavers.

As noted above, this system has been only partially successful in securing organs for transplantation. In the light of the fact that the demand for cadaver organs is likely to increase, the time has come for a reexamination of current public policy regarding the procurement of such organs.

Although many of those involved in organ procurement are making heroic efforts to increase the supply of organs from cadaver donors, there are a number of factors that severely inhibit the ability of the present system to take advantage of the supply of tissues potentially available from cadavers. Both economic and legal fears impede the present system of voluntary donation.[5,7] Moreover, there is a real danger that unless something is done to improve the efficacy of the voluntary system, advocates of a free-market solution will attempt to create a for-profit system to meet the large demand for organs.[6]

Among the factors that diminish the effectiveness of the current voluntaristic approach to cadaver donation are the lack of trust on the part of physicians and hospital administrators in the legal authority of donor cards, the failure of the public to sign and carry donor cards, the failure of hospital personnel to locate donor cards, and most important, the failure of physicians and nurses to inquire about the possibility of organ donation in the absence of a written directive on the part of the deceased.[7]

There would appear to be a number of incentives that work against the efficacy of the current voluntaristic policy in obtaining cadaver organs. First of all, many people simply find the subject of death and organ donation upsetting and distasteful. Although surveys show that the public is willing to support organ donations,[8] it is difficult to transform willingness into concrete realization on a donor card or driver's license.

Secondly, most physicians and nurses do not want to inquire about organ donation. The highly emotional circumstances under which such requests are made make it uncomfortable for both families and medical personnel to communicate about the subject of donation. Moreover, at least some health professionals doubt that family members are able to give informed, voluntary consent in the context of the sudden death of a loved one.[5]

Finally, many hospitals fear adverse legal and financial consequences from their involvement with organ procurement. Many hospital administrators refuse to allow their staff to become involved with a procedure that carries some risk of legal complications and no promise of financial return.

Current federal policy is aimed at improving the present system by centralizing the collection of information concerning donors and recipients and by encouraging further efforts at public and professional education.[29] However, these efforts are not likely to prove useful in improving the supply of organs available from cadaver sources, since they do not address the major factors hindering the efficacy of the current system.

There is a public-policy option available at both the federal and state levels, however, that might increase the supply of organs available from cadavers. Legislation could be enacted that would require a routine inquiry of available family members as part of the existing procedures in each state for discontinuing life support measures in hopeless situations. Such a law would mandate that no one on a respirator who might serve as an organ donor could be declared legally dead (assuming that the medical requirements for such a declaration had been met) until a request for donation had been made of any available next of kin or legal proxy. The request would have to be made by a physician, nurse, or physician's assistant with no connection to the determination of the actual occurrence of death, in order to assure the public that declarations of death would be made without regard to the need to obtain organs for transplantation. If family members or guardians were not available, organs could be re moved only if a donor card or other similar legal document existed.

A policy of "required request" directly addresses the major obstacles in procuring cadaver organs for transplantation. Such a policy requires that hospital personnel routinely consider the need for transplantable tissues. It ensures that the burden of decisions concerning donation is equitably allocated among all families whose relatives might serve as organ donors. A policy of routine required request standardizes the process of routine inquiring about organ donation in such a way that it lessens the psychological burden on both health professionals and family members at time of great stress and emotional upheaval. Moreover, it removes the option not to inquire, which is often chosen under the present system because of fears concerning legal and financial consequences. Finally, a policy of required request preserves the right of individuals to refuse consent, since voluntary choice remains the ethical foundation on which organ donation rests.

The benefits to society in terms of an increase in the supply of cadaver organs for transplantation would appear to outweigh the loss of clinical freedom inherent in a required-request policy for cadaver organ donation. In view of the desperate needs of those who are now awaiting organs and the large number of persons who will be able to benefit from transplantation in the years to come, the loss of this freedom would seem to be a small price to pay.

REFERENCES

1. Van Thiel DH, Schade RR, Starzl TE. After 20 years, liver transplantation comes of age. *Ann Intern Med* 1983; 99:854-6.

2. Iglehart JK. Transplantation: the problem of limited resources. *N Engl J Med* 1983; 309:123-8.

3. Kolata G. Organ shortage clouds new transplant era. *Science* 1983; 221:32-3.

4. *Final report of the task force on liver transplantation in Massachusetts.* Prepared for the Department of Public Health, State of Massachusetts, 1983.

5. Caplan AL. Organ transplants: the costs of success. *Hastings Cent Rep* 1983; 13(6):23-32.

6. Chapman DE. Retailing human organs under the Uniform Commercial Code. *John Marshall Law Rev* 1983; 16:393-417.

7. Overcast TD, Evans RW, Bowen LE, Hoe MM, Livak CL. Problems in the identification of potential organ donors. *JAMA* 1984; 251:1559-62.

8. The Gallup Organization. Attitudes and opinions of the American public towards kidney donations. Prepared for the National Kidney Foundation, Washington, D.C. 1983., (GO 8305).

9. Koop CE. Increasing the supply of solid organs for transplantation. *Public Health Rep* 1983; 98:566-72.

13. Mandated Choice for Organ Donation: Time to Give It a Try

Aaron Spital

The successful development of transplantation is one of the most miraculous accomplishments of modern medicine. Unfortunately, the ability to deliver this medical miracle is limited by a severe and steadily worsening shortage of organs.[1] According to the United Network for Organ Sharing, as of 31 March 1996, more than 45,000 persons in the United States were on the national waiting list for transplantation[2]; this list grows by several hundred each month. It is estimated that eight of these people will die each day while waiting for transplantation.[3] Even more tragic is the realization that many of these deaths are preventable. Because only about 40 percent of potential cadaveric organ donors become actual donors, large numbers of life-saving organs are continuously being lost.[4] Clearly, something is wrong with our current organ procurement system.

OUR CURRENT ORGAN PROCUREMENT SYSTEM

In the United States, explicit consent is required before organs may be removed and used for transplantation. The Uniform Anatomical Gift Act, which has been passed in some form in all states and the District of Columbia, provides the legal framework for this process.[5-7] This statute gives all competent adults legal authority to decide for themselves whether or not they wish to become organ donors after their deaths. Unfortunately, relatively few people take advantage of this law and record their wishes about posthumous organ dona-

Originally published in *Annals of Internal Medicine* 125, no. 1 (1 July 1996): 66-69. Reprinted by permission.

tion.[8,9] Furthermore, even when such directives are available, organ procurement organizations still ask the family of the deceased for consent, despite the clear stipulation of the Uniform Anatomical Gift Act that the decedent's wishes must be honored.[5-7,10] In effect, the law is simply ignored, and the question of organ donation after death is almost always left for the family to decide.

The need to obtain family consent is a major barrier to organ procurement.[1,8,11-14] Because most organ donors are young people who die unexpectedly, the family is often devastated and in shock. Under these circumstances, clear thinking may be impossible. The need to consider organ donation at such a terrible time places additional stress on the family. Furthermore, family members are often unaware of their loved one's wishes, which makes the question of donation even more difficult for them to answer.[9,13,15,16] The need to ask for permission is also stressful for hospital personnel who fear aggravating the family's pain. Considering this mixture of grief, confusion, and anxiety, it is not surprising that more than 50 percent of families say no.[4] Indeed, despite suggested techniques designed to increase the number of families who say yes, such as delaying the request for organ donation until after the notification of death,[17,18] a recent study concluded that "the major impediment to procurement was the low rate of family consent."[4]

TOWARD GREATER INDIVIDUAL CONTROL THROUGH MANDATED CHOICE

The high rate of family refusal contrasts sharply with public opinion polls that show widespread support for organ donation.[9,15] This suggests that if the stress accompanying the decision-making process could be avoided, the rate of consent would increase. This goal could be accomplished by eliminating the need for families to consider donation at the emotionally charged time of a relative's death. Instead, adults could decide for themselves at their leisure whether or not they wish to become organ donors upon their deaths. By further ensuring that each person's wishes would be known and honored, favorable public sentiment toward organ donation should translate into increased rates of organ procurement.

This proposal to transfer control away from the family and back to the individual is consistent with the intent of the Uniform Anatomical Gift Act, which states that the wishes of the individual are paramount.[5-7] Furthermore, the Council on Ethical and Judicial Affairs of the American Medical Association recently concluded that "the individual's interest in controlling the disposition of his or her own body and property after death suggests that it is ethically preferable for the individual, rather than the family, to decide to donate organs."[14] Similar views have been expressed by many philosophers and ethicists,[19-23] and several surveys suggest that most of the public agrees.[13,24-26]

How can such an individualistic approach be achieved? Mandated choice has been proposed as an alternative method for obtaining consent, which is designed to accomplish precisely this.[1,5,8,10,13,14,22,27-30] Under mandated choice, all competent adults would be required to decide and record whether or not they wish to become organ donors upon their deaths. This could be accomplished by asking about organ donation on driver's license applications, tax returns, or official state identification cards. The application or tax return would not be accepted until the question of donation was answered. A change of mind could easily be communicated with a written directive at any time. However, a person's decision would be binding and could not be overridden by the family unless that person had made a provision granting his or her family veto power.

There are several advantages to this approach.[1,8,13,14,22,27-30] First, by eliminating the need to obtain family approval, the added stress now experienced by many families and health care workers when confronting the question of organ donation would be removed, and the family consent barrier would fall; in fact, many families might be comforted to know that their relatives' wishes were clear and would be honored. Second, mandated choice would take advantage of favorable public attitudes because all competent adults would decide about organ donation for themselves in a relaxed setting, where thinking is likely to be clear. Third, because all adults would be forced to consider this issue, mandated choice might be the most effective method for increasing public awareness of the great value of organ donation, and this might further stimulate participation. Fourth, mandated choice would eliminate occasional delays resulting from the need to obtain family consent that can jeopardize the quality of organs. Finally, mandated choice would preserve altruism and voluntarism, which are the philosophical foundations of our current system for obtaining consent. Indeed, mandated choice would promote autonomy because, more than any other system, it would ensure that a person's wishes would be honored, whatever they may be.

Making good decisions about complicated issues requires careful consideration; therefore, the question of organ donation should not be sprung upon people at motor vehicle bureaus. This issue should be considered in a setting that provides ample opportunity for reflection and discussion with family and friends, and these deliberations should take place before a decision is made. Therefore, regardless of how preferences are recorded under mandated choice, all adults should be informed long before their decisions are recorded that they will have to decide about organ donation for themselves and why. This information should be coupled with ongoing educational programs that outline the great value of organ donation and dispel fears that inhibit participation.[15,18,27] Mandated choice is designed to complement these vital programs, not to replace them.

Several authors have expressed concern that requiring people to decide about organ donation is coercive.[4,31] However, as Katz[28] has pointed out, "since the gain to the public . . . is likely to be substantial . . . we as a society can legitimately decide to tolerate the negligible intrusion on an individual's privacy presented. . . ." In addition, mandated choice is not coercive with regard to the choices a person makes, and it ensures that those choices will be honored.[13,14] This assurance also suggests that the fear that mandated choice would generate public resentment and an actual decline in the rate of consent is unlikely to occur. Two recent studies support this conclusion. Among a random sample of 1,000 adults in the United States, 65 percent said they would support mandated choice.[8] In a subsequent national survey, a nearly identical number (63 percent) said they would sign up to donate their organs under this plan; furthermore, of the 30 percent who had previously decided to donate, 95 percent said they would still do so under mandated choice.[13] These and other studies[9] also refute the claim that a widespread fear of being declared dead too soon would greatly inhibit participation.[4]

ROLE OF THE FAMILY

Mandated choice has been criticized as being insensitive to families.[31,32] In fact, it is kinder to families than is our present system because it eliminates the need for devastated families to confront the emotionally wrenching issue of organ donation during their most trying moments.[1,8,13,14,29,33] The concern that most families would not tolerate being excluded from the final consent process is not well substantiated. As previously noted, surveys have shown that most of the public believes that the individual, rather than the family, is best suited to decide about organ donation and that when advance directives exist, families should not be able to override the wishes of their loved ones.[8,13,24-26,29] These data indicate that most people in the United States believe that with regard to posthumous organ donation, individual autonomy should be respected. Therefore, once family members and medical personnel realize that the best way to protect autonomy, including their own, is to know and honor a person's wishes, they would probably be willing to accept advance directives as binding. It is hoped that self-determination about organ donation would eventually become accepted as routine, just as mandated autopsy is in deaths in which foul play is suspected.

Although mandated choice would give ultimate control regarding organ donation to the individual, this does not mean that the family is unimportant. Family discussions about this sensitive issue have always been of great value, and they always will be. Such discussions may provide useful insights that can help people explore their own feelings as they try to decide whether or not to donate. These exchanges also serve to inform family members of each other's wishes. This knowledge may avoid the distress that might otherwise occur if organs were taken from recently deceased persons who had previously agreed to donate but had not notified their families of their wishes. Furthermore, although most people in the United States seem to believe that adults should decide about organ donation for themselves, a significant minority believe that their families are better suited for this task. Under mandated choice, these people could include a provision granting their families veto power.[33] However, even in these cases, a personal decision should still be made and recorded because this information would be very helpful to families trying to decide. Finally, all families should be informed of any plans for organ retrieval, treated with the utmost respect and sensitivity, and offered as much support as they need to help them deal with the enormous trauma caused by the unexpected loss of a loved one.

POTENTIAL EFFECT ON PUBLIC COMMITMENT TO ORGAN DONATION

Because the purpose of mandated choice is not only to protect individual autonomy but also to increase public commitment to organ donation, it is important to estimate the potential impact that implementing this system would have on the rate of consent before an actual trial is undertaken. As noted above, in a recent Gallup poll of 1,002 randomly selected adults in the United States,[13] 63 percent said they would sign up to donate their organs if mandated choice became law. Furthermore, because devoting thought to organ donation correlates with a positive response,[13] and because mandated choice forces everyone to consider this issue, this system may actually encourage the 13 percent who were undecided to say yes. If so, under mandated choice, as much as 75 percent of the U.S. adult population would become committed potential organ donors.

CONCLUSIONS

Our current organ procurement system is inadequate. The need to obtain family consent is at least in part to blame and results in a daily loss of life-saving organs. To rectify this tragic situation, we need to redirect our focus away from the family and back to the individual, the one who is best suited to decide the disposition of his or her own body after death. Mandated choice appears to be an acceptable method for achieving this goal and was recently endorsed by the Presumed Consent Subcommittee of the United Network for Organ Sharing[27] and the Council on Ethical and Judicial Affairs of the American Medical Association.[14] Of course, whether or not mandated choice would actually increase public commitment to organ donation remains to be seen. There have been no actual trials of this proposal (Cate F., personal communication), and the problems with public opinion polls are well known. However, the results of these polls are encouraging enough to recommend that a pilot study of mandated choice be undertaken as soon as possible. With so many lives at stake, we cannot afford to simply continue our current inefficient approach to organ procurement. It is time to try something new.

REFERENCES

1. Spital A. The shortage of organs for transplantation. Where do we go from here? *N Engl J Med.* 1991;325:1243-6.

2. Patients waiting for transplants. *United Network for Organ Sharing Update.* 1996;12:26-7.

3. Fox MD. The transplantation success story [Editorial]. *JAMA.* 1994;272:1704.

4. Siminoff LA, Arnold RM, Caplan AL, Virnig BA, Seltzer DL. Public policy governing organ and tissue procurement in the United States. Results from the National Organ and Tissue Procurement Study. *Ann Intern Med.* 1995;123:10-7.

5. Medical technology and the law: organ transplantation. *Harvard Law Review.* 1990;103:1614-43.

6. Lee PP, Kissner P. Organ donation and the Uniform Anatomical Gift Act. *Surgery.* 1986;100:867-75.

7. Overcast TD, Evans RW, Bowen LE, Hoe MM, Livak CL. Problems in the identification of potential organ donors. Misconceptions and fallacies associated with donor cards. *JAMA.* 1984;251:1559-62.

8. Spital A. Consent for organ donation: time for a change. *Clin Transplant.* 1993;7:525-8.

9. The Partnership for Organ Donation. *The American public's attitudes toward organ donation and transplantation.* Boston; 1993.

10. Iserson KV. Voluntary organ donation: autonomy . . . tragedy. *JAMA.* 1993; 270:1930.

11. Caplan AL. Organ transplants: the costs of success. *Hastings Cent Rep.* 1983;13:23-32.

12. Kokkedee W. Kidney procurement policies in the Eurotransplant region. *Soc Sci Med.* 1992;35:177-82.

13. Spital A. Mandated choice. A plan to increase public commitment to organ donation. *JAMA.* 1995;273:504-6.

14. Strategies for cadaveric organ procurement. Mandated choice and presumed consent. Council on Ethical and Judicial Affairs, American Medical Association. *JAMA.* 1994;272:809-12.

15. Prottas JM, Batten HL. The willingness to give: the public and the supply of transplantable organs. *J Health Polit Policy Law.* 1991;16:121-34.

16. Tymstra T, Heyink JW, Pruim J, Slooff MJ. Experience of bereaved relatives who granted or refused permission for organ donation. *Fam Pract.* 1992;9:141-4.

17. Garrison RN, Bently FR, Raque GM, Polk HC Jr, Sladek LC, Evanisko MJ, et al. There is an answer to the shortage of organ donors. *Surg Gynecol Obstet.* 1991;173:391-6.

18. Perkins KA. The shortage of cadaver donor organs for transplantation. Can psychology help? *Am Psychol.* 1987,42:921-30.

19. Childress JF. Ethical criteria for procuring and distributing organs for transplantation. *J Health Polit Policy Law.* 1989;14:87-113.

20. Cohen C. The case for presumed consent to transplant human organs after death. *Transplant Proc.* 1992;24:2168-72.

21. Peters DA. A unified approach to organ donor recruitment, organ procurement, and distribution. *Journal of Law and Health.* 1989-1990;3:157-87.

22. Veatch RM, Pitt JB. The myth of presumed consent: ethical problems in new organ procurement strategies. *Transplant Proc.* 1995;27:1888-92.

23. Walthe ME. Mandated choice for organ donation [Letter]. *JAMA* 1995;273: 1177.

24. Corlett S. Public attitudes toward human organ donation. *Transplant Proc.* 1985;17(6 Suppl 3):103-10.

25. Harris RJ, Jasper JD, Lee BC, Miller KE. Consenting to donate organs: whose wishes carry the most weight? *J Appl Soc Psychol.* 1991;21:3-14.

26. Manninen DI, Evans RW. Public attitudes and behavior regarding organ donation. *JAMA.* 1985;253:3111-5.

27. Dennis JM, Hanson P, Hodge EE, Krom RAF, Veatch RM. *An evaluation of the ethics of presumed consent and a proposal based on required response.* United Network for Organ Sharing Update. 1994;10:16-21.

28. Katz BJ. Increasing the supply of human organs for transplantation: a proposal for a system of mandated choice. *Beverly Hills Bar Journal.* Summer 1984;18:152-67.

29. Spital A. Mandated choice. The preferred solution to the organ shortage? *Arch Intern Med.* 1992;152:2421-4.

30. Veatch RM. Routine inquiry about organ donation—an alternative to presumed consent. *N Engl J Med.* 1991;325:1246-9.

31. Prottas J. Mandated choice for organ donation [Letter]. *JAMA.* 1995;274:942-3.

32. Murray TH, Youngner SJ. Organ salvage policies: a need for better data and more insightful ethics. *JAMA.* 1994;272:814-5.

33. Glasson J, Orentlicher D. Mandated choice for organ donation [Letter]. *JAMA.* 1995;273:1176-7.

14. Who Are the Donors in Organ Donation? The Family's Perspective in Mandated Choice

Ann C. Klassen and David K. Klassen

Voluntary donation of cadaveric organs for transplantation is often referred to as "the gift of life." Indeed, for transplant recipients, this second chance at life ultimately depends on the receipt of an organ, which, without a doubt, is a gift of great value. The most unusual aspect of this gift, however, is that the giver and the recipient can never meet; moreover, setting the rules for this gift-giving depends on a host of others—family, medical professionals, and society as a whole. More than thirty years after the advent of cadaveric transplantation, the essential ethical dilemmas of organ donation show no signs of disappearing. They are, in fact, intensifying as transplantation becomes more successful.[1-3]

The medical potential for cadaveric solid organ donation exists in less than 2 percent of hospital-based deaths in the United States.[4] Most persons in the transplantation community are painfully aware that even the recovery of every usable organ could not keep pace with the ever-increasing demand. The supply of cadaveric organs has actually increased substantially over time; from 1988 to 1993, the number of cadaveric donors increased from 4,083 to 4,844, a 19 percent increase. However, in the same period, the number of waiting-list registrants increased from 16,026 to 33,496, an increase of 109 percent.[5]

Strategies to change the number of potential organs currently include efforts to expand the definition of eligible donors, identify nonhuman sources of organs, and even divide single organs among multiple recipients. Difficult as these new technological solutions to the shortage may be to achieve, many find it more frustrating that a very "low-tech" barrier to organ availability

Originally published in *Annals of Internal Medicine* 125, no. 1 (1 July 1996): 70-73. Reprinted by permission.

remains unsolved. Despite legislation mandating donation requests (so-called Required Request laws), recent evidence indicates that fully half of potential donations are refused by next of kin when requested in hospital settings.[4] Should we feel that the glass is half full because many families do donate or that the glass is half empty, as many in the transplantation community believe? Is family refusal an unnecessary barrier to cadaveric organ procurement?

The potential to eliminate the family's role in donation is the focus of efforts such as mandated choice for organ donation.[6] Using a system of universal registration, advocates of mandated choice propose to record the wishes of as many persons as possible about donation of their own organs and to retrieve this information in the event of death with donation potential.

Proponents of such efforts put forth two concepts that require examination: (1) Increasing the number of organs procured is currently an important societal need in the United States, and (2) forcing persons to declare their wishes about organ donation before death would result in the procurement of more organs by providing previously unknown evidence of donation choices at time of death with which to either persuade or override the wishes of next of kin.

SOCIAL MANDATE TO INCREASE DONATION

In most discussions of the organ shortage, the mandate to increase donation is taken for granted. However, it is not as uniformly accepted in the United States as many in the transplantation community assume. Over the past several years, transplantation has become more common and yet, if anything, more controversial, as a treatment of end-stage organ failure. As potential recipients increase in number and are recruited from older or sicker populations, ethical issues such as cost-benefit and equity of access remain unresolved.

Even among those who believe that the social benefits of transplantation justify the costs, a wide range of cultural and religious beliefs about brain death, whole-body burial, and end-of-life decision making remain. For many families, these beliefs are not part of formal religion; they may be articulated only when the families experience the unusual series of events that compose a donation situation and realize they cannot consent to organ procurement.

Many technical aspects of solid organ procurement have a strong effect on the family and structure of the end of life. The emotional effect of these events differs for each family, and these differences should be fully respected.

Neurologically devastated patients who are potential donors must be given a series of rigorous tests until full brain death has been established. Deterioration to full brain death sometimes takes as long as forty-eight hours after the family has been told that the patient is devastatingly ill (the only exceptions to full brain death occur in the protocols for non-heart-beating donation). Some families that express initial interest in organ donation cannot endure this wait and request that their relative be extubated before final determination of brain death, thereby making donation impossible. Other families, often the parents of young children, cannot bear to lose the opportunity to hold their child as support is withdrawn and heartbeat and respirations stop, and find that they cannot allow their child to be taken for procurement surgery.

Yet some proponents of cadaveric donation have used tones of zealousness when expressing their commitment to increasing donation. The decision to donate has been described as "generosity"[6] and the "preservation of life,"[7] and nondonating families are described as "those who would deny life to another"[8] by choosing "objection and decay,"[7] a result of "invalid" or "mistaken beliefs."[9]

Such language sets the stage for the mistrust that many feel about the current transplantation and donation process. For example, to the many persons whose beliefs are not compatible with organ donation for whatever reason, hearing their decision to choose whole-body burial described as "life-saving organs continuously being lost"[10] can be extremely upsetting. To families experiencing the devastating loss of a spouse or child, especially under the shocking and often violent situations typical of brain injury and death, the ability to even hear about a total stranger's need for organ transplantation is, in our opinion, a truly amazing act of altruism.

It is true that for some families, the decision to donate brings a degree of comfort by giving them the power to create a positive medical outcome (albeit for a stranger) in a situation in which they are otherwise helpless. But if families lose their role in the decision, would this positive feeling still occur?

Proponents of mandated choice, however, take the position that persons waiting for transplantation could be the rightful owners of all potential donors' organs "by eliminating the need to obtain family approval."[10] Although it is claimed that eliminating the family's need to make a decision "leads to kinder treatment than our present system,"[10] promotion of mandated choice is clearly based on recipient—not donor—needs, and discussions of hospital staff and donor family issues have been limited.

MANDATED CHOICE WILL INCREASE DONATION

The second and major argument is that a more uniform system of mandated choice will basically remove families from any decision-making role, thereby increasing the number of organs donated. This argument is based on the assumption that families do not know their relatives' true views on donation. However, flaws in this argument must be addressed.

First, despite legislation such as the Uniform Anatomical Gift Act, family acceptance of the procurement process has remained vital to a successful system of altruistic organ donation, even when the patient's wishes on donation are known.[11,12] This is consistent with the substantial amount of research in the area of end-of-life decision making. This research has shown that communication and consensus between caregivers and the family are critical, even in situations in which advance directives exist. Information about patient preference is most persuasive when decisions are being made about treatment of the patient before death, such as pain management and use of life-saving interventions. It is not uniformly accepted by caregivers that the patient's choice should predominate over the family's wishes once the patient has died. Therefore, overriding family wishes may not reduce stress on caregivers but actually aggravate it.

Indeed, mandated choice, if it introduces additional conflict into the already emotionally stressful arena of trauma, brain death acceptance, and organ recovery and allocation, could simply turn public opinion further against transplantation. The unfortunate reality of cadaveric organ donation is that it is the family, not the deceased patient, who comes home from the hospital; talks to their friends, neighbors, and community about their experience at the hospital; and shapes public opinion about organ donation among those they know. Can the transplantation community afford to go against the wishes of a family for its own apparent gain, even if it is legally entitled to?

A second problem in this area is that there is no evidence that lack of knowledge about patient wishes is a primary cause of family refusal, or that information retrieved from a national database would convince a family that they were carrying out their relative's wishes if they were previously unaware of such information. Studies of families who refuse to donate have been limited; we are currently studying 400 families approached for donation. Among families refusing to donate, we have not found that a substantial number refuse solely because they could not verify the deceased person's wishes. Often, in fact, they have no question that their relative's views and values match their own. Regret about not donating appears to be no more frequent than regret about donating.

Arguments for mandated choice assume that the rates of consent for organ donation would be higher among persons when they register than among their family members at the time of death. For example, Spital[13] cites a survey in which 63 percent of respondents reported that they would donate under mandated choice and compares this to an actual family consent rate of only 50 percent in another study.[4] However, this is a modest difference, given what we know in behavioral research about the weak link between expressed intentions and actual behavior. Siminoff and colleagues[4] note that this link is likely to be especially weak when "surveys ask respondents to speculate on behavior for which they have no experiential basis." Few of us have lost a member of our family in a situation of brain death; it is fairly safe to say that few of us could accurately predict our behavior in such a situation.

It is more logical to believe that if forced to make a choice, many persons who refuse to donate a relative's organ would also register as a nondonor. Children, who currently supply 27 percent of donated organs,[5] would presumably not register their choices; therefore, as in the current system, their parents' wishes would prevail. Nonregistrants, like nondonors, would tend to be from "hard-to-reach" segments of the population such as lower socioeconomic groups, minorities, and non-English-speaking persons.

The proponents of mandated choice do not even begin to discuss the legal and administrative burden this system would create. The United States has no uniformly successful system of centralized registration of persons, those we do attempt as a society, such as the census, are done for reasons far less controversial than organ donation and still do not achieve anywhere near 100 percent compliance. Yet it is naively assumed that the United States will, through legislation, fund and create a system in which a hospital emergency department in the middle of the night would be able to identify a patient and retrieve donor status information from a nationally centralized information source. The costs and complexity of such a system would be enormous and must be weighed against the potential social benefit.

There is, in fact, limited information that can be used to test the efficacy of mandated choice. In eighteen states, departments of motor vehicles retain data indicating a donation choice of persons registered to drive. In several states, this information is routinely available in situations of organ request.[14] To date, most Organ Procurement Organization personnel use this information to promote donation; that is, it is offered by procurement staff to potential donor families when the family is undecided and the driver is registered as a donor. Under mandated choice, would information on a driver's registration as a nondonor also be honored?

In Virginia and Texas, a partial system of "mandated choice" currently exists: Licensed drivers are required to register their donation decision. In Virginia, three options are available: donor, nondonor, and undecided. However, anecdotal information from organ procurement personnel indicates a paradoxical moral dilemma associated with this system that did not exist when a pro-donor decision was recorded voluntarily. Knowing that this information may exist, Organ Procurement Organization personnel feel that they must retrieve it, make the family aware of it, and honor a recorded nondonor status whether or not the family has already consented to donation.

In the first six months of the program, approximately 1,000,000 Virginia drivers were asked to declare a donor preference. Forty-five percent registered as nondonors, 24 percent were undecided, and only 31 percent registered as donors (data supplied by the Virginia Department of Motor Vehicles). These data support the hypothesis that many persons who are not opposed to donation still want to leave their family the "right to refusal" and are therefore unwilling to commit to a binding pro-donation decision beforehand. This information also matches what Organ Procurement Organization personnel tell us: Forced choice before death leaves the family with no options for considering the donation in light of the circumstances of death and perhaps agreeing to donate.

Could information such as that obtained through mandated choice be used to override family wishes to a greater extent than we currently do with situations in which we have a donor preference, such as organ donor cards or drivers licenses? Could we use this information to persuade families to change their choices? Or is the best system, as many have suggested, a system of public education supporting family decision and discussion in which families are made aware of donation decisions and reach consensus on them through discussion before critical illness and death?

Discussion of organ donation should certainly be encouraged within families, and persons should be allowed to record a full range of legally binding medical decisions, including the desire to donate organs, in case of devastating injury. The imperative to do this should be to improve the quality of death, for the benefit of both the patient and the family. Forcing people to commit to a specific, isolated end-of-life decision is coercive and shortsighted. It will not win any new converts to organ donation, and it may alienate those who are neutral.

What proponents of mandated choice fail to acknowledge is that under current required request laws, we already mandate that a choice be made about organ donation at death. This is the point at which families have the most information about how the decision will be made a reality. We also offer those who are ready the opportunity to make a choice earlier, through voluntary registration. However, a substantial proportion of our society expresses reluctance to commit to organ donation, both during their own lives and at the time of a relative's death, when the final decision must be made. If the answer to a donation request is no, perhaps we should find out why, rather than mandating more requests.

We do not believe that mandated choice shows a clear promise of radically changing the organ shortage, certainly not enough to justify its moral, societal, and financial costs. Thus, the recommendation to "redirect our focus away from the family and back to the individual"[11] hardly seems persuasive. We remain convinced that understanding the causes of family refusal of cadaveric donation requests offers more legitimate ways to increase donation rates than does ignoring families at their moment of devastating loss.

REFERENCES

1. Fox RC, Swazey JP, Watkins JC. *Spare Parts: Organ Replacement in American Society.* New York: Oxford Univ Pr; 1992.

2. Joralemon D. Organ wars: the battle for body parts. *Med Anthropol Q.* 1996;9:335-56.

3. Lock M. Transcending mortality: organ transplants and the practice of contradictions. *Med Anthropol Q.* 1995;9:390-9.

4. Siminoff LA, Arnold RM, Caplan AL, Virnig BA, Seltzer DL. Public policy governing organ and tissue procurement in the United States. Results from the National Organ and Tissue Procurement Study. *Ann Intern Med.* 1995;123:10-7.

5. Annual Report of the US Scientific Registry for Organ Transplantation and the Organ Procurement and Transplantation Network; 1993.

6. Spital A. The shortage of organs for transplantation. Where do we go from here? *N Engl J Med.* 1991;325:1243-6.

7. Dukeminier J Jr, Sanders D. Organ transplantation: a proposal for routine salvaging of cadaver organs. *N Engl J Med.* 1968;279:413-9.

8. Stuart FP, Veith FJ, Cranford RE. Brain death laws and patterns of consent to remove organs for transplantation in the United States and 28 other countries. *Transplantation.* 1981;31:238-44.

9. Veatch RM. Routine inquiry about organ donation—an alternative to presurned consent. *N Engl J Med.* 1991;325:1246-9.

10. Spital A. Mandated choice for organ donation: time to give it a try. *Ann Intern Med.* 1996;125:00-00.

11. Overcast TD, Evans RW, Bowen LE, Hoe MM, Livak CL. Problems in the identification of potential organ donors. Misconceptions and fallacies associated with donor cards. *JAMA.* 1984;251:1559-62.

12. Prottas J. Encouraging altruism: public attitudes and the marketing of organ donation. *Milbank Mem Fund Q Health Soc.* 1983;61:278-306.

13. Spital A. Mandated Choice. A plan to increase public commitment to organ donation. *JAMA.* 1995;273:504-6.

14. Klassen AC. *Study Design to Evaluate the Effects of State Department of Motor Vehicle Organ Donor Programs on Rates of Organ Donation: Technical Report.* Office of Science and Epidemiology, Health Resources and Services Administration, Fall, 1994.

15. Presumed Consent: The Solution to the Critical Donor Shortage?

Laurie G. Futterman

What the evolutionary structure of the Metaphysics of Quality shows is that there is not just one moral system. There are many. There is the morality called the "laws of nature," by which inorganic patterns triumph over chaos; there is morality called the "law of the jungle," where biology triumphs over the inorganic forces of starvation and death; there is morality where social patterns triumph over biology, "the law"; and there is an intellectual morality, which is still struggling in its attempts to control society.[1]

The concept of exchanging body parts through transplantation is part of early medical lore. Previously considered experimental, transplantation for end-stage organ disease is now the standard intervention for patients who no longer respond to conventional medical or surgical therapies. Since its inception and application, organ transplantation has been scrutinized by medical professionals and by the public.

Extraordinary advances in science and medicine such as transplantation of human tissues bring about previously unimaginable societal benefits, but also create profound implications involving autonomy and belonging, opposing moral considerations, and legal concerns. In a situation in which technology is changing faster than our values, the issue of salvaging organs from the dead to meet the escalating need of human organs for transplantation has evolved into an intricate web of interdisciplinary concerns and value conflict, in which right and wrong are only opinions.

This organ supply-demand disparity and the call for its resolution have

Reprinted by permission of *Alternative Therapies in Health and Medicine, American Journal of Critical Care* 4, no. 2 (September 1995): 383-88.

become major challenges to the transplant community and to those in political and bioethical arenas.[2-33]

Permission of those who have rightful authority over the body after death is required for the lifesaving uses of human organs. Because wills regarding posthumous disposal of organs are rare, donation can only be presumed when death occurs. As a result, the next of kin is typically given the responsibility of making the decision, taking into consideration all personal variables. Ethicists have long debated the rightful authority over the dead and the "morally correct" way to impose this right.

Medical, ethical, and legal constraints have created a gap between the human organ supply and demand. An increase in organ supply that is sufficient to meet current needs does not appear feasible within the present voluntary or request-for-consent framework. Most alternative solutions to the organ donation system fall short of societal and/or legal acceptance. Zealous transplant policy reform alone will not solve the crisis; it can only provide a framework within which all concerned groups can be motivated to collaborate. The answer may be found in a combination of effective public policies that are sustainable and reflect noble moral and ethical thinking. These policies would be bolstered by public education and would have the commitment of the healthcare fraternity for its preservation and success.

The purpose of this article is to dramatize the failure of required request legislation to increase the organ needs for transplantation, and to demonstrate the critical need for policy reform that assuages medical-legal concerns and differentiates autonomy and belonging from moral obligations and altruism. A presumed consent or mandated choice policy would eliminate the obstacles of professional reluctance and family opposition, ubiquitous in the required request structure, and must be tested.

In 1993 the number of organ transplants exceeded 18,000.[2] National, annual patient survival after vascular organ transplants ranged from 70 percent to 93 percent. Although more than 33,000 patients continue to wait for some type of organ, thousands die annually, while they are waiting.[2] As the benefits of organ transplantation increase and the barriers fall, the demand for transplantation grows, far exceeding its limited resources.[2,4,5,9,19] Despite a decline in traumatic deaths as a result of improved safety laws, as well as an increased percentage of donors with medical contraindications, approximately 15,000 to 20,000 persons still succumb to brain death annually. Of this group, 10,000 to 12,000 are medically qualified as organ donors but only 15 to 20 percent become donors.[2]

Research findings indicate that the organ supply-demand disparity stems not from a lack of donors but rather from failure to obtain permission to recover viable donor tissues and organs.[34] If transplantation is to remain a feasible option for patients with end-stage organ disease, society must reevaluate its philosophy toward organ donation. Healthcare professionals who deal directly with the public must be afforded security to fulfill their commitment to the consent process, and to the management and retrieval of donor organs.

HISTORICAL REVIEW

Before the 1950s there were no official provisions for the removal of organs or tissues from living or deceased persons for transplantation. Currently, some form of legislation, although varied, exists in all fifty states.[20] In response to demands to rectify previous deficiencies in the early systems of voluntary donation, various legislative proceedings were drafted and passed. The Uniform Anatomical Gift Act was enacted in 1968 and provided a simplified process through which people eighteen years of age or older could make a gift of their own organs or those of a relative. This act was later amended to mandate that on any hospital admission the patient's desire for organ donation would be noted (called routine inquiry) in the admitting record and that on the diagnosis of impending death, a hospital representative would be required to discuss the option of organ donation with the next-of-kin (called required request).[10,11,20-27,34]

The Uniform Determination of Death Act was passed in 1981 and clearly defined death as either (1) irreversible cessation of circulatory and respiratory functions or (2) cessation of all functions of the entire brain, including brain stem. This act prohibits the physician from declaring brain death in and procuring organs from the same patient.[10,11]

In 1986 the Omnibus Budget Reconciliation Act was passed. This legislation emphasized that federally and state-funded healthcare institutions were required to have a written protocol pertaining to the identification of potential donors, notification of a designated organ procurement organization, and a framework for the clinical management of the potential donor.[10,11,19]

The effectiveness of our voluntary system of organ donation has been limited. Inherent problems in the policy permit a significant number of patients to die in hospitals under circumstances that would otherwise enable organ donation. These problems can be largely attributed to three factors: the citizen, the medical profession, and the donor family.

Americans consider disposal of their body to be a fundamental right; however, few exercise control over this right. Citizens must be assured that others will intervene only in the absence of a clearly expressed will. Natural hesitation to confront one's mortality is a major reason that only 15 percent of the public sign and carry an organ donor card, request notation on their driver's license, or make some provision in a living will.

Paradoxically, when proper documents can be located, almost all organ procurement organizations require additional approval from the next of kin (despite the provisions of the Uniform Anatomical Gift Act) and may even overrule the patient's preference if the family refuses donation so as to prevent conflict, legal action, or adverse publicity.

Inadequate efforts by healthcare professionals to request donation from families has received most of the blame for loss of potential organs. A large percentage of healthcare professionals who are responsible for the required request do not fully understand the consent process; they are poorly educated about organ donation and brain death issues and are often uncomfortable requesting a donation from the bereaved family. In hospitals in which required request is written policy, haphazard compliance with existing laws is well-known.

At least one third of families, having sustained the tragic and sudden loss of a loved one, refuse donation. However, surveys indicate that opposition to donation is less frequent before the family has actually been confronted with the request for donation than after the request has been made.[20-45]

NEED FOR CHANGE

The American society, as well as nurses and physicians who care for the critically ill, expects the healthcare system to consistently cure illness and preserve life.[31] These expectations can lead to confusion and turmoil in groups caring for the terminally ill or injured.

Failure of Required Request Legislation

Successful interactions between healthcare professionals and the bereaved family depend in part on professionals' understanding of their role and the role of other team members involved in the procurement process. In several studies a significant number of healthcare professionals are shown to be unaware of their institution's policy on brain death and organ donation or to lack adequate knowledge of related medical criteria.[28-34,46]

The absence of an assumed consent policy by our society reflects the sensationalized fear and mistrust of the medical community, as well as the struggle between posthumous autonomy, belonging, and moral obligation. Lingering frustration over failure of required request legislation and the suboptimal use of human organ resources spurred the development of "alternative" procurement proposals. Because most alternative organ donation proposals have some aspect that is unacceptable to present societal norms and values, none has yet been initiated.[9,10,12,14-17,19-34,47,48]

Alternative Solutions

Mandated Choice

Mandated choice would require all adults (eighteen years or older) to express their written preference or objection to organ donation before death.[11,12,48] The success of this popular strategy, however, is contingent on an educated and informed public regarding the purpose and importance of organ donation.

Routine Salvage

Routine salvage, a communal policy, would eliminate the need for consent. Proponents argue that like homicide laws and required autopsies, laws governing procurement of organs to save lives should be justified despite family objections. Certain states have amended their Uniform Anatomical Gift Act to allow for "tailored" routine salvage, "reasonable search," or "no known objection," if and when symbolic demonstration of donor preference can be established and reasonable attempts to locate the family are unsuccessful after four hours.[17,34,49,50]

Financial Incentives, Live Unrelated Donor Compensation, and Preferred Status

Despite its drastic nature, a market in organs has been proposed to increase organ donation and supply. Proposals such as future contracts,[34] rewarded giving,[51] and direct financial gain imply some form of organ commerce. Although the sale of any human tissue is prohibited by law in the United States, financial inducements for donation are being debated.[13,34,48,52-58] Preferred status involves rewarding organ donors by providing them with some type of non-monetary recognition for their willingness to donate (e.g., higher status if they, or a family member, need organ transplantation in the future).

Xenografting

The use of animals as a source of organs has also been suggested, but public criticism regarding "experimentation" on the critically ill and animal rights issues is vigorous. Immunologic barriers preclude xenografts as a feasible alternative to human allografts, but research efforts are continuing.[59,60]

Altering Brain Death Criteria

Brain death, a relatively new concept, and its direct equation with death of the person, has allowed clinical transplantation to advance.[61,62] As an attempt to increase the availability of human organs for transplantation, alteration of brain death criteria is suggested to expand the pool of organ donors. Modification of brain death criteria (now accepted as total cessation of cortical and brainstem function) to include patients in a persistent vegetative state and/or anencephalic infants would redefine brain death as the absence of cortical function only.[63-65] Consideration of anencephalic infants as potential organ donors has been declared ethically permissible within strict guidelines. However, public debate continues to preclude any transition to a higher brain death standard and its application.[48,66]

Use of Minors as Living Organ Donors

Use of organs from living minors is another alternative that may expand the organ donor pool. Although this alternative seems innocuous, the use of minors as organ donors is fraught with risk and issues of understanding, voluntarism, and coercion.[48]

Extended Donors and Donors with No Heart Beat

Organs procured in situations that compromise tissue integrity and postoperative function (e.g., after declaration of cardiorespiratory death or from suboptimal donors) are a viable but last option.[67]

Use of Condemned Prisoners

Organ donation from executed prisoners has been suggested but has been deemed unethical, unless the prisoner made the decision to donate before conviction.[48]

Presumed Consent and Mandated Choice

The reemergence of presumed consent and mandated choice as solutions to the organ donor shortage shifts the responsibility of organ donation from donor families to donors, who have ample opportunity during their lifetime to object, or consent, to organ donation.

Regardless of the origin of consent, the term "donor" implies giving, which transcends any legal or moral duty. Therefore, an altruistic contribution is reflected by the absence of objection rather than the presence of consent. Adoption of this principle allows physicians to remove organs from cadavers for transplant purposes without having to search for explicit consent, unless an objection was expressed and registered by the donor or the donor's family.

Although presumed consent, or an opting-out policy, respects individual autonomy, it reflects and communicates moral responsibility more so than a consenting policy. Presumed consent makes donation routine, which minimizes emotional burdens by limiting the inquiry to objections. The burden of requesting donation by healthcare professionals and the anxiety of decision making by distressed families are eliminated. Furthermore, delays stemming from long family searches that can jeopardize organ integrity are avoided. The right to refuse is preserved for people who do not wish to donate.

Technical complexities of this system that still remain to be resolved include (1) establishing the burden of inquiry and participation; (2) lack of an effective mechanism for registering objections, with reliable means of entering, updating, and honoring data; and (3) absence of a vehicle by which the public can be made aware of their opting-out prerogative. In addition to securing the individual's right to object, unequivocal legal immunity must be ensured for the healthcare professionals who act in good faith. Furthermore, presumed consent, although logical and meritorious in theory, would lure lawyers and body-snatching movie productions into our already litigious and media-sensationalized society.[10,19,34-45,48]

At least thirteen European countries, the leading organ procurement countries worldwide, operate under presumed consent legislation. In half of these countries physicians approach families to obtain consent, whereas in the others, physicians proceed with routine organ salvage if there is no prior objection.[43-45]

In Belgium individuals register their decision regarding donation in a computerized central registry accessible only to the transplant centers. Physicians may act according to their own ethics, within the limits of the recorded decision of the donor and the right of the family to object. This physician freedom is one of the crucial components of the program's success.[35,44,45]

To accept a presumed consent policy, a society must first remodel the attitudes of healthcare professionals and the public they serve toward the moral good of organ donation. Lewin's theory for planned change,[68-69] which consists of unfreezing, moving, and refreezing phases, enables individuals to recognize, accept, and value the need for change. Age, cultural, educational, and economic differences, individual perception and management of bereavement stressors, and ease of the donation process affect willingness to comply and must be considered.[3-34]

Media and role models, as well as meetings and discussions among civic, social, and academic leaders, can be effective means of propagating pro-donation and transplant information.[15] A centralized data bank, using driver's license numbers, could be maintained by the United Network for Organ Sharing to register and update consent or dissent of respondents. Procurement and transplant centers could then access this information easily and determine donor status with or without family intervention.

A centralized database is being implemented in an aggressive campaign in Louisiana, using the driver's license bureau to provide the medical community with a more accurate means of identifying potential donors. When this system is established, hospitals will have access to the database through local organ procurement organizations.[70]

Furthermore, a new Pennsylvania law, PA Act 102,[67] requires hospitals to call the regional organ procurement organization regarding every patient death to determine the suitability for organ donation. The law calls for a rejuvenated driver's license program in which drivers are asked to indicate whether they wish to be an organ donor. Police and emergency personnel are asked to make every effort to recover and bring the driver's license to the hospital. This law also states that consent from next of kin for donation is not necessary when evidence of the patient's wish to donate organs is documented.[67]

CONCLUSION

Until the hospital doctor can look down on his dying patient whose life as he knows he cannot save and see in him the chance of life for the patients of his colleagues; until donor organs are recognized by all of us as the pieces of human tissue that they are, waiting to be burned or buried a few days after death; and until opting out legislation has been introduced to this country, making available for transplantation all viable organs unless the deceased in his lifetime has recorded his dissent, this tragic waste of life will continue.[57]

Organ and tissue transplantation has progressed from a bizarre notion to an established lifesaving reality. Despite advances in living-related organ transplantations and the retrieval of certain organs from donors with no heart beat, incessant demands for organ transplantation have all but depleted the supply of human organs. Isolated state legislative modifications of organ donation policies have been attempted but have not engendered a global response. Healthcare professionals are not prepared to interact with a hesitant society and are less than enthusiastic about complying with required request mandates.

Presumed consent implies that a person is considered to be a potential organ donor unless or until an objection is made. Implementing an organ donation policy based on presumed consent, where donation is no longer perceived as burdensome, may result in more positive donation interactions and fewer wasted organs. However, a number of obstacles remain before presumed consent mandates can be effective. Changes in a social policy must be preceded by the acknowledgment and acceptance of the need for the change by the public. The valuing of organ transplantation and donation by the individual should occur first as a result of moral duty and then autonomy, directed by information and education. A change model such as Lewin's[68,69] may provide the framework for successful modification of one the most debated and challenging societal issues[48]: presumed consent for organ donation.

REFERENCES

1. Pirsig R. *Lila.* New York, NY: Bantam Books; 1991:158-161.

2. *1994 Annual Report of the United States Scientific Registry of Transplant Recipients and the Organ Procurement and Transplantation Network.* Richmond, Va: US Department of Health and Human Services. No 240-93-0051 and 240-93-0052.

3. Scott R. The human body: belonging and control. *Transplant Proc.* 1990;22:1002-1004.

4. Robertson JA. Supply and distribution of hearts for transplantation: legal, ethical, and policy issues. *Circulation.* 1987;75:77-86.

5. Benjamin M. Supply and demand for transplantable organs: the ethical perspective. *Transplant Proc.* 1992;24:2139.

6. Turcotte JG. Supply, demand, and ethics of organ procurement: the medical perspective. *Transplant Proc.* 1992;24:2140-2142.

7. Quah SR. Social and ethical aspects of organ donation. *Transplant Proc.* 1992;24:2097-2098.

8. Keyserlingk EW. Human dignity and donor altruism: Are they compatible with efficiency in cadaveric human organ procurement? *Transplant Proc.* 1990;22:1005-1006.

9. Whittaker M. Bequeath, bury or burn? *Nurs Times.* 1990;86(40):34-37.

10. Rodgers SB. Legal framework for organ donation and transplantation. *Nurs Clin North Am.* 1989;24:837-850.

11. Miller M. A proposed solution to the present organ donation crisis based on a hard look at the past. *Circulation.* 1987;757:20-27.

12. Grenvik A. Ethical dilemmas in organ donation and transplantation. *Crit Care Med.* 1988;16:1012-1018.

13. Marsden C. Ethical issues in cardiac transplantation. *J Cardiovasc Nurs.* 1988;2:23-30.

14. Prottas JM. Encouraging altruism: public attitudes and the marketing of organ donation. *Milbank Q.* 1983;1961:278-303.

15. Caplan AL. Professional arrogance and public misunderstanding. *Hastings Cent Rep.* 1988;18:34-37.

16. Robbins RA. Signing an organ donor card: psychological factors. *Death Stud.* 1990;14:219-229.

17. Menzel PT. The moral duty to contribute and its implications for organ procurement policy. *Transplant Proc.* 1992;24:2175-2178.

18. Hessing DJ, Elffers H. Attitude toward death: fear of being declared dead too soon, and donation of organs after death. *OMEGA.* 1987;1 7:115-124.

19. Spital A. The shortage of organs for transplantation: Where do we go from here? *N Engl J Med.* 1991;325:1243-1246.

20. Cutler JA, David SD, Kress CJ, et al. Increasing the availability of cadaveric organs for transplantation: maximizing the consent rate. *Transplantation.* 1993;56(1):225-227.

21. Denvey P. Organ donation and required request legislation. *J Pediatr Nurs.* 1990;5:288-289.

22. Veatch RM. Routine inquiry about organ donation: an alternative to presumed consent. *N Engl J Med.* 1991;325:1246-1249.

23. Mann JE. Obligations of the health care community in organ procurement. *Transplant Proc.* 1990;22:1012-1013.

24. Caplan AL, Virnig B. Is altruism enough? Required request and the donation of cadaver organs and tissues in the United States. *Crit Care Clin.* 1990;6:1007-1018.

25. Rudy LA, Leshman D, Kay NA, Ballenger OM. Obtaining consent for organ donation: the role of the health care profession. *J S C Med Assoc.* 1991;87:307-310.

26. Norris MK. Required request: Why has it not significantly improved the donor shortage? *Heart Lung.* 1990:19:685-686.

27. Kubler-Ross E. *On Death and Dying.* New York, NY: Macmillan; 1969.

28. Batten HL, Prottas JM. Kind strangers: the families of organ donors. *Health Aff* 1987;6:35-47.

29. Vernale C. Critical care nurses' interactions with families of potential organ donors. *Focus Crit Care.* 1991;18:335-339.

30. Adams MM. Support to organ donor families. *Genesis.* 1989;1:2.

31. Stark JL, Reily P, Osicki A. Attitudes affecting organ donation in the intensive care unit. *J Heart Lung.* 1984;13:400-401.

32. Kiberd MC, Kiberd BA. Nursing attitudes towards organ donation, procurement, and transplantation. *Heart Lung.* 1992:21:106-111.

33. DeYoung S, Temmler L, Adams EF, Just G. Brief, organ referrals: Would nurses do more if they knew more? *J Contin Educ Nurs.* 1991:212,219-221.

34. Murray TH, Youngner AJ. Organ salvage policies: a need for better data and more insightful ethics. *JAMA.* 1994:272:814-815.

35. Michialsen P. Organ shortage: What to do? *Transplant Proc.* 1992:24:2391-2392.

36. Cwiek MA. Presumed consent as a solution to the organ shortfall problem. *Public Law Forum.* 1984:4:81-99.

37. Ward ED. Can opting out legislation solve the shortage of donor organs? *Br J Hosp Med.* 1990;43:80.

38. Benoit G, Spira A, Nicoulet I, Moukarzel M. Presumed Consent Law: results of its application/outcome from an epidemiological survey. *Transplant Proc.* 1990;22:320-322. 39.

39. Council on Ethical and Judicial Affairs, American Medical Association. Strategies for cadaveric organ procurement: mandated choice and presumed consent. *JAMA.* 1994:272:809-812.

40. Sadler BL. Presumed consent to organ transplantation: a different perspective. *Transplant Proc.* 1992:24:2173-2174.

41. Cohen C. The case for presumed consent to transplant human organs after death. *Transplant Proc.* 1992;24:2168-2172.

42. Cantaluppi A, Scalamogna A, Ponticelli C. Legal aspects of organ procurement in different countries. *Transplant Proc.* 1984;XVI: 102-104.

43. Gnant MF, Wamser P, Goetzinger P, et al. The impact of the presumed consent law and a decentralized organ procurement system on organ donation: quadruplication in the number of organ donors. *Transplant Proc.* 1991;23:2685-2686.

44. Roels L, Vanrenterghem Y, Waer M, et al. Three years of experience with a "presumed consent" legislation in Belgium: its impact on multi-organ donation in comparison with other European countries. *Transplant Proc.* 1991;23:903-904.

45. Thomas G, Ryall M, Taber SM. Ethical dilemmas in transplantation. *Transplant Proc.* 1992;24:2099.

46. Futterman LG. *Does Education Affect Attitudes of Health Care Professionals Toward Organ Donation?* Miami, Fla: Barry University; 1994. Thesis.

47. Fentiman L. Organ donations: the failure of altruism. *Issues Sci Technol.* 1994;121(1):43-48.

48. Council on Ethical and Judicial Affairs. *Code of Medical Ethics: Current Opinions With Annotations.* Chicago, Ill: American Medical Association; 1994:25-31.

49. Dickens BM. Legal aspects of transplantation: judicial issues. *Transplant Proc.* 1992;24:2118-2119.

50. State of Texas Civil Statutes, §11B, chap 173, Acts of the 47th Legislature; House Bill 271 (1991):1-3.

51. Dossetor JB. Rewarded gifting: Is it ever ethically acceptable? *Transplant Proc.* 1992;24:2092-2094.

52. Blumstein JF. The case for commerce in organ transplantation. *Transplant Proc.* 1992;24:2190-2197.

53. Cantarovich F. Current risks of organ commerce. *Transplant Proc.* 1992;24:2091.

54. Sells RA. Consent for organ donation: What are the ethical principles? *Transplant Proc.* 1993;25:39-41.

55. Sells RA. Some ethical issues in organ retrieval, 1982-1992. *Transplant Proc.* 1992;24:2401-2403.

56. Kittur DS, Hogan MM, Thukral VK, McGaw LJ, Alexander JW. Incentives for organ donation? *UNOS Update.* 1992;8:8-10.

57. Sells RA. Organ commerce: ethics and expediency. *Transplant Proc.* 1990;22:931-932.

58. Thomas G, Ryall M, Taber SM. Ethical dilemmas in transplantation. *Transplant Proc.* 1992;26:2099.

59. Cooper DKC. Is xenotransplant a realistic clinical option? *Transplant Proc.* 1992;24:2393-2396.

60. Hammer C, Suckfull M, Saumweber D. Evolutionary and immunological aspects of xenotransplantation. *Transplant Proc.* 1992;24:2397-2400.

61. Frist WH, Fanning WJ. Donor management and matching. *Cardiol Clin.* 1990;8:55-59.

62. Wikler D. Brain-related criteria for the beginning and end of life. *Transplant Proc.* 1990;22:989-990.

63. Ivan LP. The persistent vegetative state. *Transplant Proc.* 1990:22:993-994.

64. Downie J. The biology of the persistent vegetative state: legal, ethical and philosophical implications for transplantation. *Transplant Proc.* 1990;22:995-996.

65. Walters JW. Anencephalic infants as organ sources: should the law be changed? Yes: the law on anencephalic infants as organ sources should be changed. *J Pediatr.* 1989;115:825-828.

66. Winslow GR. No: the law on anencephalic infants as organ sources should not be changed. *J Pediatr.* 1989;115:829-832.

67. Benenson E. Comprehensive organ donor law goes into effect: Penn hospital required to call down program on all deaths. *UNOS Update.* 1995;11(3):24-25.

68. Lancaster J. Change Theory: an essential aspect of nursing practice. In: Lancaster J, Lancaster W, eds. *The Nurse as a Change Agent.* St Louis, MO: CV Mosby; 1982:5-8.

69. Mauksch I, Miller MH. *Implementing Change in Nursing.* St Louis. CV Mosby; 1981.

70. Benenson E. Louisiana Registry. *UNOS Update.* 1994;10(12):24.

ADDITIONAL REFERENCES

Burdick JF. Preferred status for organ donors. *UNOS Update.* 1994;10(7):15,16.

Caplan A, Siminoff L, Arnold R, Virnig B. Increasing organ and tissue donation: What are the obstacles, what are our options? *Proceedings of the Surgeon General's Workshop on Increasing Organ Donation.* Washington, DC: 1991;199-232.

Kass LR. Organs for sale? Propriety, property, and the price of progress. *Public Interest.* 1992;Spring:65-86.

Solving the Organ Donor Shortage: A Report of the Partnership for Organ Donation. Boston, Mass: Partnership for Organ Donation, Inc. 1990.

Peters TG. Life or death: the issue of payment in cadaveric organ donation. *JAMA.* 1991;265:1302-1305.

Prottas JM. Buying human organs—evidence that money doesn't change everything. *Transplantation*. 1992;53:1371-1373.

Siminoff LA, Arnold RNI, Caplan AL, Virnig BA, Seltzer DL. Public policy governing organ and tissue procurement in the United States. *Ann Intern Med*. 1995;123:10-17.

Tymstra TJ, Heyink JW, Pruim J, Slooff MJ. Experience of bereaved relatives who granted or refused permission for organ donation. *Fam Pract*. 1992;9:141-144.

16. The Myth of Presumed Consent: Ethical Problems in New Organ Procurement Strategies

R. M. Veatch and J. B. Pitt

The acute shortage of organs for transplantation has led to considerable interest in laws that are designed to increase the number of organs procured. These laws are often referred to as "presumed consent" laws. Such laws are alleged in many popular and scholarly articles to exist in several European countries and Singapore, among other places. The reasoning behind recent arguments in favor of adopting a so-called presumed consent law in the United States is that if we can presume the consent of the deceased to organ procurement there will be a substantial increase in the yield of organs.

THE DIFFERENCE BETWEEN CONSENT AND SALVAGING

The problem with this approach, however, is that, with a few exceptions, the existing laws never actually claim to presume consent, nor can they rightly be said to do so. They simply authorize the state's taking of the organs without explicit permission. It therefore seems wrong to call them presumed consent laws. They are, in effect, what used to be called *routine salvaging* laws.[1] We believe the time has come to be more careful in distinguishing between policies of presumed consent and those of routine salvaging. While the net outcome may be the same under either kind of policy, the underlying assumptions about the relation of the individual to society are radically different.

It is our hypothesis that those who support a societal right to procure

Originally published in *Transplantation Proceedings* 27, no. 2 (April 1995): 1888-92. Reprinted by permission of Appleton & Lange, Inc.

organs without consent find it embarrassing to speak bluntly about taking organs without consent, hence they adopt the *language* of presuming consent even when there is no *basis* for such a presumption. In doing so, they preserve the appearance of the preferred gift-mode and the guise of respect for individual choice. (This desire for euphemistic language is also seen in the persistent practice of referring to persons from whom organs are taken as *donors* even in cases, such as small children, in which these people could never have actually made a gift or donation.) We shall suggest that important matters of societal relations are at stake in distinguishing between policies that allow the procurement of organs on the presumption that people would consent and those that simply take organs without consent. One form of society gives central place to the individual, holding that his or her person can be used by the state only with some form of consent. That has been the society of liberal Western culture, particularly the United States. It underlies the gift-mode and the doctrine of consent that has been central not only to organ procurement, but to the practice of medicine in general, for decades.

Another form of society gives more central authority to the state, authorizing it to use the individual for important societal purposes even without individual consent. It underlies routine salvaging, or the taking of organs without consent. For the purposes of this article, we are not pressing for one form of policy or the other. It is possible that the time has come for elevation of the state by adopting a routine salvaging law. That seems to be the rationale behind new movements toward enhancing communitarianism and stressing the common good in social policy.[2] It is also possible that the importance of the individual continues to require procuring organs in the gift or donation mode in which organs may be taken only with proper permission. The conflation of these two is, we shall suggest, a dangerous prospect indeed.

THE STATE OF THE LAW

Countries with Routine Salvaging Laws (With No Claim of Presuming Consent)

It is striking that it is so common for commentators to refer to these laws as "presumed consent" laws. For example, according to Gerson, the French law on organ procurement adopted in 1976 is one which presumes the consent of persons who do not, during their lifetime, expressly refuse to have their organs taken upon their death.[3] However, on examination of the law itself, one is hard pressed to find any mention of presuming consent, overt or implicit. The law states that, "An organ to be used for therapeutic or scientific purposes may be removed from the cadaver of a person who has not during his lifetime made known his refusal of such a procedure."[4] Although the law offers a provision for those willing and able to record their dissent, it is not clear why we should conclude that the rationale behind the opting out system it establishes is based upon the presumed consent of the decedent rather than the primacy of the state. Gerson, citing an article by Cantaluppi, also attributes presumed consent laws to Austria, Belgium, (the former) Czechoslovakia, Finland, Italy, Norway, Spain, and Switzerland, among other countries[4] (p 1019, note 35). *Not one* of these laws mentions anything about presuming consent, directly or indirectly.[5-13] Among the other countries that have laws authorizing organ procurement without claiming to presume consent are Cyprus,[14] Hungary,[15] Singapore,[16] Syria,[17] and the former Yugoslavia.[18] Some of these have been referred to in the literature as countries with presumed consent laws, yet none of them actually claims to presume consent in its legislation.

Laws with an Explicit Presumption of Consent

By contrast we have located a few laws and proposed laws that do actually state a presumption of consent or, its equivalent. For example, the Colombian law on organ procurement states that, ". . . there shall be a legal presumption of donation if a person during his life time [*sic*] has refrained from exercising his right to object to the removal from his body of anatomical organs or parts during his death . . ."[19]

Within the United States at least two states have recently considered laws that would properly be called presumed consent laws. In Maryland, a bill proposed on March 10, 1993, had it not been defeated, would have allowed for the presumption of consent of those who did not opt out. It read, "in the absence of specific objection by an individual expressed during that individual's lifetime, or by any of the individual's next of kin immediately following the individual's death, the individual is deemed to have consented to the donation of the individual's body or any part of the individual's body for and of the purposes specified . . ."[20] In Pennsylvania, a subchapter entitled, "Presumed Anatomical Gifts," of a proposed amendment to an act, reads, "Organs and tissues may be removed, upon death, from the body of any Commonwealth resident by a physician or surgeon for transplantation or for the preparation of therapeutic substances, unless it is established that a refusal was expressed. . . ."[21] Both of these proposed law changes adopt the language of presuming consent. This, of course, begs the question of whether consent can actually be presumed in these jurisdictions at all.

WHY CONSENT CANNOT VALIDLY BE PRESUMED

Although the difference between the European laws that do not presume consent and the New World laws and proposals that do presume it may seem small, matters of fundamental importance are at stake. It is important to see why consent cannot validly be presumed in the present cultural environment.

To presume consent is to make an empirical claim. It is to claim that people *would consent* if asked, or, perhaps more precisely, that they would consent to a policy of taking organs without explicit permission. The reasoning behind true presumed consent laws is that it is legitimate to take organs without explicit consent because those from whom the organs are taken would have agreed had they been asked when they were competent to respond.

That, however, is a claim which, if it is to be made with authority, must be corroborated with empirical evidence. Social survey evidence makes clear that if we assume people would agree to having their organs procured if they were asked, we would be wrong at least 30 percent of the time. A recent 1993 Gallup poll shows that only 37 percent of Americans are "very likely" to want their organs transplanted after their death, and only 32 percent are "somewhat likely." Furthermore, only 55 percent are willing to grant formal permission for organ removal. It should also be noted that although 55 percent are *willing* to grant permission, only 28 percent have *actually* done so (The Gallup Organization. Inc, conducted for The Partnership for Organ Donation, Boston, MA. February 1993, pp 4, 15). In other words. only about half of the Americans who are willing to grant permission have taken the proactive steps necessary to do so, creating a large number of *false negatives*. We might expect that if ours were an opting out system, we might also see a large number of *false positives*. Based even on the larger figure of 69 percent who would be either "very likely" or "somewhat likely" to want their organs to be transplanted, it is clear that there can be no basis for presuming consent. Claiming such a presumption is an ill-informed notion at best; it is an outright deception at worst.

Perhaps even more pertinent to this discussion are the relative proportions of Americans who would agree to the system of presumed consent itself, as the ethos of the presumed consent mode would seem to demand. One recent survey shows that only 38 percent of Americans agree with presumed consent, defined as a system in which doctors routinely remove organs from deceased persons unless the person indicated a wish to the contrary while alive.[22] Another survey shows that number to be only 7 percent.[23]

To gain a better understanding of the issues involved, a comparison with the presumption of consent to treatment in an emergency room is helpful. When people suffer accidents or heart attacks that render them incapable of consenting to medical treatment, they are rushed to an emergency room where they are treated by the hospital team. They are treated without explicit consent. This policy is defended on the grounds that consent is presumed.[24] Under these circumstances such a presumption allows us to preserve the notion that people can receive medical treatment only with their consent.

In the case of the emergency room treatment of the patient incapable of giving explicit consent, the presumption of consent is surely valid. Were we to conduct a survey of the population asking its members whether they would want such a presumption made, agreement would be close to unanimous. To be sure, some small group would object. A patient who is a Jehovah's Witness may refuse blood products; a Christian Scientist may refuse treatment altogether. This reveals that on occasions the presumption of consent in the emergency room may be an erroneous presumption (it will, on occasion, yield *false positives*). But it will be accurate an overwhelming percentage of the time, and the presumption is therefore justified.

By contrast if we presume consent in the case of organ procurement, we will be wrong at least 30 percent of the time. (It is interesting to ask exactly what percentage of people would have to agree to a policy when surveyed before we can presume that individuals being treated by that policy would have consented. One's first instinct might be to assume that a majority must indicate endorsement of the policy, but that surely is wrong. It would lead to erroneous presumption of consent as much as half the time. One possibility is to take a figure of 95 percent approval in a survey as sufficient to presume that any one individual would have consented, if asked. That would mean 5 percent of the time we would have erred in presuming the individual would have consented. Even then the rights of individuals would be violated 5 percent of the time.) In a society that affirms the right of the individual not to have his or her body invaded without appropriate consent, procuring organs on the basis of a presumption of consent will violate that right at least 30 percent of the time.

WHAT IS AT STAKE

What is at stake is something very fundamental: the ethics of the relation of the individual to the society. A pioneer in the study of contemporary medical ethics, Paul Ramsey, introduced the issue in distinguishing between organ procurement in the modes of "giving" and "taking."[25] In liberal Western society certain rights are attributed to the individual. Among these is the right to control what is done with one's body. Hence, in Western culture medical treatment is acceptable only with the consent of the individual or the individual's appropriate surrogate. Research on a human subject is ethically acceptable only when consent is obtained. According to the Nuremberg Code, such voluntary consent is absolutely essential. An individual is in a position whereby he or she has the authority to give to society by authorizing medical research and now by authorizing procurement of organs for transplant, research, therapy, and other purposes.

The alternative is the mode of "taking" or what Dukeminier and Sanders called "routine salvaging." In this model the central authority has claims over the individual without relying on the individual's consent or approval. In the model of presumed consent, the individual is before the state; in the alternative the individual is subordinate. This underscores the problems associated with casual misuse of the term, "presumed consent." Many authors merely confuse routine salvaging for presumed consent, claiming that they are the same thing.[26,27] Others have implied that their versions of so-called presumed consent can be justified by the concept of eminent domain.[28,29] However, eminent domain involves the taking of private property for public use, and has no bearing on questions of consent. Clearly a system which validly presumes the consent of persons does not—cannot—rely upon notions of eminent domain.

Choosing the language of legitimating organ procurement is, in effect, choosing how we want to see the individual in relation to the state. Those who use the language of presumed consent are trying to hold on to the liberal model in which gift-giving is the foundation of organ procurement. In cases in which consent can validly be presumed, presumed consent seems consistent with such an orientation. However, in cases in which the evidence makes clear that consent cannot be presumed, this language is simply a disguise for the less acceptable reality of state authority over the individual.

This in itself, of course, does not make routine salvaging wrong; it is, however, deceptive if one advocates such a relationship in the name of the more liberal mode of gift-giving and consenting. Such deception is a moral affront to members of a society built upon respect for the rights of the individual.

It is worth speculating why there is this strong propensity to use the language of presuming consent when the apparent intention is to take organs without consent. One possibility is that, at least in countries reflecting liberal political philosophy's affirmation of the rights of the individual, it is more comforting to use the language of gift-giving and consent. It leaves the impression of the priority of the individual. Thus there is a strong tendency to use the language of the gift mode (words such as "donor"), even in cases in which the source of the organs may be a small child who never could have made an actual donation and in cases in which a medical examiner rather than the individual whose organs are being taken is the one approving the procurement. The language of consent is a more comfortable language, one that may be necessary to win approval of policies that de facto authorize procurement without donation.

THE POLICY IMPLICATIONS:
ALTERNATIVES TO PRESUMING CONSENT

Routine Salvaging

There are a number of alternatives to persisting in calling organ procurement "presumed consent" in cases where there is no explicit individual permission. One would be to follow Dukeminier and Sanders and bluntly call it "routine salvaging." That at least is an honest policy. That would be appropriate if one wanted to refer to a policy that is grounded not in a presumption of individual consent, but in a belief that the society had a right to procure organs without individual consent.

Routine Salvaging with Opting Out

Most versions of routine salvaging policies include a provision that permits individuals to opt out by executing a document explicitly asking not to have organs procured.[30-33] These policies place the burden on the individual actively to signal a desire not to have organs procured. Such policies, however, are still not presuming the consent of the those who fail to opt out (or at least there is no valid basis for presuming that those who fail to opt out would consent if asked). Some people might not even know about the organ procurement policy or its opting out provisions. Surveys show that persons of lower education are far less likely to consent to organ donation, yet it is precisely this group of people who would run the highest risk of not knowing the proper procedures for opting out of the system.[23] Others might be overwhelmed by other concerns so that they simply never execute the necessary document. Many people do not execute economic wills during their lifetimes. If they do not, their assets will be dispersed at the time of their deaths according to default state policy. It would be a mistake, however, to presume that all who die intestate have consented to or favor the state's default provisions. It would be more appropriate to say that because of their inability or lack of willingness to complete a will, such persons have unfortunately not been able to secure their own preferences. A routine salvaging policy with opting out shows more respect for the wishes of the individual than does a straight salvaging law without such a provision, but it still involves the taking of organs. It replaces the gift-mode with one of taking without asking for permission.

Required Request of Next of Kin

Another option is the type of law that requires hospitals to request permission of the next of kin in cases in which the deceased has not explicitly expressed his or her preferences for or against organ procurement.[34,35] Such policies are an uneasy intermediary between the gift and salvaging modes. They imply that the state needs permission, but not the permission of the deceased.

There are both practical and theoretical problems with required request of the next of kin. At the practical level, there are doubts that such required requests significantly increase the yield of organs.[36,37] There may even be backlash refusals of relatives to cooperate if they feel they have been treated crassly in a moment of family crisis. At the theoretical level, if the moral foundation of procuring organs is the consent of the individual whose organs are procured, then next-of-kin approval is, at best, a poor substitute. It may be the best available alternative in cases in which there is no knowledge of the deceased's wishes, but the better course, ethically and practically, for those who rest organ procurement in the approval of the individual whose organs are going to be procured, would be a policy that maximizes the opportunity for the individual to record his or her wishes, not one that rests on the wishes of a family member.

Required Response

An option that preserves the gift mode (and the correlative affirmation of respect for the integrity of the individual) is a policy we have called required request[38] and routine inquiry,[39] but might better be referred to as required response. The United Network for Organ Sharing Ethics Committee's Presumed Consent Subcommittee has recently endorsed "required response" as an alternative to presuming consent.[40] It would provide for organized requests for individuals to consent or refuse to consent to organ procurement and would require some response from the individual. A number of mechanisms have been suggested for obtaining such responses. This is not the place to develop such proposals in detail. This article will simply list some mechanisms that have been proposed. Asking for a decision to donate and requiring a response might be done as in the past during the drivers' license renewal process or could be included on the federal income tax return. The latter policy has the advantages of reaching almost all adults (the only people who can exercise a gift of organs), providing for a single federal list of those willing to donate, and providing for yearly updates. The new feature would be that people would be required to answer the question. For any required response mechanism, it would probably be wise to permit an "I don't know" response. Such responses would trigger requests from next of kin, just as would be necessary for minors and others who are not mentally competent to make a gift of an organ.

If this approach to organizing and encouraging the giving of organs is unacceptable, then the alternative would appear to be some version of routine salvaging, presumably with opting out. However, until there is empirical evidence that the presumption of consent is warranted, those who favor the state's procurement without some explicit permission should affirm their communitarianism and acknowledge that their policy commits them to the view that the state has the right to take organs without permission. They should refrain from the misleading language of "presumed consent," which implies the gift mode, but cannot be justified unless there is evidence that essentially all people (or all people whose explicit opting out cannot be located at the moment of crisis) would consent to such an arrangement if they were asked. That presumption is warranted for life-and-death emergency room treatment, but not presently for procuring organs.

REFERENCES

1. Dukeminier J, Sanders D: *N Engl J Med* 279:413,1968.
2. Callahan D: *What Kind of Life: The Limits of Medical Progress.* New York: Simon and Schuster, 1990.
3. Cantaluppi. Cited by Gerson W: *NYU J Int Law Politics* 19:1013,1987.
4. Farfor J: *Br Med J* 1:497, 1977.
5. *Int Dig Health Legislat* 37(l):332,1986 (Austrian Law of June 1, 1982).
6. *Int Dig Health Legislat* 38(3):523,1987 (Belgian Law of June 13, 1986).
7. *Int Dig Health Legislat* 3(3):477,1982 (Czechoslovakian Mandatory directives of February 27,1978).
8. *Int Dig Health Legislat* 36(4):971,1985 (Finnish Law of April 26, 1985).
9. *Int Dig Health Legislat* 28(3):621,1977 (Italian Law of December 2, 1975).
10. Puca A: *Trapianto di Cuore E Morte Cerebrale del Donatore.* Torino, Italy: Edizione Camilliane, 1993, pp 128-133; 201-224.
11. Lov om tansplantasjon og avgivelse av lik m.m. February 9, 1973.
12. Ley de Octubre 1979, no. 30/79, art. 5.3.
13. *Int Dig Health Legistat* 36(1):50, 1985 (Swiss Regulation of September 17, 1984).
14. *Int Dig Health Legislat* 40(4):836, 1989 (Cyprus Law of May 22, 1987).
15. *Int Dig Health Legislat* 40(3):588, 1989 (Hungarian Law of February 17, 1988).
16. Republic of Singapore, "Human Organ Transplant Bill," *Government Gazette Bills Supplement* October 31, 1986, pp 1-10.
17. *Int Dig Health Legislat* 38(3):530, 1987 (Syrian Law of December 20, 1986).
18. *Int Dig Health Legistat* 42(1):46, 1992 (Yugoslavian Decree of October 18, 1990).
19. *Int Dig Health Legislat* 41(3):436, 1990 (Colombian Law of December 20, 1988).
20. Md State Senate Bill 428, § 4-509.2.
21. General Assembly of the Commonwealth of Pa. proposed amendment to Title 20, Chapter 86, Subchapter C.
22. Organ Donation Study. United Network for Organ Sharing Executive Summary. February 15, 1992.
23. Manninen DL, Evans R: *JAMA* 253:3111, 1985.
24. Applebaum PS, Lidz CW, Meisel A: *Informed Consent: Legal Theory and Clinical Practice.* New York: Oxford, 1987, pp 66-69.
25. Ramsey P: *The Patient as Person.* New Haven: Yale, 1970.
26. Silver T: *Boston University Law Review* 68:681, 1988.
27. Spital A: *N Engl J Med* 325:1243, 1991.
28. McNeil DR: Hamline *J Public Law Policy* 9:343, 1989.
29. Stuart FP, Veith FJ, Cranford RE: *Transplantation* 31:238, 1981.

30. Kennedy I: *J Med Ethics* 5:133, 1979.

31. Steinbrook R: *J Health Polit Policy Law* 16:504, 1981.

32. Steuer JD, Bell SK: *Crit Care Nurse* 9:466, 1989.

33. Schotsmans P: In Land W Dossetor JB (eds): *Organ Replacement Therapy: Ethics, Justice and Commerce.* Heidelberg: Springer-Verlag Berlin, 1991.

34. NY State Task Force on Life and the Law: The Required Request Law March, 1986.

35. Caplan A: *N Engl J Med* 311:981, 1984.

36. Caplan AL, Welvang P: *Clin Transplant* 3:170,1989.

37. Ross SE, Nathan H, O'Malley KF: *J Trauma* 30:820, 1990.

38. Veatch RM: *Death, Dying and the Biological Revolution* (revised ed). New Haven: Yale, 1989 p 216.

39. Veatch R: *N Engl J Med* 25:1246, 1991.

40. Dennis JM, Hanson P, Hodge E, et al.: UNOS Update 10(2):16, 1994.

17. Join the Club: A Modest Proposal to Increase Availability of Donor Organs

Rupert Jarvis

I.

In a health service where rationing has become a fact of life, nowhere is the problem of demand outstripping supply more obvious than in the field of organ transplants. For reasons not entirely obvious, despite the fact that the majority of Britons believe that cadaver donation of organs is both ethically acceptable and practically desirable, still only a minority actually possess donor cards, and even fewer carry them:

> a Gallup poll for the British Kidney Patient Association, quoted in *The Guardian* (9.5.90), found that 73 percent of respondents would agree to their kidneys being used for transplantation, although only 27 percent actually had a donor card and only seven percent were carrying one on them at the time.[1]

The problem is not that there are insufficient numbers of organs potentially suitable for transplantation, but that these organs, far from being made available for transplant, are destroyed, leaving those in need of a transplant either to improve their quality of life, as in the case of a kidney transplant, or as a life-saving measure, in the case of a heart transplant still waiting. At one and the same time, the organs necessary to save or immeasurably improve actual, identifiable lives[2] are themselves in existence, and yet people are dying for the want of them: "Organ supply is the major limiting factor in organ transplantation."[3] That is to say, the number of lives saved as a result of transplants

Originally published in the *Journal of Medical Ethics,* 1995;21:199-204. Reprinted by permission of BMJ Publishing Group.

could—if donor organs were more readily available to transplant surgeons—
be considerably higher.

Nor is the problem a medical one: since the introduction of immunosuppressive drugs such as cyclosporin, which vastly lessen the dangers of rejection, the actual process of transplantation is not a particularly unusual or dangerous one. Although the operations are long and complex, they are, at least
in centers largely dedicated to such procedures, relatively routine. In the best
B-movie tradition, we have the technology.

The upshot of this is clear enough: given that demand for resources
exceeds the (presently available) supply, there is a need to ration the available resources by prioritizing demand to decide who is to receive the benefits offered by a transplant operation, and who is to go without. Such overt
rationing, particularly when it is applied to identifiable individual patients, is
often held to be highly distasteful both by health care professionals and by
the lay public, since it seems to sit uneasily alongside a duty to care. It is not
my present purpose to examine the interesting question of whether a health
care professional can or should act as a gatekeeper to resources. Instead, I
shall look briefly at some problems associated with the current parameters by
reference to which transplant organ availability is rationed, and examine two
suggested remedies to the current shortage of organs available for transplant.
I shall then suggest some desiderata of any proposed solution to the problem,
and apply them to one further possible solution.

II.

There is a familiar suggestion that any finite health care resources for which
there is excessive demand could be rationed by one or more of the more or
less quantifiable, non-medical parameters, such as age, desert, or social
utility. The latter two are, fortunately, not often suggested except in the context of a thought experiment, while the former is more usually dressed up in
the guise of ability to benefit, which I discuss below. I take it that there is
little doubt that it would be unjust to ration access to transplant services by
such factors as desert or social utility, or any other non-medical category,
such as class, ethnic origin,[4] or gender. What would be unjust about a policy
that used such criteria to ration is that it would violate the to Aristotelian principle of distributive justice, that only those cases that are relevantly dissimilar should be treated differently. It is abundantly clear that class or social
utility are utterly irrelevant to considerations of prioritizing demand for
transplant services.

If such non-medical criteria are of no use in rationing, then what of the
traditional concept of ability to benefit from the treatment? Even a cursory
review of the literature reveals that of the various criteria, this is the one most

nearly agreed upon, and it seems reasonable that this should be so: to take an extreme example, there is neither point nor justification in treating someone for a condition which is not present. More realistically, it seems reasonable to suggest that those patients whose chance of survival is significantly lower for one reason or another, for example the existence of another condition which prejudices their chance of surviving the operation, should not receive as high a priority in the queue for donor organs as those whose ability to benefit is greater. This is to say that an assessment of the relationship between a proposed transplant's risks and benefits to an individual could be used to determine access to transplant services.

The 'Free Rider'

While this looks like an elegant and reasonable solution to the rationing problem, it is not. As a means of *ordering* a queue it has a certain merit, particularly that it takes account only of those differences which are relevant to the particular case. However, perhaps unfortunately from the point of view of finding a tool for rationing, there are still many, many more people who could benefit *somewhat* from a transplant operation than there are available donor organs for them. The problem of the inequality between supply and demand, then, is not to be resolved simply by applying the criterion of the patient's ability to benefit. It is inadequate as a tool of rationing since it allows far too many in through the gates. While it may serve to reduce the total number of those waiting for transplants by a small amount, it leaves us a long way from a satisfactory account of how to ration donor organs.

A third problem with the current system by which donor organs are rationed is that it takes no account of, indeed it encourages, the "free rider": the individual who hopes to benefit from the cooperation of others even though he does not himself contribute to the socially desired end. Although it is in each individual's interest that donor organs should be available, it is in nobody's interests to make *his/her own* organs available: the choice to donate postmortem is an entirely altruistic one. We therefore have the current situation where demand is not matched by supply, and individual patients who could benefit from a transplanted organ are denied that treatment owing to a lack of suitable organs available for transplant.

III.

If that is the problem, what have been the suggested solutions? Two main strands have emerged, one of which has received little support. They can be labeled respectively opting-out, and cash payments for organs.

The first proposed solution has already been implemented in a number of countries, including Denmark, Austria, Sweden, France, Israel and Switzerland. It involves a "presumed consent polic[y], where physicians can take required tissues and organs unless either the deceased carries a card to prohibit this, or the next of kin object."[5] It therefore places the burden of decision on the individual, who is required to make a conscious effort to opt out of the scheme if s/he wishes to do so.

Hint of Coercion

Mason and McCall Smith suggest that this policy "smacks of 'body-snatching' and carries with it a hint of coercion . . . [and they] cannot foresee a British government risking such a major policy change."[6] Although I do not disagree with their conclusion, it is worth being clear what exactly is coercive about such a scheme.

The notion of consent, properly voluntary and adequately informed, is absolutely central to modern medical ethics, and readers of the journal will not need to be reminded of its salient features. But it is worth reminding ourselves that "the notion underlying 'giving one's consent' is 'feeling together' —that is 'agreeing' and hence 'giving approval or permission.' "[7] In the increasingly abstruse discussion of informed consent, it is easy to lose sight of the fact that underlying the whole question is the notion of agreeing—of deciding *together*. Given that the notion of agreement *between* is internal to the idea of consent, it is clear why true consent cannot go by default: we cannot assume that in the absence of any contra-indications, a brainstem dead patient would not have minded his/her organs being removed for transplant. If consent is as important to the ethical practice of medicine as it is held to be, then an opt-out scheme is not a possibility.

It may of course be that an individual's wishes are held to be irrelevant in the face of the public good, and that the general utility would be promoted by the removal of cadaveric organs without express permission, but that is another matter entirely. Utilitarian considerations of the problem of the shortage of potential donor organs, as Harris has shown, give very different—and often strikingly counterintuitive—results.[8]

Market in Organs

The other solution to the drastic shortage that is conventionally proposed, usually but not exclusively as a thought experiment,[9] is to create a market in organs. The purchase of organs from live donors has yet to be legalized, although the practice is by no means unknown[10] and proposals to allow cadaveric organs to be purchased have so far failed to be realized. But once a demand among the rich has been identified and the means to satisfy that demand devised by the poor, it becomes increasingly difficult to stop the development of a market. It is therefore imperative to be absolutely clear whether that market is an acceptable one or not before it gains a foothold.

Since 1989, the sale of organs has been outlawed in Britain by the Human Organ Transplants Act, in line with the principle of English common law that the body is not to be treated as property. Abouna et al. considered the notion of paid organ donation and found it to be

> a flawed, short-sighted, and self-defeating approach to a complex problem. Paid organ donation has a serious negative impact on many of the medical, moral, and ethical values intimately connected with organ transplantation including the donor, the recipient, the local transplant programs, the medical profession, society, and the international community.[11]

The problems with paying live donors for organs are too well known to rehearse in any great detail here, but mainly concern danger to, and exploitation of, both donor and recipient in the face of commercial pressures, and a fall-off in voluntary donation. These undesirable consequences are in addition to the conceptual problems concerned with treating the body or its parts as property.

Paying Next of Kin

A variant of the policy is sometimes proposed, which advocates paying the deceased donor's next of kin.[12] Although this avoids the problem of danger to the donor, a moment's reflection reveals that it is even less attractive an option than paid donation from live donors. Not only are the same conceptual difficulties present, but

> the selling of cadaver organs is, at root, directed to the enticement of the next of kin. Put this way, the proposition can only be seen as appealing to the basest of human instincts and as something with which the medical profession should have no truck.[13]

As lawyers from the city where Burke and Hare once plied their horrid trade, Mason and McCall Smith are only too well aware of what lies at the bottom of this particular slope.

Allied to this suggestion is the notion of "required request" which has been embodied in federal law in the USA since October 1987, whereby physicians are *obliged* to ask the relatives of suitable deceased patients for permission to harvest organs for transplant. This policy seems objectionable for two reasons. Firstly, and most importantly, it makes the wishes of the surviving relatives determinative rather than those of the individual whose organs are being sought; secondly, it risks creating the impression in the minds of the relatives that a patient's ventilation is being discontinued simply because his/her organs are needed by somebody else, thus eroding trust in the intensivists.

It should also be clear that our pre-reflective notions of justice are outraged by the possibility of a market in donor organs. The NHS is founded on a principle of equity of access to care irrespective of income or wealth, and this is hardly likely to be served by establishing a means by which the already limited supply of donor organs for transplants can be further diminished by financially enabled queue-jumping.

IV.

If these traditional solutions to the problem fail, then what more can we offer? Or is there nothing more that we can do except commission bigger and louder advertisements exhorting the public to carry donor cards? Before we can answer that question, we need to have an idea of the sort of answer we are looking for. I suggest that there are six desiderata of any proposed solution.

Firstly, and most obviously, any putative solution must address the problem of shortage by better matching supply of donor organs to demand for them. This might be achieved either by increasing the supply, for instance by a successful campaign to encourage donation, or by reducing the demand by, for instance, the development of acceptable alternative therapies.[14]

Secondly, the solution must satisfy the requirements of justice, which I glossed above, following Aristotle, as treating only those cases that are relevantly dissimilar in different ways.

Derived from this general condition but specific to current understandings of health care provision in Britain, no individual should be excluded from the transplant program on the grounds of inability to pay for the treatment. As I argued above, this condition rules out the creation of a market in donor organs.

Fourth, in accordance with our conception of the individual as a rational free agent, our putative solution should be founded in an autonomous choice. Although it would be easy (in theory) to ensure an adequate supply of donor organs if no account were taken of individuals' wishes—by Harris-like selected sacrifice, for example—our basic intuitions about the place of autonomy in our lives rules out such coercive practices. It can, of course, be argued that all laws are in some measure coercive, and that therefore any legislative solution to the problem will inevitably infringe the autonomy of some. Notwithstanding this, in a liberal society coercion, particularly over a matter as important as bodily integrity, is to be shunned.

Although the fifth condition is not central in the way that the first four are, it nonetheless seems desirable in a solution that should address the problem of the free rider. Of course, if a proposal can be tabled that appears to fit the other desiderata but still allows some individuals to benefit from, without participating in, the scheme, then we would not on those grounds alone reject it. Even so, a solution that eliminates the possibility is to be preferred to one that does not, *ceteris paribus*.

Finally, and equally non-centrally, it would be desirable although in no way necessary, if the solution were to encourage altruism.

V.

I now turn to another possible solution to the problem which I shall outline briefly and examine with these desiderata in mind. It is worth noting in passing that this solution relies on a decision that takes place behind a Rawlsian veil of ignorance, and might therefore be presumed to yield a prima facie just result.

I suggest that legislation governing organ donation be amended such that all and only those who identify themselves as potential donors (perhaps by a card similar to the one currently in use, or by registration on a central computer) are eligible themselves to receive transplant organs.[15]

It will be immediately apparent that this solution is a form of the closed, co-operative agreement beloved of social contract theorists: that is, its members receive a benefit in return for the agreed, mutual sacrifice of one or more of their interests. That is the positive side of the contract, as embodied by the principle that *all* those who participate stand to benefit. The negative aspect of exclusion is captured in the condition that *only* those who undertake to sacrifice their own interests are eligible for the benefits.

Thoroughly Attractive Option

This is a particularly compelling example of a social contract, however, because of an unusual feature. Many hypothetical contracts focus on the trade-off between two interests that are seen as exclusive (standardly, my—presumed—wish to rape and pillage and my own desire for the security to be free from being myself raped and the victim of pillage). This contract, however, trades a—if not *the*—central interest, one's interest in remaining alive, against one's postmortem interest in having one's organs removed. This latter is at best *de minimis*: my interests in my organs after death can hardly be said to be enormous. We are presented, then, with what seems to be a thoroughly attractive option: by sacrificing our minimal postmortem interests we guarantee our inclusion on the waiting list for the donor organ which might save or vastly improve the quality of our own life. That is, we make possible the satisfaction of our own most compelling interest by renouncing one which is of little or no concern to us.

Adoption of this scheme would, I suggest, address the problem of shortage on two fronts simultaneously. Firstly, by excluding those who do not elect to join the scheme, it will reduce legitimate demand for donor organs. It should be noted that the reduction thus effected will probably be minimal, which is surely a good thing, in that it seems preferable that supply be better matched to demand by increasing supply rather than by eliminating or reducing demand.

Secondly, and more importantly, the supply of donor organs would at the same time increase as a result of an upturn in the number of registered potential donors. It hardly seems fanciful to suggest that the vast majority of people would elect to join the scheme, since it is so clearly in their interests to do so, with the potential gain (life) being infinite and the potential loss (postmortem dissection which, depending on the manner of their death, they might well have to undergo anyway) being zero. Unlike the "survival lottery" proposed by Harris, nobody is going to be sacrificed in order to save others. Under this scheme, the potential for benefit and loss is separated by the moment of death: *only* benefits can accrue to the living, and losses—if it makes sense to speak of postmortem losses—can only occur after death.

The proposed scheme appears to satisfy the requirements of justice, in that differences in access to a particular treatment are grounded in considerations, and those and only those who elect potentially to contribute to the system stand to benefit from it. In this way the problem of the free rider is eliminated by the exclusion of those who do not—at least potentially—contribute.

The contract scheme would also have the (marginal) benefit of promoting—albeit self-regarding—altruism, which is taken to be a morally desirable end in and of itself. Moreover, this alignment of the individual's self-regarding interests with the public good is a strength as far as the scheme's likely successful implementation is concerned. Given a moderate version of the social contract theorist's premise, that people tend to act in what they perceive to be their own best interests, it follows that a scheme under which acting in one's best interests is concomitant with, and necessarily entails acting in, the best interests of the population at large will inevitably tend to promote the public good.

Conceptual, ethical and aesthetic problems arising from the commercialization and objectification of body parts are avoided since the scheme makes no reference to money or any market principles. Similarly, since there is no question of purchasing organs, there is no danger of individuals being excluded from a transplant program on the grounds of their inability to pay. Nor, moreover, is there the financial inducement to sell organs as a live donor in order to alleviate financial hardship.

Finally, the proposal seems no more coercive than any other arrangement which offers a valued future goal as a reward for some sacrifice. Indeed, the coercion involved looks to be particularly thin, given that all the benefits accrue to the individual while s/he is alive while the costs are exacted exclusively after his/her death. The responsibility to register as a potential donor—and therefore as a potential recipient—rests with the individual alone. Voluntary exclusion, therefore, is a real possibility, although it would carry with it obvious costs. But the choice remains a real one.

VI.

The scheme seems to me to be self-evidently in the interests of all of us jointly and each of us severally. However, it is worth pointing out that there is one possible injustice that could arise from its successful implementation. Imagine that ten years hence, the registration scheme has been adopted and has been found to be a success. Transplant specialists are now no longer restricted with respect to their choice of recipients by the availability of donor organs, but by medical criteria. In fact, so successful has the scheme been in encouraging voluntary cadaver organ donation, that there is a surplus of organs suitable for transplant: more hearts, lungs, kidneys and livers are being donated than are required to transplant into those individuals registered as potential donors, who are the only ones who have a legitimate claim on them.

Imagine also that there are a number of people *outside* the registration scheme who objected to, balked at, or simply never got around to registering as potential organ donors. A certain percentage of these people will suffer renal failure, or develop cardiopulmonary conditions that could be alleviated by a transplant. But, because of their failure to join up, they have no legitimate claim on the—available—donor organs. They would be dying only because of an inflexibility in the law.

I think this situation would indeed offend our sense of justice. We would be right to be sickened if it were to come about. But this does not show that the scheme is at fault, merely that it may, if it is very successful, need to be flexible in its implementation. Perhaps it would be fairer to say that those who register as potential organ donors will be given *first refusal* on any organ available for transplant. Perhaps there is another proviso that could be added. That seems a matter for the legal draftsman, and not the philosopher.

But note that the kind of injustice that we are considering here arises from an oversupply of donated organs, rather than the shortage that is the status quo. If this is a kind of injustice (and I suggest that it is easily avoided in the manner I have sketched above) then it is a very different sort from the one we have presently. And it is not only different, but considerably less offensive.

REFERENCES AND NOTES

1. West R. *Organ transplantation.* London: Office of Health Economics, 1991: 10.

2. One of the remarkable features of transplant surgery that makes resource allocation in this field such a compelling problem is that the opportunity costs of any decision are clear and immediate. If Mr McHenry and Mr. McTavish both need the same donor heart—which is of a particularly rare blood group and weight—in order to survive beyond the end of the year, then the surgeon knows, even as s/he is saving Mr. McHenry's life in the operating theater, that s/he is—in all likelihood—depriving Mr. McTavish of his last chance. Unlike many fields of health care resource allocation, where one Positron Emission Tomography (PET) scan represents an opportunity cost of so many theoretical, anonymous, hip replacements, in transplant surgery the cost can be traced to one particular individual.

3. See reference (1): 9.

4. Ethnic origin may become a relevant medical factor where tissue matching is dependent on it. In such a case, however, since the difference is a relevant one, it justifies discrimination on those grounds.

5. See reference (1): 7.

6. Mason J, McCall Smith R. *Law and medical ethics* (3rd ed). London: Butterworths, 1991: 312.

7. Ayto J. *Bloomsbury dictionary of word origins.* London: Bloomsbury, 1990: 132.

8. Harris J. The survival lottery. *Philosophy* 1975; 50:81-87.

9. Cohen L. The ethical virtues of a futures market in organs. In: Land W, Dossetor J. *Organ replacement therapy: ethics, justice, commerce.* Berlin: Springer Verlag, 1991: 302-310.

10. See reference (9): 164-172.

11. See reference (9): 165.

12. Pliskin J. Cadaveric organs for transplantation: is there a need for more? *Journal of forensic sciences* 1976; 21: 83.

13. See reference (6): 313.

14. The implantation of an entirely artificial mechanical heart into Arthur Cornhill at Papworth Hospital in August 1994 provides some hope that such alternatives may no longer be the reserve of science fiction. We may be moving forward from the time when "the artificial heart is . . . only seen as a bridge until a suitable donor can be found." (See reference (1): 12.)

15. Note that "being eligible to receive" does not necessarily entail "will receive." Obviously, any eligibility will be subject to suitable organs being available. Moreover, there is a case for applying a risk/benefit assessment even *within* the contractual scheme. However, as I argued above, any such assessment would be useful only to *order* a waiting list, not to govern admittance to it. Simple application of risk/benefit analysis is inadequate to resolve rationing problems.

PART THREE
Commodification

Patients who die waiting for a transplant do so not because of a shortage produced by natural limits or human indifference, but rather due to an inefficiency of existing organ procurement policies. In Part Two, we examined many different proposals to maximize the efficiency of procurement policies. While some of the practices have proved moderately successful in the United States and abroad, the considerable scarcity of transplantable organs remains. As a result, many in the transplant community have began to re-examine the 1984 National Organ Transplant Act, which forbids "any person to knowingly acquire, receive, or otherwise transfer any human organ for valuable consideration for use in human transplantation, if the transfer affects interstate commerce." Since the mid-1980s, more and more members of the transplant community have supported financial incentive programs, asserting that money and morals can mix in human transplantation.

There are two main arguments that support this belief. One, a libertarian argument, holds that individual autonomy protects that right to dispose of body parts in any fashion. The second, a more consequentialist position, holds that sale of cadaveric body parts is an acceptable method if it secures more organs to save human lives. Some people believe in the validity of both philosophies while others cannot justify the mixing of money and morals for any reason. Clearly, organ commodification remains a very controversial subject and changing attitudes may very well reflect a societal uncertainty about values.

Among the first proposals to alleviate organ shortages by means other than altruism was a program of "reward gifting," a plan to increase cadaveric donations by offering a $1000 "death benefit" incentive to the families. Thomas Peters submits that such a tangible incentive would increase donation and result in saving many of the lives now lost due to long waiting lines. However, Edmund Pellegrino asserts that Peters's dismissal of altruistic motivation in donation could have wide-reaching detrimental effect on the future supply of donated organs. Pellegrino believes that any system of cadaveric donation based on financial compensation is inherently ethically questionable and stresses the importance of continued reliance on education and altruism to meet our nations organ needs.

Andrew Barnett and colleagues agree with Dr. Pellegrino's dismissal of compensatory arrangements to increase organ donation. However, rather than relying on education and altruism to remedy the shortages, they argue that a market-based system of cadaveric organ procurement is the most practical and ethical means for increasing available organs. Creating fair markets for scarce organs based on the laws of supply and demand, the authors contend, would address both the problems of potential donors refusing to donate and that of their never having been asked. They present a model for a working organ market and systematically address and dismiss a host of ethical concerns over such a system.

Issues of incentive, compensation, and markets for cadaveric organ donation prove particularly distasteful to Arthur L. Caplan and colleagues. They envision significant risks to autonomy and fairness posed by calls for commodification that likewise threaten fundamental values for human life, respect, and self-esteem. Furthermore, the coercive nature of money would make notions of informed consent impossible. The authors contend that in addition to the ethical liabilities of such practices, practical problems such as the opposition of many religious groups to commodifying the body would lead to a decrease in available organs and the eventual failure of such a system.

Reflective of our shifting values in the face of dire organ shortages, the transplant community continues to push the envelope of what is ethically acceptable in the face of equally enthusiastic denunciations of such practices. Members of the International Forum for Transplant Ethics call for the allowance of regulated kidney sales from living donors. By opening the debate on live unrelated donation for money (obviously, only organs that one can live without—kidney, bone marrow, parts of the bowel, and, infrequently, lobes of the liver, lung, and pancreas) the authors suggest a practice that only a few years ago would have been met with unanimous professional condemnation. In their proposal, live organ sales would not replace current procurement and allocation, but rather would supplement existing practices. They justify lifting the ban on live organ donation, indicating that "our own feelings of disgust" are not substantial reason to deny life-saving treatment to the suffering and dying. Common concerns over live donation are discussed and dismissed, while explaining how such a policy would prove beneficial to donor, recipient, and society.

The shifting values in the transplant community are particularly well illustrated in this set of articles. Many noted scholars have reversed their original rejection of organ commodification in favor of a seemingly more practical solution to organ shortages. For example, N. Tilney's article with Arthur Caplan (1993) summarily dismissed financial relationships in cadaveric organ procurement. Yet five years later, as a member of the International Forum for Transplant Ethics and a co-author of the above paper, he calls for the lifting of bans on live organ sales bans. Such changes of heart are not uncommon. Robert A. Sells, also a member of the International Forum for Transplant Ethics and also a co-author of the above paper, denounced live organ sales in a 1985 letter to the *Lancet*. Since the early 1990s one can see many similar changes in attitude within the transplant community with respect to economic incentives and organ use.

The controversies that arise from commodification of organ procurement will indeed continue to fill the bioethics literature. Equally controversial are ongoing debates about the role economics and money should play in organ distribution. If a right to health care is acknowledged, is an expensive heart or liver transplant a part of that right? Are we fundamentally entitled to a new heart even if we cannot pay the costs for it and may not have contributed to a health plan or the tax base? With 12,039 kidney transplantations being done in 1996 (UNOS) in the United States at an average cost of $30,000 you don't need an accounting degree to realize that organs are not the only scarce resource in modern transplantation. Money is as well. Unfortunately or not money plays an important role in access to organ transplants. It is a role that Roger W. Evans sees as critical given competing health and social needs. Unequal access to transplantation, Evans asserts, will persist until some form of universal access to health care is created.

However, Norman Daniels believes that the rationing of health care services by ability to pay is ethically unacceptable under any circumstances. He goes on to explain how transplantation is no different from other kinds of health care and, like other kinds of health care, we can not limit access by ability to pay without widespread negative consequences. Furthermore, he reminds us that limiting transplantation only to those who can pay may result in a significant decrease of donations by those who cannot.

The Evans and Daniels articles exemplify what remains an ongoing debate over bottom-line economics, values, and the ethical issues attendant to organ transplantation. While we often say that all life is of equal value and that all life is precious these sentiments often clash with the economic realities faced by those who seek transplants but lack the insurance or the out-of-pocket resources to pay for them.

Arthur L. Caplan
Daniel H. Coelho

18. Life or Death: The Issue of Payment in Cadaveric Organ Donation

Thomas G. Peters

In 1989, 1,878 people died while awaiting organ transplantation. Public awareness programs, professional education, and legislation have not increased organ donation; the motive for consent in organ donation remains altruism. I shall argue that because of an ever larger number of patients listed as candidates for lifesaving organs, the policy of a death benefit payment to motivate families of potential organ donors should be studied. A death benefit of $1000 paid through organ procurement organizations would not necessarily be coercive. Laws now prohibiting organ brokerage and assuring fair organ allocation would continue unchanged. A death benefit payment may most favorably affect the socially disenfranchised through increased organ transplantation in minority populations. Because so many salvageable lives are now lost, only because organs cannot be obtained, pilot programs to determine the impact of death benefit payment to the enabling (consenting) next-of-kin should be initiated. If organ recovery increases sufficiently, a nationwide program could save thousands of lives.

BACKGROUND

During 1989, the United Network for Organ Sharing (UNOS) listed 18,946 new patients as candidates for vascularized organ transplants (W. K. Vaughn, PhD, United Network for Organ Sharing, written communication, July 1990). By February 1990, at least 1,094 of these newly listed patients died waiting for a transplant. This 5.8 percent mortality figure included those

---

Originally published in *JAMA* 265, no. 10 (March 13, 1991): 1302-1305.

patients waiting for a kidney or pancreas (1.7 percent died waiting) or a life-saving heart, liver, or heart-lung combination (14 percent died waiting). With the current success of transplant procedures, the shortage of donor organs was primarily responsible for needless death.[1,2]

The 1,094 deaths of newly listed patients, however startling, actually understate the number of patients who died while waiting for a transplantable organ, because many patients waiting for an organ were listed prior to 1989. Since October 1987 when UNOS began a national waiting list of patients, data compiled quarterly disclose an increasing number of patients on the waiting list, a steady but small increase in transplant operations, and an alarming number of patients who die waiting (Table).[3] Actually, 1,878 people died during 1989 while each was on the active national list to receive a cadaveric vascularized organ. These patients could have been saved by organ transplantation. For the last three years, the number of organ donors has not increased, staying at approximately 4,000 donors annually in the United States.[3,4] The issue in transplantation today is, therefore, that lives are being lost because cadaveric organ recovery is not currently meeting the need.

Many important guidelines about organ donation were promulgated during a period when organ recovery meant freeing one or two patients from dialysis therapy, not necessarily saving anyone's life.[5,6] For many years transplant professionals have known that lifesaving organs are often not obtained because procurement personnel are turned down by family members of the potential donor.[7,8] Altruism (the major motivational guideline), professional and public education, and legislative efforts[5,9-12] have not worked universally to increase organ donation commensurate with the need. Experienced organ procurement coordinators have dealt with families who might consent to organ donation from the brain dead family member, but refuse because there is no financial incentive for the decision to permit organ recovery. The concept of a death benefit paid to the donor family so that organ recovery might be more positively viewed should now emerge as a matter to examine and debate. Several active organ procurement organizations should test the concept of death benefit payment in the field. If a greater number of organs are procured, a nationwide program should be adopted so that a compassionately administered, centrally controlled death benefit pay-plan to families of cadaveric organ donors is operating throughout the United States.

The main argument supporting a study of death benefit payment for organ recovery is the prospect of saving lives through organ transplantation. Topics that remain important to the question include altruism, coercion, organ brokerage, access to lifesaving organs only for those who can pay, and legal issues.

POTENTIAL ORGAN TRANSPLANT RECIPIENT LISTING: PATIENTS AND PATIENTS WHO DIED WAITING FOR TRANSPLANTS

| Time Period | | No. of Patients | | | |
Year	Quarter	Total on List	New on List	Transplant Received	Died Waiting
1987	Oct-Dec	13168	4695	2053	291
1988	Jan-Mar	14332	4411	2172	376
1988	Apr-Jun	14766	4153	2512	393
1988	Jul-Sep	15395	4484	2654	433
1988	Oct-Dec	16035	4368	2644	414
1988	Jan-Mar	16966	4764	2609	516
1989	Apr-Jun	17705	4665	2705	456
1989	Jul-Sep	18511	4728	2732	396
1989	Oct-Dec	19173	4789	2830	510
1990	Jan-Mar	20177	5169	2875	565

ALTRUISM AND COERCION

During the 1960s and 1970s, nearly all cadaveric organs recovered for transplantation were kidneys. Because of effective dialysis treatments, few patients died if a kidney was not procured. Altruism (the regard for or the devotion to the interests of others) was deemed the appropriate motive for obtaining cadaveric kidneys. Now, approximately 70 percent of all organ donors give vascularized organs other than kidneys; the hearts, lungs, and livers are lifesaving. The medical community has retained altruism as the only motive for cadaveric organ recovery, perhaps for the incorrect assumption that altruism emerges with counseling and education, that altruistic behavior should prevail in this matter, and that persons unwilling to exhibit altruistic behavior should not be coerced into any other behavior as this coercion would impinge on free personal decision making.[5,10,14-16]

When I was a newly appointed attending transplant surgeon, I was called concerning a case of fatal head trauma in a young man. The usual efforts at "altruistic counseling" about organ recovery began with the next-of-kin, an older brother. The brother stopped us abruptly—I was sure our request would be denied. "I hated that s.o.b.! Go ahead and cut him . . . take his organs! Where do I sign?" I was stunned, mostly because my own moral concepts had been attacked. But I was also wrong to believe that counseling could make an individual aware of the needs of others. He was not only filled with hatred, but also unwilling (and maybe unable) to discover any facet of altruism. Counseling and teaching—especially at the bedside of a brain dead potential donor—may be fruitless with next-of-kin who have ideas entirely alien to our own.

We in the organ transplantation field have falsely assumed that altruism should be accepted by everyone. Our own concepts of regard for the interests of others have been nurtured within the social context of plenty: we are educated, well paid, and generally able to manage circumstances to the benefit of ourselves and others. We have established societal mores about the organ recovery process so that decisions regarding organ donation are entirely altruistic. This posture eliminates any possibility that consent for cadaveric organ recovery could be motivated by something of tangible value even though we know that some population groups harbor different thoughts or feelings about organ donation.[14,17-20] Some individuals may think that we in the organ transplantation field want to take the organs of a dead person (for no payment to that person's family) to make money ourselves from those organs. We who have advocated "free choice" in altruistic organ donation have fully ignored the fact that we are imposing values on persons who may not appreciate those values at all. *We may be coercing* some families to accept concepts foreign to them at a time of great personal loss. More tragically, our unwavering belief that altruism must prevail dooms some of our own patients who could be saved.

A death benefit payment for cadaveric solid organs would be neither coercive nor result in loss of altruistic values. Payment would in no way affect the brain dead donor, as no effort to obtain organs is made prior to the time of brain death. Should the family's beliefs be so strongly negative concerning organ removal, a modest sum of $1,000 in the form of a death benefit would not be so great a financial temptation to deter strongly held beliefs. On the other hand, should a negative attitude of a potential donor's family be superstition, reaction to "the establishment," or belief that the disadvantaged in society are again being exploited, such a level of remuneration may be enough to help the family toward considering donation favorably.[8,12,17,19,20] A death benefit payment may also foster the belief that society dealt fairly with the family in this matter. Most important, a death benefit payment may increase donation in populations now giving the fewest organs, needing them the most, and being underserved by the present donation system.[8,17,19-22] We should not lose sight of the good of altruism, and we should promote it to an even greater extent. While a death benefit should be offered to all families of potential organ donors, with the understanding that payment would be made after completion of solid-organ recovery, no family would be compelled to accept payment for recovered organs.

ORGAN BROKERAGE

There may be concerns that payment for organs would begin or extend a process of organ brokerage or commercialization. On the contrary, reimbursement could be designed so that undesirable practices of payment were essentially eliminated. If there were a standard amount of $1,000, paid only through the controlled organ acquisition process as a death benefit to the consenting next-of-kin, those paying large sums (as occurs today in some areas of the world) would be viewed as paying far too much. Were payment to have the desired effect of increasing the number of organs donated, there could ultimately be a surplus of organs such that, at least for kidneys, export to foreign countries might occur. This could reduce the real brokerage for kidneys now condoned in certain transplant centers willing to participate in commercial transactions, actually buying organs from unrelated living donors (Sells,[23] the Council of the Transplantation Society,[24] and *Am Med News.* April 20, 1990:3).

PAYMENT WOULD FAVOR THE RICH

A death benefit payment to the donor family would in no way favor those who could better afford costly medical care. Any organ obtained, whether or not the donor family accepted the death benefit payment, would go into the organ procurement organization and national organ allocation system in which all recipients are now registered and treated alike. That system is based on matching, time waiting, and medical need. The matching process involves immunologic determinations that are related, at least in part, to race. Renal allograft survival is strongly related to recipient race,[25] and donor-recipient matching within the same race has been associated with better results in some centers[26] since antigen expression differs among different populations. As matters stand now, transplants are least available for certain patients such as multiparous, transfused, immunologicaly sensitized black women. Black cadaveric donors, who might match with such recipients, are being lost with the current organ donation process.[8,17,19,21] If a financial incentive to organ donation were productive within this or any minority group, payment to donor families would most likely favor minority populations while not adversely affecting others.

PAYMENT WOULD BE ILLEGAL

Both state and federal law prohibit buying and selling organs. The National Organ Transplant Act (NOTA) makes it illegal to "acquire, receive, or transfer any human organ for valuable consideration."[27] Similarly, the Uniform Anatomical Gift Act (UAGA), as revised in 1987 and adopted in some form in ten states, makes it a felony to "knowingly for valuable consideration purchase or sell" cadaveric organs for transplantation.[28] However, the principal legal, moral, and ethical issue should be preservation of life. The 1987 UAGA permits all persons involved in transplantation (recovery surgeons and their teams, operating room personnel, donor hospital staff involved in donor care, transplant coordinators, transplant surgeons, transplant physicians) to be paid; resource use is also reimbursed. Why, then, would a sum of $1,000 per donor (payment for the enabling decision to obtain a lifesaving resource) be considered objectionable only because the money goes to the donor family? The cost per lifesaving and health-restoring organ would be small. Reasonable and legal payment to all who participate in the process of organ donation is now assured except for donor family members, who are the most important participants in the process.

Laws to increase organ supply have been enacted previously with the advice of the transplantation community.[6,27,28] Laws could be amended in such a manner to allow organ procurement organizations to administer and direct a one-time death benefit to the donor family. Such an amendment to both the NOTA and UAGA could pronounce an exemption for such a benefit. This would not permit development of a "market" for organs, or the sale of an organ to an identified recipient since these are currently illegal practices. The amount and source of the benefit would be controlled by law, and bartering for organs would continue to be prohibited. A death benefit would, in my judgment, increase the supply of donor organs that would continue to be distributed under otherwise current laws and allocation policies.

THE PAYMENT PROCESS

The death benefit payment to the family would be wholly administered by organ procurement organizations now defined under the NOTA of 1984.[27] Payment would be offered to the individual who legally enables organ donation in any case where solid-organ recovery for transplantation is completed. In general, the enabling individual is defined by law as the spouse, adult son or daughter, parent, brother or sister, or legal guardian (in that order). The organ procurement organization would then be reimbursed exactly as reimbursement for all other costs now occurs. Cost accounting in the organ procurement organization would treat the death benefit payment to the enabling family member no differently than it treats payment to the recovery surgeon, charter aircraft owner, or any other individual involved in the organ procurement and distribution process.

The death benefit, while potentially costing $4 million annually, would not necessarily have a significant impact on overall cost of organ acquisition. If more organs were obtained through death benefit payment, the increased efficiency and use of nonexpendable resources (fixed costs) would promote an economy of scale diminishing some costs per organ recovered. Few organ procurement organizations are busy enough that they have made the best use of their fixed resources. In addition, it is clearly recognized that successful renal transplantation is far more cost-effective than continued dialysis treatment. Any pilot project to study the fiscal effects of a death benefit payment to families of organ donors should take into account the cost savings resulting from increased renal transplantation vs dialysis therapy.

OTHER ISSUES

Other questions remain. Why not extend the same consideration of payment to families of tissue donors? Most tissue donors, while valuable in the care of many patients, do not so identifiably save another human life. This is, in part, due to the processing, storage, and marketing of tissue. Many organizations manage tissue donation and banking that are not centrally controlled, as all organ procurement organizations are. Fiscal reimbursement patterns and regulations are different for organs and tissues. In addition, most cadaveric organ donors give tissue, and payment for organs would not likely have a positive impact on tissue recovery. Payment should not be offered to families of tissue-only donors.

Wouldn't payment lead to "bad organs," as in tainted blood from paid blood donors of the past? No, because cadaveric organ donation has stringent criteria, which would not differ simply because a death benefit is paid. And, cadaveric organ recovery is a one-time event, not a habitual income-producing situation as in the skid-row blood donor.

What about payment for consent, not just recovery of usable organs? In organ recovery, we should not spend money for goodwill or for consent when the decedent is unsuitable to give lifesaving organs. We should be spending dollars to *save lives*. The life is saved by a recovered organ, not a consent to consider organ recovery. Unfair? Perhaps, but the focus must remain on saving lives that are now lost because next-of-kin cannot be fiscally rewarded in a manner that might increase organ recovery.

CONCLUSIONS

Payment for organ donation has been judged anathema by some families of organ donors, but the general public may accept such a concept nearly twice as often as would families who have donated a loved one's organs.[14] Probably some degree of sorrow visits families because a loved one was an organ donor, and some negative family reaction to organ donation will happen from time to time no matter what motivates organ donation. I do not believe, however, that a death benefit payment is a "philosophic slippery slope," especially if payment to donor families is studied before its full implementation. Should studies show that some form of death benefit payment expands the organ donor pool, lives will be saved. If pilot studies prove that death benefit payment does not increase organ recovery, massive human tragedy will not result. Reversion to the current system would ensue, or other methods to increase organ donation could be similarly studied. In the case of death payment to the enabling next-of-kin, I believe the risk to society is extremely small and the potential benefit to those patients who may be saved is considerably greater.

I have argued that we in the organ transplantation field have wrongly adhered to certain moral values of our own, and have coerced others at times of personal tragedy to accept our views. We may have held our philosophic values so dear, in fact, that the very patients whom we place on the waiting list for transplantable organs are dying because we continue to promote only these values. The legal sanctions to organ brokerage must be maintained, and the organ allocation system must be used fairly for all patients in need of a transplant. Payment to families for cadaveric organs might bring into the present system more organs for the underprivileged who are not adequately served now. Our concerns must focus not on some philosophic imperative such as altruism, but on our collective responsibility for maximizing life-saving organ recovery. Unless proven otherwise by soundly designed pilot programs, I submit that a death benefit payment would save lives that now are lost, lives that should be more important to us all than adherence to concepts and rules that we have promulgated ourselves.

REFERENCES

1. Evans RW, Manninen DL, Garrison LP, Maier AM. Donor availability as the primary determinant of the future of heart transplantation. *JAMA*. 1986;255:1892-1898.

2. Starzl TE, Demetris AJ, Van Thiel D. Liver transplantation. *N Engl J Med*. 1989;321:1014-1022.

3. Strawn J. *UNOS Monthly Activity Reports*. October 1987 to April 1990.

4. Evans RW. Organ donation: facts and figures. *Dialysis Transplant*. 1990;19:234-240.

5. Caplan AL. Sounding board: ethical and policy issues in the procurement of cadaver organs for transplantation. *N Engl J Med*. 1984;311:981-983.

6. Rettig RA. The politics of organ transplantation: a parable of our time. *J Health Polit Policy Law*. 1989;14:191-227.

7. Chatterjee SN, Payne JE, Berne TV. Difficulties in obtaining kidneys from potential postmortem donors. *JAMA*. 1975;232:822-824.

8. Hanto DW. Midwestern regional report. *Chimera*. 1990;1: 12-13.

9. Caplan AL. Professional arrogance and public misunderstanding. *Hastings Cent Rep.* April/May 1988:34-37.

10. Caplan AL. Letter. *Hastings Cent Rep.* March/April 1989:45.

11. Overcast TD, Evans RW, Bowen LE, Hoe MM, Livak CL. Problems in the identification of potential organ donors. *JAMA.* 1984;251:1559-1562.

12. Sutton EC. Organ donation legislation: the role of the physician. *Med Staff Couns.* 1989;3:43-50.

13. Peters TG, Vaughn WK. Organs for transplantation: analysis of 27 000 cadaveric donor organs. *South Med J.* 1990;83:889-892.

14. Batten HL, Prottas JM. Kind strangers: the families of organ donors. *Health Aff.* Summer 1987:35-47.

15. Diethelm AG. Ethical decisions in the history of organ transplantation. *Ann Surg.* 1990;211:505-519.

16. Englehardt HT. Special report: Shattuck Lecture—allocating scarce medical resources and the availability of organ transplantation. *N Engl J Med.* 1984;311:66-71.

17. Callender CO, Bayton JA, Yeager C, Clark JE. Attitudes among blacks toward donating kidneys for transplantation: a pilot project. *J Natl Med Assoc.* 1982;74:807-809.

18. Johnson LW, Lum CT, Thompson T, Wilson J, Urdaneta ML, Harris R. Mexican-American and Anglo-American attitudes toward organ donation. *Transplant Proc.* 1988;20:822-823.

19. Manninen DL, Evans RW. Public attitudes and behavior regarding organ donation. *JAMA.* 1985;253:3111-3116.

20. Miles MS, Frauman AC. Public attitudes toward organ donation. *Dialysis Trans.* 1988;17:74-76.

21. Hagle ME, Rosenberg JC, Lysz K, Kaplan MP, Sillix D. Racial perspectives on kidney transplant donors and recipients. *Transplantation.* 1989;48:421-424.

22. Rostand SG, Kirk KA, Rutsky EA, Pate BA. Racial differences in the incidence of treatment for end-stage renal disease. *N Engl J Med.* 1982;306:1276-1279.

23. Sells RA. Commerce in human organs: a global review. *Dialysis Transplant.* 1990;19:10-17.

24. The Council of the Transplantation Society. Commercialization in transplantation. *Transplantation.* 1986;41:1-3.

25. Kramer NC, Peters TG, Rohr MS, Thacker LR, Vaughn WK. Beneficial effect of cyclosporine on renal transplantation. *Transplantation.* 1990;49:343-348.

26. Fernandez-Bueno C, Samimi F, Reinmuth B, Baker JR, Peters TG. Improved results in cadaveric renal transplantation for black recipients. *Transplant Proc.* 1988;20:398-400.

27. National Organ Transplant Act, Pub L No.98-507, 3 USC §301.

28. Uniform Anatomical Gift Act §4,8A ULA 15(1987).

19. Families' Self-Interest and the Cadaver's Organs: What Price Consent?

Edmund D. Pellegrino

It is tragic for an eligible recipient to die for want of a lifesaving organ. The profession and society are under a clear moral compulsion to seek ways to prevent such deaths. But it would be equally tragic, even in order to save lives, to resort to such a morally dubious and destructive policy to increase the supply of donated organs as Peters suggests. His proposal that a $1000 death "benefit" be offered to motivate families to consent to removal of organs from their deceased relatives is logically, ethically, and practically flawed.

In his sincere and understandable commitment to save lives, Peters follows an oversimplified line of reasoning: people die waiting for organ transplants. Organs are scarce because we have relied on altruism to motivate donors. Therefore, self-interest must replace altruism as a motive. With the obstacle of activism out of the way, Peters believes that an adequate supply, and even a surplus, of organs can be expected; that minority groups would benefit; that the "coercion" he sees in our reliance on altruism would be eliminated; and that altruism itself would be preserved.

Peters' argument is based on a faulty interpretation of altruism. Altruism is not a value imposed on donor families. No one can be coerced into altruism because altruism requires a free and conscious recognition of other persons in the way we conduct ourselves.[1,2] It is a fundamental virtue of, good societies and good persons. It is not valid only in a context of plenty. Physicians are not free unilaterally to eliminate altruism from decisions to donate organs. To create a deliberate conflict between altruism and self-interest is to reduce our freedom to make a gift to a stranger.[3] This, as Titmuss[3(pp12-13)] shows

Originally published in *JAMA* 265, no. 10 (March 13, 1991): 1305-1306.

in his study of the commercialization of blood donation, has serious destructive effects, ethical and nonethical, on the whole of a society.

Peters' proposal also seriously undermines the consent process. Ethically, the family does not have proprietary rights over a relative's dead body. That body is not an object to be scavenged even for good purposes. The body is the last reminder of a once-living person and, as such, it is entitled to a certain dignity. To give valid consent for organ removal, family surrogates should reflect the deceased person's wishes and values—not their own. The death benefit clearly legitimates family interests over the deceased's. It can even come to be seen as an entitlement tempting physicians and families to withdraw or withhold treatment sooner than might ordinarily be the case. Poor families will be subject to more duress and manipulation than the well-to-do, and this is discriminatory.

Once commercialization of consent becomes accepted, many new questions can logically be raised. If the family can benefit from consent, why shouldn't the donor receive $1,000 for agreeing to donate his or her organs in anticipation of death? What will keep the price from escalating if an insufficient number of organs are procured? If experience in other commodities is any guide, a black market of covert payments exceeding the going rate is certain to arise.

Who should the broker be—the physician, the organ transplant agency, or the hospital? Will not their interests in reimbursement, and in dominating the market and the income from doing transplants, conflict with the interests of both recipients and donors? Won't the poor be losers again—through manipulation of the consent of donors' families, or through their lack of insurance, as recipients?[4,5] Will the family's property rights override expressed, but not legally formalized, objections of the dead person while alive? Could an experimental trial be of any use at all since the ethical issues are not resolvable by public acclaim or acceptance?

Some may reject these as "slippery slope" questions. But history painfully reminds us that the slippery slope is no ethical illusion but a recurrent reality. Once a moral barrier is broken, it is difficult to contain abuses by regulation or law. Peters is right to be concerned and to seek ways to relieve the scarcity of lifesaving organs for donation. For patients to die waiting for an available lifesaving organ is an indictment of the level of altruism in our society, but not a sufficient reason for eliminating altruism itself. A policy that resorts to monetary inducements, that replaces altruism by selfish self-interest and that manipulates consent by monetary incentives, has too many ethical liabilities to be acceptable either as a policy or an experiment. Frustrating as the effort may be, we cannot abandon the effort to increase the supply of organs by education and appeals to altruism.

REFERENCES

1. Nagel T. *The Possibility of Altruism.* Princeton, NJ: Princeton University Press; 1978:144-146.

2. Blum L. *Friendship, Altruism, and Morality.* Boston, Mass: Routledge & Kegan Paul; 1980:9-11.

3. Titmuss R. *The Gift Relationship: From Human Blood to Social Policy.* New York: Pantheon Press; 1971:245-246.

4. Beauchamp TL, Childress JL. *Principles of Bioethics.* New York: Oxford University Press Inc; 1989:110-111.

5. Frankfurt H. *The Importance of What We Care About.* New York: Cambridge University Press; 1989:26-28.

20. Improving Organ Donation: Compensation versus Markets

Andrew H. Barnett, Roger D. Blair,
and David L. Kaserman

A number of proposals have recently emerged suggesting monetary compensation for cadaveric organ donors or their surviving family members as a method of encouraging greater donation rates.[1] If successful, such compensation schemes would save thousands of lives annually by expanding the currently inadequate supply of transplantable organs.[2]

Several necessary conditions must exist for cadaveric organ donation to occur. Potential donors are generally brain-dead, heart-beating cadavers less than fifty-five years old and free of infection. All major organs other than the brain must be functioning while they are temporarily sustained on the heart-lung machine. As a result, most organ donors are relatively young persons who have been involved in an accident in which severe head injury occurred. Despite these rather demanding requirements, there appear to be a sufficient number of deaths under these circumstances to satisfy the annual demand for transplantable organs if collection rates could be improved.

The recent compensation proposals represent a drastic departure from the medical profession's long-standing policy advocating continued reliance on altruism for organ supply and opposing payment of any kind to organ donors. Such proposals stem from a recognition that, from a truly ethical point of view, the primary objective of saving patients' lives should dominate our natural desire to impose our own moral or philosophical attitudes on others. In the case at hand, this means that, on ethical grounds, physicians (and others) should abandon their traditional support for the current altruistic organ procurement policy if some alternate policy can reasonably be expected to increase the number of organs available for transplantation. Assuming that such an alternative system exists, defenders of the current system are effectively sacrificing patients' lives in order to indulge their own penchant for altruistic behavior (by others).

Given the (ethical) view that patients' well-being should dominate our policy selection, the important question then becomes: How can we best organize the organ procurement system to achieve our primary objective—saving patients' lives—while not violating any fundamental ethical principles. In this paper, we argue that, while compensation of organ donors within the existing organ procurement system would certainly increase the number of organs collected (and, thereby, represent an improvement over the current system), it is less likely to generate an adequate supply of transplantable organs than a true market system in which cadaveric organs are purchased by profit-seeking firms that specialize in organ acquisition. Therefore, we evaluate here how our system of donor compensation would perform relative to a market system of procurement. In addition, we argue that alleged ethical concerns that have been voiced concerning donor compensation[3] (and, by implication, a market system) are misguided or are ethically dominated by the needs of potential transplant recipients.

While much of our discussion is couched in terms of ethics, it is important to remember that this is not simply an abstract philosophical debate. Human lives are at stake. Every day that the current organ shortage is allowed to persist, more treatable patients are condemned to unnecessary suffering and premature death.

COMPENSATION VERSUS MARKETS

The current altruistic procurements system exhibits a number of serious flaws—both economic and ethical (Blair and Kaserman 1991). Among these, two particular shortcomings stand out as important factors contributing to the organ shortage. First, this system provides little incentive for donation to occur. Organ procurers must appeal exclusively to a sense of community and benevolence on the part of families of the recently deceased. Second, and probably more important, the current system provides little or no incentive for attending physicians, nurses, or organ procurement officers to solicit organs from families of the deceased. Asking a grieving family to donate the organs of their deceased relative is a decidedly unpleasant task. This undertaking is so unpleasant, in fact, that many physicians and nurses simply do not ask, or when they ask they do so only half-heartedly.

The crucial question then becomes: Why does organ donation fail to occur in most cases? Is it because of refusal to donate or is it because of the failure to ask? What little empirical evidence is available suggests it is the latter. When individuals were asked in a 1985 Gallup poll if they would be willing to donate the organs of recently deceased relatives, fully 73 percent indicated they would.[4] Consequently, it appears that the principal cause of the current shortage is a widespread failure to request donation from potential organ suppliers, not a refusal to donate.

Unfortunately, compensation under the current collection system fails to address this important problem. A market system of organ procurement, however, would provide a profit incentive for organ procurement firms to actively seek out potential organ donors and negotiate a mutually agreeable supply contract. Thus, the market system corrects both problems with the current altruistic system—lack of incentive to donate and lack of incentive to ask—while compensation solves only one (and, apparently, the less important one). Therefore a market for organs, with procurement prices set by the forces of supply and demand, has important advantages over compensation.

Because the issue of organ markets is so emotionally charged and often misunderstood, let us be clear what market advocates propose, and, equally important, what they do *not* propose. They do not advocate buying organs from living donors. In fact, an active market for cadaveric organs could eliminate the need for living donors altogether. Market advocates do not propose auctions in which desperate recipients bid against each other for life-sustaining organs. Indeed, given an equilibrium price that clears the market, a shortage of organs will not exist, and such bidding would be entirely unnecessary. Finally, market advocates do not propose organ brokers hawking human organs on street corners. Orders from transplant centers would simply be filled by organ procurement firms at the market price as the needed organs become available.

What most market advocates do propose is a process that separates procurement from distribution. The distribution of organs, once collected, could be organized exactly as it is today. Third parties—private insurance companies and the Health Care Financing Administration—would continue to pay the cost of transplantation, including any organ procurement costs. Once an organ is purchased by a transplant center, surgeons (not market forces) would still determine which donors receive which organs. In fact, the United Network for Organ Sharing allocation formula could still govern these decisions, although the need for such an allocation system would be greatly reduced. The only difference would be that many more organs would be available for transplantation, and the lengths of waiting lists and expected waiting times would fall dramatically.

The procurement function itself, however, would be governed by market forces. Organ procurement firms would be allowed, in the case of spot markets, to pay the states or surviving family members of organ donors for collected organs, or, in the case of a futures market, to pay the potential donor today for the right to remove needed organs at death. Moreover, the altruism inherent in this exchange would still remain, because recipients would still receive the same benefits (improved health or life) that exist under the current system. In effect, the organ exchange would be much like giving money to charities or the church, where such gifts are motivated by both altruism and the reduced taxes achieved. In other words, payment, in itself, does not rule out the altruistic motive. Organs collected could then be sold to transplant centers at a price dictated by supply and demand.[5] These centers, in turn, would place their orders for needed organs with the organ procurement firms.

Because they could sell the organs collected, procurement firms would have an economic incentive to collect as many organs as could profitably be sold. This opportunity to earn profit from the sale of organs provides a strong incentive for these firms to formulate procurement strategies that more effectively encourage donation (or sale). A likely part of such a strategy would include employment of procurement experts trained to approach potential donors in the least offensive way. Procurement firms would also have an incentive to construct compensation packages that maximize benefits to a donor's estate or surviving family members, and, thereby, encourage maximum donation rates.

Proposals for introducing markets where they have not been used before often encounter myths and misconceptions about how markets work. In this case, there may be some concern that market procurement of organs could lead to "battles at the bedside," as competing procurement firms vie for valuable organs. Obviously, this concern does not apply to a futures market, because such a market involves purchasing options from healthy individuals that would allow future harvesting of the individual's organs if they should be rendered terminal by some accident or illness. On the other hand, in the case of spot markets, some measures may be required to limit or prevent bedside bargaining. For example, hospitals may auction collection rights to competing organ procurement firms for one year. Such an auction would allow a procurement firm exclusive rights to harvest organs at a given hospital but only for a limited period of time. Further it would require the licensed procurer to purchase that right in a competitive auction.

When markets allocate scarce resources, a buyer pays for resources received and a seller receives compensation for the resources supplied. The payment made by buyers encourages them to conserve the scarce resource and recognize the social value it represents. The greater the degree of scarcity, the higher the price and the greater the incentive to conserve. The compensation to suppliers encourages them to provide the good; and, of course, the greater the scarcity, the higher the price and the greater the incentive to supply. In short, demand and supply determine prices so that the quantity demanded is approximately equal to the quantity supplied. With freely functioning markets, shortages simply cannot persist.[6]

Moreover, a market for organs would be more flexible than either the current system or a system of compensation in making relatively scarce organs more available.[7] Organs with an unusual HLA antigen makeup or a comparatively rare blood type would command a relatively high market price (where demand warrants such a price). This price, in turn, would encourage a greater quantity supplied thereby reducing the extreme waiting times currently experienced for such organs. This ability of markets to reflect relative scarcity in the prices that are determined represents a subtle but important advantage over its system of compensation that sets reimbursement levels the same for all donors.

Providing compensation for organ donors under the current collection system accomplishes only part of what a true market for organs achieves. Namely, compensation provides an additional incentive for donors to agree to supply the available organs when asked. It does not, however, increase the incentive to seek out donations.[8] In all likelihood, providing compensation would reduce the current shortage by an unknown amount. But it is unlikely to entirely eliminate that shortage, because it fails to provide an increased incentive to request donations (or sales). As a result, while compensation may reduce the organ shortage, a market system of procurement would eliminate it. Consequently, by the ethical criteria of saving patients' lives, a market system is clearly superior to compensation.

ETHICAL ISSUES OF AN ORGAN MARKET

Critics of the market mechanism often raise ethical objections to the creation of the market for cadaveric organs. These objections, however, are either totally specious or at best poorly reasoned. Among these ethical objections are (1) economic coercion of the poor, (2) access to transplants by the poor, (3) premature termination of care of potential organ donors, and (4) a potential deterioration in the quality of organs harvested. We will examine each of these arguments in turn.

Economic Coercion of the Poor

First, it has been alleged that the market system is coercive, that is, that the poor will be forced to do something they would prefer not to do. This line of reasoning, however, fails to recognize how the market system operates. The essence of coercion is to induce an action through force or threat, while the market system relies upon a totally voluntary exchange. Voluntary exchange between a willing buyer and a willing seller normally makes neither party worse off and usually makes both parties better off.[9] Otherwise, voluntary exchange would not occur. If a poor person does not value the payment received more than he or she values burying the body intact, then he or she simply refuses the market offer. In a free market, one cannot be forced to do something that one does not voluntarily choose to do.

Some may object that a poor person may feel compelled to sell his or her organs due to the family's impoverished circumstances when, in fact, he or she would prefer not to do so. The market is not the source of the problem. The economic circumstances of the poor may induce them to do many things that they would not do otherwise, but one cannot condemn the market for the choices made. Poor people do a wide variety of things that they would not do if they were not poor: work in coal mines, neglect their children while working two jobs, join the military, drop out of school, sell family heirlooms, and a host of other undesirable actions. But are we prepared to ban all such activity in the paternalistic pursuit of what we think is right for them? If we are going to proscribe some particular set of market transactions because we deem them coercive, what general principles can we rely upon to identify those specific transactions that poor people should be allowed to make and those that poor people should not be allowed to make? In other words, what fundamental criteria can we apply to separate those market transactions that are acceptable from those that are unacceptable for those of limited means? Advocates of the current altruistic organ procurement policy who base such advocacy on avoidance of economic coercion must be prepared to specify such criteria if their argument is to be seriously considered.

Focusing only on the market for organs and pursuing the coercion argument to its logical conclusions, one way to prevent economic coercion of the poor is to prohibit them from participating in this market. In other words, we can permit the poor to be as altruistic as they want to be, but deny them the opportunity to sell their organs. We simply pass a law that says that anyone with income less than X dollars cannot be compensated for organ donation. In this way, low-income individuals cannot be coerced by market forces. The details of determining who is sufficiently wealthy to be eligible to sell his or her organs would have to be worked out, but the principle has obvious merit to those concerned with relieving the poor from economic coercion—poor people will not be coerced, they will remain poor, and the rich will get richer. Such a policy obviously serves neither society at large nor the poor.

Transplant Accessibility for the Poor

The second ethical concern for the poor is in their role as consumers rather than as suppliers. The fear is that if organs are sold, only the wealthy will be able to afford transplants. This is a curious argument given the expense of transplant operations. A liver transplant, for example, costs around $250,000 (Clark, Robinson, and Wickelgren 1988). In the absence of government aid, such an operation is clearly inaccessible to anyone without substantial medical insurance or extraordinary wealth. Simply adding the market price of the liver to the cost of the operation is not going to make the transplant less accessible to anyone.

Implicit in this particular concern for the poor is the assumption that market clearing organ prices will be high. But there is a large potential supply of cadaveric organs and opening the market is likely to lead to a substantial response that would result in low prices for the needed organs. Moreover, to the extent that more organs are made available for transplant, there is the opportunity to make transplants more accessible for everyone. In addition, the use of market forces for organ collection does not require the use of market forces for their subsequent allocation. The system for distributing organs can remain in the hands of transplant surgeons and centers, just as it is today.

If, as a society, we are dissatisfied with the distribution of available organs, we can adopt redistributive policies that will give the poor a better chance of receiving a needed transplant. In fact, shifting renal patients from dialysis to transplants would allow the End Stage Renal Disease program to reduce its budget by purchasing kidneys for potential recipients because transplantation is a much less expensive treatment modality. Thus, accessibility of transplants to the poor would actually improve under a market system of procurement.

Premature Termination of Care

Finally, some have expressed concern that there might be incentives for the premature termination of care under a market system of procurement. Consider how this could occur. An accident victim is in a coma and is not expected to live very long. If the family pulls the plug on this patient, it can receive the market price of the organs a week or so earlier than otherwise.[10] The incentive to pull the plug early created by the market, then, is the interest that could be earned on the money for a week or two. This is a trivial sum compared to the cost of treatment, which provides a much more substantial incentive for premature termination of care. But, one may argue, this situation could involve a case in which the patient could be kept alive for quite some time. This simply means that the interest on the price that the organs will command is a bit larger, but the incremental costs of the medical care needed to sustain life over this prolonged period will then be astronomical. These costs will provide a much larger incentive for premature termination of care. Once again, the market for organs is not the culprit.

Finally, the attending physician (who has no financial stake in the decision to terminate care) must first determine that death has occurred. That is, the family's decision to terminate treatment is conditioned on the physician first determining that the patient is brain dead. The existence of an organ market (or compensation), then, is much like the presence of a will. Someone will benefit financially from the patient's death but it cannot be the physician who is in charge of the patient's care. Thus, concerns over premature termination of care are ill-founded. They stem from a misperception of the way in which an organ market would work.

Reduced Organ Quality

We live in an age when there are justifiable concerns about AIDS and other diseases that are difficult to detect. In fact, federal health officials have proposed a national system to track organs and tissues from the time of donation to the time of transplant in order to reduce the risk of transplanting an AIDS-infected organ.[11] One potential problem with a market system for organ procurement is that it provides the donating family with an incentive to lie about the donor's health habits, for example, being an intravenous drug user. Critics may point to the case of blood supplies and the problems with blood quality that have surfaced. When we examine the general problem of organ quality, however, it appears that the market mechanism does not exacerbate the problem and may serve to diminish it.

First, the market will generate a far greater supply of transplantable organs than the current system based on altruism. As a result, transplant surgeons can be more selective in which organs they will actually use in a particular case. In other words, even if the average quality of organs harvested were to fall, it does not follow that the average quality of the organs transplanted will fall. Given a larger supply of organs, enhanced screening procedures can lead to enhanced organ quality.

Second, the analogy to blood supply is not apt. Paying for blood may induce infected people to offer their blood for sale, but organs come from cadavers. It's highly unlikely that paying for organs will lead to a greater supply of dead people with infectious diseases. Moreover, problems with the blood market have arisen largely because blood suppliers have been given liability exclusion from malfeasance. As a result, those in a position to control quality have had little incentive to do so.

Firms supplying organs, however, should be held responsible for the quality and safety of what they supply. Liability rules ought to emerge that provide organ procurement firms with the proper incentives to insure quality through screening procedures.

CONCLUSIONS

The facts are simple. Transplantable cadaveric organs are plentiful relative to the need for organ transplants.[12] Nonetheless, many patients die because harvestable organs are not available for use in their treatment. Our problem is not one of an inherent organ shortage mandated by nature but, rather, one of a contrived shortage created by existing organ procurement policies. Most analysts agree that payment for organs would encourage donations. And all agree that more donated cadaveric organs would save lives. Yet many medical practitioners steadfastly hold that monetary incentives for organ donors and, even more so, organ markets are unethical or immoral.

Many opponents of financial incentives for cadaveric organ donation argue that compensation introduces some potentially troublesome ethical issues. Our discussion here touches on some of the more prevalent arguments in this area and shows them to be seriously flawed.[13] By the same token, however, refusal to offer financial incentives yields a severe organ shortage and that shortage, in turn, condemns many patients to death. The current policy thus forces us to make decisions about who will receive treatment and who will die. These decisions (or "tragic choices") certainly pose some difficult ethical questions. They are, however, wholly unnecessary. By adopting a more rational organ procurement policy that relies upon the powerful forces of supply and demand, the need for such decisions can be reduced if not completely eliminated.

Consequently, it is far from obvious that opposition to organ markets constitutes the moral high ground. Instead, it is clear to us that, due to the many lives that could be saved, a market for organs is morally and ethically superior to the current altruistic procurement system.

While we continue to debate ethics, potential transplant patients suffer and die. While we extol the virtues of benevolence and decry greed, patients go without treatment that could significantly improve their health and save their lives. If the first priority of medical practitioners is to sustain life, not to formulate moral and ethical dictates for society, then many in the medical community are guilty of neglecting their primary responsibility.

Finally, it is important to recognize that the current altruistic system of organ procurement has been in place now from more than thirty years. During that time, it has never once yielded an annual supply of transplantable organs sufficient to meet the demand. Thus, cries for improved education and greater altruism designed to prolong the current system fail to recognize the historical failure of that system and effectively condemn even more patients to death.

As a society concerned with the health of our citizens, we simply must consider alternative procurement policies. And, as we do, we must evaluate all possible alternatives and weigh their likely performances against one another. Given the tremendous inertia that public policy typically exhibits, it is imperative that we select carefully and in light of the best information available. The "road not taken" may otherwise prove regrettable.

NOTES

1. See, for example, Peters (1991). The idea of paying organ donors is not new. It has a long history in the literature. See Brams 1977; Freier 1978-79; Cohen 1989; Hansmann 1989; Kaserman and Barnett 1991; Barney and Reynolds 1989; Schwindt and Vining 1986; and Blair and Kaserman 1991.

2. Peters (1991) estimates that, in 1989, 1,878 patients died as a result of the shortage of transplantable organs. The actual number of deaths that could be avoided by fully resolving the organ shortage, however, is understated by this estimate, because only those patients who died while on official waiting lists are included. Excluded from this count are the thousands of additional patients who die annually, who for a variety of reasons were never placed on these lists, but who, nonetheless, could have been saved by an organ transplant. See Randall (1991). Some (perhaps most) of these patients are excluded due to the shortage itself. If transplantable organs were readily available, the criteria for admitting patients to waiting lists would be considerably less severe. Good examples of this are the discussions of rationing of available donor livers in Moss and Siegler (1991) and Cohen and Benjamin (1991).

3. See, for, example, Pellegrino (1991). Others raising similar ethical concerns include Titmuss (1971) and the Council of the Transplantation Society (1985).

4. See "Developments in the Law . . ." (1990).

5. There are good economic reasons to believe that this equilibrium market price would be low. See Blair and Kaserman (1991).

6. The superiority of the market mechanism as an instrument for allocating scarce resources among competing uses was affirmed by Pope John Paul II in a major encyclical issued on May 2, 1991: "The free market is the most efficient instrument for utilizing resources and effectively responding to needs." See Rosen (1991).

7. We are grateful to the anonymous reviewer who pointed this out to us.

8. Compensation may cause some potential donors to seek out organ procurement officials. It provides no added incentive, however, for these officials to intensify their efforts to seek out and approach potential donors.

9. This, of course, assumes no serious information problems or addictive properties of the good exchanged. Such problems, however, are not present in organ sales.

10. By leaving the patient on the respirator, however, the family also runs the risk of making the organs worthless for transplantation due to infection.

11. See Altman (1991). The author points out that few patients have been HIV-infected through transplant surgery.

12. Estimates are currently emerging that we may actually be collecting around 50 percent of available cadaveric organs. See, for example, Nathan, et al. (1990). These figures are considerably higher than the earlier estimates of 15 to 20 percent. Nonetheless, the fact remains that a very large increase in supply is feasible and such an increase would substantially reduce (and, over a period of several years, eliminate) the existing organ shortage.

13. For a more complete critical evaluation of both the economic and ethical arguments against a market system of cadaveric organ procurement, see Blair and Kaserman (1991).

REFERENCES

Altman, L. K. 1991. Citing AIDS, Officials Propose Tracking Transplants. *New York Times* (December 15):18.

Barney, D. L., and R. L. Reynolds. 1989. An Economic Analysis of Transplant Organs. *Atlantic Economic Journal* 17:12.

Blair, R. D., and D. L. Kaserman. 1991. The Economics and Ethics of Alternative Cadaveric Organ Procurement Policies. *Yale Journal on Regulation* 8:403.

Brams, M. 1977. Transplantable Human Organs: Should Their Sale Be Authorized by State Statutes? *American Journal of Law & Medicine* 3:183.

Clark, M., C. Robinson, and I. Wickelgren. 1988. Interchangeable Parts. *Newsweek* (September12):61-63.

Cohen, C., and M. Benjamin (and the Ethics and Social Impact Committee of the Transplant and Health Policy Center, Ann Arbor, Mich.) 1991. Alcoholics and Liver Transplantation. *Journal of the American Medical Association* 265:1299-1301. [Chapter 29 this volume]

Cohen, L. R. 1989. Increasing the Supply of Transplant Organs: The Virtues of a Futures Market. *George Washington Law Review* 58:1.

Council of the Transplantation Society. 1985. Commercialization in Transplantation: The Problems and Some Guidelines for Practice. *Lancet* 715.

Developments in the Law: Medical Technology and the Law. 1990. *Harvard Law Review* 103:1621.

Freier, D. T. 1978-1979. Organ Selling for Transplantation. *Progressive Clinical and Biological Research* 38:141.

Hansmann, H. 1989. The Economics and Ethics of Markets for Human Organs. In *Human Organs, Organ Transplantation Policy: Issues and Prospects,* ed. J. F. Blumstein and F. A. Sloan. Durham, N.C.: Duke University Press.

Kaserman, D. L., and A. H. Barnett. 1991. An Economic Analysis of Transplant Organs: A Comment and Extension. *Atlanta Economic Journal* 19:57-63.

Moss, A. H., and M. Siegler. 1991. Should Alcoholics Compete Equally for Liver Transplantation? *Journal of the American Medical Association* 265:1295-1298.

Nathan, H. M., et al. 1990. Estimation and Characterization of the Potential Organ Donor Pool in Pennsylvania: Report of the Pennsylvania Statewide Donor Study. Presented at the American Society of Transplant Surgeons Annual Meeting, Chicago.

Pellegrino, E. D. 1991. Families' Self-Interest and the Cadaver's Organs. *Journal of the American Medical Association* .265:1305-1306.

Peters, T. G. 1991. Life or Death: The Issue of Payment in Cadaveric Organ Donation. *Journal of the American Medical Association* 265:1302-1305.

Randall, T. 1991. Too Few Human Organs for Transplantation, Too Many in Need . . . and the Gap Widens. *Journal of the American Medical Association* 265:1223-1227.

Rosen, G. R. 1991. Pope John Paul II Upholds Capitalism with Social Justice. *IMF Survey* (May 27): 169.

Schwindt, R., and A. R. Vining. 1986. Proposal for a Future Market for Transplant Organs. *Journal of Health, Politics, Policy and Law* 11:483-500.

Titmuss, R. M. 1971. *The Gift Relationship.* New York: Pantheon.

21. Financial Compensation for Cadaver Organ Donation: Good Idea or Anathema?

A. L. Caplan, C. T. Van Buren, and N. L. Tilney

The transplant community is currently awash in a sea of proposals calling for the creation of financial incentives in the United States as a solution to the shortage of cadaver organs and tissues.[1-6] Although the plans vary in detail, all imply that monetary incentives will increase donation. African Americans are a particular target of financial compensation schemes as they are underrepresented in the overall pool of cadaver donors relative to their numbers in the general population.[7] Because they and other minorities may be in low income categories, financial incentives are sometimes touted as likely to be attractive.[8,9] Advocates of paying for organs often argue that since some poor persons face the potential burden of uncovered medical expenses, funeral costs, or both, the prospect of compensation might encourage them to agree to organ or tissue donation, should the situation ever arise.[10] Those favoring reforms to make it legal to pay for cadaver body parts sometimes support the morality of such policies by noting that since other parties involved in transplantation, from procurement organizations to surgeons, make money from the procedure, it should not be illegal for donor families also to be compensated.[8,11]

We believe that existing law and public policy should not be modified to permit compensation. A national policy, regional efforts, or pilot projects which permit payment, either direct or indirect, for cadaver organs may further reduce already marginal numbers of donors and may very likely be deleterious for those currently awaiting transplants. There are important ethical and pragmatic reasons for not changing the present policy.

Originally published in *Transplantation Proceedings* 25, no. 4 (August 1993): 2740-42. Reprinted by permission of Appleton & Lange, Inc.

ETHICAL PROBLEMS WITH COMPENSATION SCHEMES

The argument for permitting a market in cadaver body parts is that respect for personal autonomy allows those who wish to do so to sell their organs after death. Individuals should be free to decide how to dispose of their bodies and their parts, whether they choose burial, cremation, or donation or sale for medical purposes. This rationale does not seem persuasive and may even destroy the environment in which personal autonomy can flourish. Allowing the sale of the human body reduces people to objects. Offering compensation towards life insurance, cash rebates, estate tax discounts, or payment for funerals contingent upon a favorable decision about the disposition of cadaver remains indicates that medicine and the law are willing to turn the body into a commodity to allow more transplants to be performed. The message conveyed is that it is permissible, even desirable, to treat the body as an object of sale and profit; this is not likely to nurture mutual respect or esteem amongst the public and the professions, further diminishing the prospects for the exercise of autonomy. An obvious suggestion is that those whose organs and tissues are taken in the context of a financial reward are "sources," not donors; when the dead are treated as things, the dignity and moral standing of the living, and thus, their autonomy, are imperiled. Conversely, one could argue that once the donation occurs, particularly of multiple organs, the body is treated as "a thing," often with total failure by the procurement team to maintain the individual dignity of the donor. Indeed, it is fortunate that the public does not question the practical implications of donation, believing in the integrity of their physicians. The assumption leading to "opting out" legislation in some European countries accentuates this point.

Fairness must also be considered by those who advance markets in body parts in the name of personal autonomy. The problems associated with the poor in gaining access to health and welfare services are all too real. If the only way our society, or any other, can find to pay the costs of medical care or funerals for the indigent is to offer remuneration for their body parts, should such a society be viewed as humane, decent, or fair? In this context, efforts of the transplant and medical communities to procure organs from such individuals could also be construed as a conflict of interest.

Calls for the reform of existing federal and state laws to permit payment for cadaver body parts are especially disturbing at a time when many poor persons may face enormous fiscal obstacles in gaining access to transplants.[12-13] As Medicaid programs in some states do not pay for some types of transplants, the underinsured and the uninsured are sometimes forced to resort to public begging to be considered as a recipient. In particular, the position that financial incentives will be especially attractive to the poor, and will help redress the underrepresentation of African Americans in the existing donor pool, is indifferent to the history of this group in the United States, for whom making the body an object carries special moral significance. For centuries this population were bought and sold as chattel. As slaves, their bodies were often used by physicians without consent for experimentation and after death for autopsy and teaching purposes (*Southern History* 48:331, 1982). Indeed, the last time the federal government and private agencies paid for funeral expenses for poor African Americans was when the bodies of those who died in the notorious Tuskegee Syphilis study were sought for autopsy.[14,15] Thus, the attitudes of this segment of the population about payment for organs and tissues may be influenced by these historical realities in a way that none of those calling for markets and compensation in the name of autonomy have acknowledged, much less taken into account (*St. Petersburg Times*, January 6, 1992: 1A, 6,7).

PRACTICAL PROBLEMS WITH COMPENSATION

Little empirical evidence beyond anecdotal accounts has been introduced by proponents of compensation schemes that families themselves raise the issue of money or compensation at a time when they actually have to face requests to make cadaver organs and tissues available for transplantation.[10] In practice, families often do not donate because they do not want their relative to undergo further "suffering"; they cannot yet accept his/her death; they cannot cut through their shock and grief to make an altruistic decision. Indeed, as suggested, significant numbers of Americans may become so angered, offended, and insulted by offers of money or financial rewards as to resist donation[16,17] (and *St. Petersburg Times*, January 6, 1992: 1A, 6,7). Other factors may also be important. The attitudes of the individuals, doctors, nurses, social workers, and chaplains, who initiate requests for donation from families that include offers of money or compensation are not known. For decades, such professionals have been taught that altruism, not sale, is the moral foundation for cadaver procurement.[18] Again, in practical terms, mention of money may only detract from an important interaction with the family of a potential donor at a particularly delicate, distressing, and emotional time.

Similarly, recent history does not support the view that the public would be comfortable with a market in body parts. A variety of state, federal, professional, and international organizations and societies have prohibited and condemned any form of commerce in cadaver organs.[19] The consistent rejection of compensation schemes by legislative bodies and professional organizations and the reluctance of courts to acknowledge a property interest in the human body illustrates that significant disquiet about allowing commercial trade in cadaver remains.[20,21]

Calls for payment for body parts ignore the fragile nature of assent among religious groups for procurement of cadaver organs. Historically, some major religious faiths have had serious reservations and doubts about the moral licitness of transplantation, supporting the use of cadaver organs only in so far as the practice is seen as humane, respectful of the dead, and as not treating the body as object, property, or commodity.[22-26] Although obviously not accepted by all, many religious traditions may vigorously oppose any position which permits the body to be seen as property owned by the individual rather than as a gift from God, and will object to treatment of the body as an object to be sold.[22-24,27]

Implementation of a system of financial incentives for cadaver organs and tissues would be no simple matter. If reimbursement were legal it would not be long before the prices sought and paid either aboveboard or on the black market would escalate.[28] If buyers set prices, financial incentive schemes might disenfranchise and disadvantage the very groups often cited by those advancing fiscal schemes: indigent recipients awaiting transplants who would not be able to compete for cadaver parts in an open market. How will the payment be made for medical expenses or funeral expenses? Are these payments to be made directly to the families or to the involved providers of these services? Who will be responsible for scrutinizing these costs? Indeed, who will be responsible for payment?

In more theoretical terms, if compensation was allowed, would physicians and hospitals become liable for failing at efforts to detect and pronounce brain death promptly to facilitate sales? Who will pay for brain death protocols to be performed when families, lured by the prospect of compensation, insist that efforts be made to see whether procurement might be possible? How long will it be before funeral directors, medical examiners, coroners, and procurement personnel begin to seek payment according to what the market will bear for their roles and services in cadaver organ and tissue procurement?

The only evidence available concerning the practical import of permitting compensation for body parts has accrued through the practice of payment to living sources[29] (and *New York Times*, June 3, 1991:7). The lessons to be derived from this experience should give pause to those who would permit a market in cadaver organs and tissues in this country. Abuses have been so blatant that many nations are moving to reform their laws to bring compensation schemes to an immediate end[30,31] (and *New York Times*, January 23, 1992:A16). Others retain their policy (at least unofficially), particularly in situations where the rich from one country buy organs from prisoners executed in another.[32]

CONCLUSION

Calls for markets, compensation, bounties, or rewards should be rejected because they pose risks to personal autonomy and fairness. They convert donors into sources, human beings into products, thus undermining the foundational values requisite for respect for others and for self-esteem. Commercial schemes risk further disadvantaging and alienating the already disadvantaged who often are underrepresented in transplant programs. Proposals to permit fiscal incentives in organ and tissue procurement should continue to be rejected by the transplant community, the medical community, and the public.

REFERENCES

1. Buttle NJ: *Med Ethics* 17:97, 1991.
2. Cohen LR: *George Washington Law Rev* 58:1, 1989.
3. Cohen LR: *Clin Transplant* 5:467, 1991.
4. Hansmann HJ: *Health Politics Policy Law* 14:57, 1989.
5. Harvey JJ: *Med Ethics* 16:117, 1990.
6. Wight JP: *Br Med J* [Clin Res] 303:110, 1991.
7. Callender CO: *Transplant Proc* 19:36, 1987.
8. Peters TG, *Physicians* W 8:14, 1991.
9. *UNOS Update* 7:1, 1991.
10. Kittur DS, Hogan MM, Thukral VK, et al: *Lancet* 338:1441, 1991.
11. Peters TG: *JAMA* 265:1302, 1991.
12. Caplan A: *Transplant Proc* 21:338, 1989.
13. Sanfilippo FP, Vaughn WK, Peters TG, et al: *JAMA* 267:247, 1992.
14. Brandt AM: *Hastings Cent Rep* 8:21, 1978.
15. Jones JH: *Bad Blood.* New York: Free Press, 1981.
16. Caplan A, Virnig B: *Crit Care Clin* 6:1007, 1990.
17. Watts M: *Lieberman Research,* 1991, pp 1-21.
18. Youngner SJ, Landefeld S, Coulton CJ, et al: *JAMA* 261:2205, 1989.
19. Council of Transplant Soc: *Lancet* 2:715, 1985.
20. Scott R: *The Body as Property.* New York: Viking, 1981.
21. World Health Organization: *Lancet* 337:1470, 1991.
22. McReavy D: *Clergy Rev* 41:164, 1956.
23. May WF: *Transplant Proc* 20:1078, 1988.
24. John Paul II: *Transplant Proc* 23:xvii, 1991.
25. Wolstenholme G, O'Connor M (eds): *Law and Ethics of Transplantation.* London: CIBA Foundation, 1968.
26. Campbell CS: *Hastings Cent Rep* 20:4, 1990.
27. Kass LR: *Hastings Cent Rep* 20:6, 1990.
28. Tufts A: *Lancet* 337:605, 1991.
29. Cheng IKP, Lai KN, Au TC: *Transplantation* 41:2016, 1991.
30. Daar AS, Sells RA: *Transplant Rev* 4:128, 1990.
31. Guttmann RD: *Transplant Rev* 6:189, 1992.

22. The Case for Allowing Kidney Sales

J. Radcliffe-Richards, A. S. Daar,
R. D. Guttmann, R. Hoffenberg, I. Kennedy,
M. Lock, R. A. Sells, and N. Tilney

When the practice of buying kidneys from live vendors first came to light some years ago, it aroused such horror that all professional associations denounced it[1,2] and nearly all countries have now made it illegal.[3] Such political and professional unanimity may seem to leave no room for further debate, but we nevertheless think it important to reopen the discussion.

The well-known shortage of kidneys for transplantation causes much suffering and death. Dialysis is a wretched experience for most patients, and is anyway rationed in most places and simply unavailable to the majority of patients in most developing countries.[5] Since most potential kidney vendors will never become unpaid donors, either during life or posthumously, the prohibition of sales must be presumed to exclude kidneys that would otherwise be available. It is therefore essential to make sure that there is adequate justification for the resulting harm.

Most people will recognize in themselves the feelings of outrage and disgust that led to an outright ban on kidney sales, and such feelings typically have a force that seems to their possessors to need no further justification. Nevertheless, if we are to deny treatment to the suffering and dying we need better reasons than our own feelings of disgust.

In this paper we outline our reasons for thinking that the arguments commonly offered for prohibiting organ sales do not work, and therefore that the debate should be reopened.[6,7] Here we consider only the selling of kidneys by living vendors, but our arguments have wider implications.

The commonest objection to kidney selling is expressed on behalf of the vendors: the exploited poor, who need to be protected against the greedy rich.

Originally published in *The Lancet* 352 (June 27, 1998): 1950-52. Reprinted by permission.

However, the vendors are themselves anxious to sell,[8] and see this practice as the best option open to them. The worse we think the selling of a kidney, therefore, the worse should seem the position of the vendors when that option is removed. Unless this appearance is illusory, the prohibition of sales does even more harm than first seemed, in harming vendors as well as recipients. To this argument it is replied that the vendors' apparent choice is not genuine. It is said that they are likely to be too uneducated to understand the risks, and that this precludes informed consent. It is also claimed that, since they are coerced by their economic circumstances, their consent cannot count as genuine.[9]

Although both these arguments appeal to the importance of autonomous choice, they are quite different. The first claim is that the vendors are not competent to make a genuine choice within a given range of options. The second, by contrast, is that poverty has so restricted the range of options that organ selling has become the best, and therefore, in effect, that the range is too small. Once this distinction is drawn, it can be seen that neither argument works as a justification of prohibition.[7]

If our ground for concern is that the range of choices is too small, we cannot improve matters by removing the best option that poverty has left, and making the range smaller still. To do so is to make subsequent choices, by this criterion, even less autonomous. The only way to improve matters is to lessen the poverty until organ selling no longer seems the best option; and if that could be achieved, prohibition would be irrelevant because nobody would want to sell.

The other line of argument may seem more promising, since ignorance does preclude informed consent. However, the likely ignorance of the subjects is not a reason for banning altogether a procedure for which consent is required. In other contexts, the value we place on autonomy leads us to insist on information and counselling, and that is what it should suggest in the case of organ selling as well. It may be said that this approach is impracticable, because the educational level of potential vendors is too limited to make explanation feasible, or because no system could reliably counteract the misinformation of nefarious middlemen and profiteering clinics. But even if we accepted that no possible vendor could be competent to consent, that would justify only putting the decision in the hands of competent guardians. To justify total prohibition it would also be necessary to show that organ selling must always be against the interests of potential vendors, and it is most unlikely that this would be done.

The risk involved in nephrectomy is not in itself high, and most people regard it as acceptable for living related donors.[10] Since the procedure is, in principle, the same for vendors as for unpaid donors, any systematic difference between the worthwhileness of the risk for vendors and donors presumably lies on the other side of the calculation, in the expected benefit. Nevertheless the exchange of money cannot in itself turn an acceptable risk into an unacceptable one from the vendor's point of view. It depends entirely on what the money is wanted for.

In general, furthermore, the poorer a potential vendor, the more likely it is that the sale of a kidney will be worth whatever risk there is. If the rich are free to engage in dangerous sports for pleasure, or dangerous jobs for high pay, it is difficult to see why the poor who take the lesser risk of kidney selling for greater rewards—perhaps saving relatives' lives,[11] or extricating themselves from poverty and debt—should be thought so misguided as to need saving from themselves.

It will be said that this does not take account of the reality of the vendors' circumstances: that risks are likely to be greater than for unpaid donors because poverty is detrimental to health, and vendors are often not given proper care. They may also be underpaid or cheated, or may waste their money through inexperience. However, once again, these arguments apply far more strongly to many other activities by which the poor try to earn money, and which we do not forbid. The best way to address such problems would be by regulation and perhaps a central purchasing system, to provide screening, counselling, reliable payment, insurance, and financial advice.[12]

To this it will be replied that no system of screening and control could be complete, and that both vendors and recipients would always be at risk of exploitation and poor treatment. But all the evidence we have shows that there is much more scope for exploitation and abuse when a supply of desperately wanted goods is made illegal. It is, furthermore, not clear why it should be thought harder to police a legal trade than the present complete ban.

Furthermore, even if vendors and recipients would always be at risk of exploitation, that does not alter the fact that if they choose this option, all alternatives must seem worse to them. Trying to end exploitation by prohibition is rather like ending slum dwelling by bulldozing slums: it ends the evil in that form, but only by making things worse for the victims. If we want to protect the exploited, we can do it only by removing the poverty that makes them vulnerable, or, failing that, by controlling the trade.

Another familiar objection is that it is unfair for the rich to have privileges not available to the poor. This argument, however, is irrelevant to the issue of organ selling as such. If organ selling is wrong for this reason, so are all benefits available to the rich, including all private medicine, and, for that matter, all public provision of medicine in rich countries (including transplantation of donated organs) that is unavailable in poor ones. Furthermore, all purchasing could be done by a central organization responsible for fair distribution.[12]

It is frequently asserted that organ donation must be altruistic to be acceptable,[13] and that this rules out payment. However, there are two problems with this claim. First, altruism does not distinguish donors from vendors. If a father who saves his daughter's life by giving her a kidney is altruistic, it is difficult to see why his selling a kidney to pay for some other operation to save her life should be thought less so. Second, nobody believes in general that unless some useful action is altruistic it is better to forbid it altogether.

It is said that the practice would undermine confidence in the medical profession, because of the association of doctors with money-making practices. That, however, would be a reason for objecting to all private practice; and in this case the objection could easily be met by the separation of purchasing and treatment. There could, for instance, be independent trusts[12] to fix charges and handle accounts, as well as to ensure fair play and high standards. It is alleged that allowing the trade would lessen the supply of donated cadaveric kidneys.[14] But although some possible donors might decide to sell instead, their organs would be available, so there would be no loss in the total. And in the meantime, many people will agree to sell who would not otherwise donate.

It is said that in parts of the world where women and children are essentially chattels there would be a danger of their being coerced into becoming vendors. This argument, however, would work as strongly against unpaid living kidney donation, and even more strongly against many far more harmful practices which do not attract calls for their prohibition. Again, regulation would provide the most reliable means of protection.

It is said that selling kidneys would set us on a slippery slope to selling vital organs such as hearts. But that argument would apply equally to the case of the unpaid kidney donation, and nobody is afraid that that will result in the donation of hearts. It is entirely feasible to have laws and professional practices that allow the giving or selling only of non-vital organs. Another objection is that allowing organ sales is impossible because it would outrage public opinion. But this claim is about western public opinion: in many potential vendor communities, organ selling is more acceptable than cadaveric donation, and this argument amounts to a claim that other people should follow western cultural preferences rather than their own. There is, anyway, evidence that the western public is far less opposed to the idea, than are medical and political professionals.[15]

It must be stressed that we are not arguing for the positive conclusion that organ sales must always be acceptable, let alone that there should be an unfettered market. Our claim is only that none of the familiar arguments against organ selling works, and this allows for the possibility that better arguments may yet be found.

Nevertheless, we claim that the burden of proof remains against the defenders of prohibition, and that until good arguments appear, the presumption must be that the trade should be regulated rather than banned altogether. Furthermore, even when there are good objections at particular times or in particular places, that should be regarded as a reason for trying to remove the objections, rather than as an excuse for permanent prohibition.

The weakness of the familiar arguments suggests that they are attempts to justify the deep feelings of repugnance which are the real driving force of prohibition, and feelings of repugnance among the rich and healthy, no matter how strongly felt, cannot justify removing the only hope of the destitute and dying. This is why we conclude that the issue should be considered again, and with scrupulous impartiality.

REFERENCES

1. British Transplantation Society Working Party. Guidelines on living organ donation. *BMJ* 1986; 293: 257-58.

2. The Council of the Transplantation Society. Organ sales. *Lancet* 1985; 2: 715-16.

3. World Health Organization. A report on developments under the auspices of WHO (1987-1991). WHO 1992 Geneva. 12-28.

4. Hauptman PJ, O'Connor KJ. Procurement and allocation of solid organs for transplantation. *N Engl J Med* 1997; 336: 422-31.

5. Barsoum RS. Ethical problems in dialysis and transplantation: Africa. In: Kjellstrand CM, Dossetor JB, eds. *Ethical problems in dialysis and transplantation.* Kluwer Academic Publishers, Netherlands. 1992: 169-82.

6. Radcliffe-Richards J. Nephrarious goings on: kidney sales and moral arguments. *J Med Philosph.* Netherlands: Kluwer Academic Publishers, 1996; 21: 375-416.

7. Radcliffe-Richards J. From him that hath not. In: Kjellstrand CM, Dossetor JB, eds. *Ethical problems in dialysis and transplantation.* Netherlands: Kluwer Academic Publishers, 1992: 53-60.

8. Mani MK. The argument against the unrelated live donor. In: Kjellstrand CM, Dossetor JB, eds. *Ethical problems in dialysis and transplantation.* Netherlands: Kluwer Academic Publishers, 1992: 164.

9. Sells RA. The case against buying organs and a futures market in transplants. *Trans Proc* 1992; 24: 2198-202.

10. Daar AD, Land W, Yahya TM, Schneewind K, Gutmann T, Jakobsen A. Living-donor renal transplantation: evidence-based justification for an ethical option. *Trans Reviews* (in press) 1997.

11. Dossetor JB, Manickavel V. Commercialisation: the buying and selling of kidneys. In: Kjellstrand CM, Dossetor JB, eds. *Ethical problems in dialysis and transplantation.* Netherlands: Kluwer Academic Publishers, 1992: 61-71.

12. Sells RA. Some ethical issues in organ retrieval 1982-1992. *Trans Proc* 1992; 24: 2401-03.

13. Sheil R. Policy statement from the ethics committee of the Transplantation Society. *Trans Soc Bull* 1995; 3: 3.

14. Altshuler JS, Evanisko MJ. *JAMA* 1992; 267: 2037.

15. Guttmann RD, Guttmann A. Organ transplantation: duty reconsidered. *Trans Proc* 1992; 24: 2179-80.

23. Paying for Organs from Living Donors

P. J. Morris and R. A. Sells

SIR,—Allegations that renal transplantation between living unrelated donors and recipients from outside Britain, where the donor has been paid for the donation, is being done at private hospitals in London cause us grave concern. Both the international Transplantation Society and the British Transplantation Society have opposed such practice and feel strongly that steps should be taken to prevent any further such operations in the UK.

The only circumstances where a kidney may be removed ethically from a living donor is when it is a gift to the recipient. Transplants between relatives are, therefore, permissible and widely practiced. In unusual circumstances living unrelated donors might be considered where there is a special relationship between donor and recipient, as, for example, between a husband and wife. But payment is an inducement for the donor to submit to the operation. People should never be operated on under such duress or as a result of bribery; such an inducement not only destroys the very special nature of the gift made by the donor but also threatens the safeguards normally used to preserve the health of both donor and recipient. For if financial gain is the object of the donation, an organ may be removed from a donor who might be unsuitable for medical reasons, and a kidney which is less than ideal may be transplanted into a recipient. These latter objections are, we believe, verified by experience with blood transfusion in countries where blood donors are paid. For this practice has led to an increased spread of disease through the vector of a blood transfusion with a deterioration in the quality of the service and a great increase in the expense of blood as a result of obligatory screening procedures.

Originally published as a letter, *Lancet* (June 29, 1985): 1510.

However, more importantly, we believe that such monetary transactions corrupt and demean the relationship between the donor and the recipient, which should be one of altruism or charity. No matter how beneficial the payments may be in improving the ultimate wellbeing and standard of living of the donor and his family, we do not believe that there is a moral defense to the sale of a donor organ. For these reasons, The Transplantation Society and the British Transplantation Society agreed in 1983 to forbid their members to participate in the transplantation of any tissues where there had been any monetary exchange between donor and recipient, as indeed have several other national transplantation societies. We look to those statutory bodies concerned with the maintenance of high standards of medical practice in Britain to do the same.

24. Money Matters: Should Ability to Pay Ever Be a Consideration in Gaining Access to Transplantation?

R. W. Evans

Most of us have puzzled from time to time over the complex issues associated with the payment of organ transplantation procedures. We have all been exposed to various commentaries suggesting that organ transplants are too expensive given other health care needs.[1-3] In addition, we have been entertained by debates concerning the experimental or therapeutic status of various organ transplant procedures.[4] In this article, I direct my attention to a single question: Should the ability to pay be a condition for gaining access to transplantation?

To answer this question, I think we must address several specific issues: (1) the problem of the medically uninsured, (2) the development of insurance coverage policies, (3) current insurer coverage policies pertaining to transplant procedures, and (4) the views of the general public concerning access to transplantation.

THE HEALTH INSURANCE DILEMMA

Today it is estimated that 37 million, or 15.5 percent of the people in the United States, are uninsured.[5] Add to this another 26 or 27 million people who are underinsured. All told, therefore, as many as 64 million people are uninsured or underinsured. This means that at least 26.1 percent of the U.S. population is at risk of not having insurance coverage for a liver or heart transplant. Kidneys, of course, are covered for over 90 percent of all U.S. cit-

Originally published in *Transplantation Proceedings* 21, no. 3 (June 1989): 3419-23. Reprinted by permission of Appleton & Lange, Inc.

izens under provisions of Medicare's End-stage Renal Disease (ESRD) Program. Not surprisingly, the majority of transplant programs in the United States today require assurance of payment for transplantation before a patient becomes a candidate. Because of previous misadventures, hospitals recognize that significant losses are incurred when payment has not been properly assured. Clearly, Caplan's "green screen" is operational. A patient who is able to pay is more likely to get a transplant than one who is not.[6]

From the patient's perspective, the ability-to-pay factor is seemingly unfair. Why should an individual in need of accepted medical care be denied that care based on ability to pay? However, the transplant hospital also has a justifiable claim—its economic losses are significant if transplants are provided at no charge to medically needy, although financially indigent, recipients. To recover losses associated with unreimbursed transplants, hospitals are forced to increase their charges to other patients, thus giving rise to higher hospital operating costs, which, in turn, ultimately threaten the viability of the hospital in an increasingly competitive marketplace. Clearly, both the patient and the transplant hospital have legitimate claims, claims that often cast the insurance industry in a negative light. For example, providers and patients have bitterly chastised both public and private insurers for failing to pay for all transplants.

What should be recognized, however, is that ability to pay is a condition of access that characterizes all of medical care in a health care delivery system such as ours.[7] Transplantation is simply a specific example, more poignant only because of the immediacy of the life and death crisis. This is not to suggest that we ignore the problem because it is so complex, but only that we understand that to solve the particular problem we must address the general issue.

Several years ago the National Task Force on Organ Transplantation addressed the economic problems associated with transplantation. Concerning the equitable access to transplantation issue, the Task Force concluded that patient financial status should not limit the availability of transplantation.[8] It was recommended that all transplant procedures recognized as medically effective should be made available through reimbursement by existing public and private insurers.

The Task Force recommendations often are contrasted with those of the President's Commission for the Study of Ethical Problems in Medicine and Biomedical and Behavioral Research that stated, ". . . equitable access to health care requires that all citizens be able to secure an adequate level of health care without excessive burdens."[9] In response to this, the Task Force concluded that[8]:

> Although opinions may differ over what constitutes an "adequate level of care"
> and "excessive burdens," life-saving procedures that are comparable in cost and
> efficiency to other procedures that are routinely funded would seem to qualify.

Thus, at every juncture, the Task Force rejected the notion that ability to pay should obstruct access to transplantation.

Although I continue to support the remarkable findings, conclusions, and recommendations of the Task Force, I think we must be cognizant of the full implications of the recommendations. I am sympathetic to the concerns of both public and private insurers, as well as legislators, who must respond to sweeping recommendations that clearly go beyond the provision of transplantation services.[10] Moreover, the problems that insurers and legislators face are essentially problems that we as a society must face—specifically, what is the value of a human life, and how are we going to pay to both save and maintain it?[10,11]

COVERAGE POLICY AND MEDICAL INNOVATION

Organ transplantation ranks among the most significant of medical innovations in the past twenty years. However, as scientific advancements yield medical progress, payment becomes essential to clinical innovation and patient management. Where primary research terminates, clinical applications take over.[12,13] Basic research gradually takes a back seat to clinical research. Initially, what qualifies as patient treatment is indistinguishable from clinical research. Insurers who are concerned primarily with the treatment of patients are only moderately responsive to the needs of researchers. In short, insurers, private as well as public, are not in the business of funding either basic or clinical research. Consequently, as innovations occur, insurers make a careful evaluation in hopes of determining when an innovation has become sufficiently acceptable to qualify as treatment. Hence, the distinction between experimental procedures and therapeutic procedures.

Insurers typically distinguish between two concepts—coverage and reimbursement. Coverage refers to what insurers are willing to pay for, whereas reimbursement refers to the amount they are willing to pay for a service.[14,15] Elsewhere, I have described at length the development of coverage and reimbursement policy by public and private insurers for heart transplantation.[16]

There is no single source of information on which to base coverage determinations, and, as a result, the insurance community at times seems inconsistent in its policies. Some insurers may cover certain procedures, and others may not. Some insurers may invoke limitations of coverage; others may not. Ultimately, it becomes evident that insurance policies are not adjudicated and applied uniformly! As time passes, insurers may look to each others' policies in an effort to offer competitive benefits packages, but all this takes time. Moreover, for costly procedures, the coverage determination process can be very protracted, since no insurer looks forward to incurring sizable losses if premiums are insufficient to cover claims.

Fig 1. Conceptual overview of the coverage and reimbursement continuum.

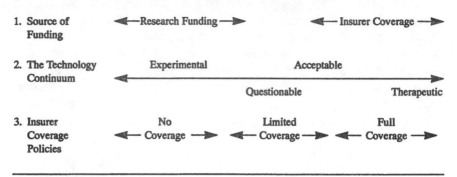

In Fig 1, I graphically summarize what I refer to as the coverage and reimbursement continuum—a composite of three overlapping continua. They are the source of funding continuum, the technology continuum, and the insurer coverage policies continuum. Along the technology continuum, I have imposed several adjectives to describe the status of a procedure or technology—experimental, questionable, acceptable, and therapeutic. As shown, experimental and questionable procedures are the subject of research funding, whereas insurer coverage is applied to acceptable and therapeutic procedures. Finally, specific coverage policies vary, but, in general, coverage is withheld for experimental procedures, whereas full coverage is made available for therapeutic procedures. For procedures that are questionable or acceptable, attention has begun to focus on limited coverage policies as a method by which insurers can ease the transition of technologies through the questionable and acceptable periods into the therapeutic stages.

COVERAGE OF ORGAN TRANSPLANTS

This discussion focuses on the specific coverage policies of Medicare, Medicaid, and private insurers. I begin with Medicare, given its dominant role in the development of coverage policy. I then proceed with a discussion of Medicaid programs and conclude with an analysis of the policies of private insurers.

Medicare

To qualify for Medicare, a person must meet at least one of the following conditions: (1) be age sixty-five or older, (2) be permanently disabled, or (3) have end-stage renal disease.[16] Given current patient selection criteria, few people age sixty-five and over qualify for Medicare coverage for extrarenal transplants. The majority of patients who qualify for Medicare coverage of heart transplants do so because of disability, although as patient selection criteria are relaxed, people age sixty-five and over could conceivably qualify for heart transplants.[17,18]

Medicare currently provides coverage for some kidney, heart, liver, and bone marrow transplants. The most liberal conditions of coverage apply to kidney transplants. Only the usual medical restrictions of the Medicare program apply, and benefits are available on an entitlement basis. In the case of heart transplantation, there are both patient and provider restrictions, and the benefits are not available as an entitlement. Liver transplant coverage is very restrictive and limited to children eighteen years of age and younger. In fact, the criteria are so restrictive that Medicare has yet to cover a single liver transplant. Finally, bone marrow transplants are covered, provided the patient has leukemia or aplastic anemia. Other medical restrictions also are applied, and benefits are not offered as an entitlement.

Medicaid

Medicaid coverage of organ transplant procedures is both inconsistent and unpredictable.[19] The definition of persons eligible for coverage varies by state. In general, eligibles fall into three categories: (1) the categorically needy, (2) the medically needy, and (3) state only coverage.[20] As these categories suggest, Medicaid coverage is not easily obtained. In 1984, approximately 8.2 percent of the population was covered by Medicaid, about 5.9 percent having Medicaid coverage alone.[21]

Data on Medicaid coverage of organ transplants have been collected periodically by the Intergovernmental Health Policy Project at George Washington University.[19] Table 1 summarizes these data for 1985, 1986, and 1988. As indicated, coverage varies according to transplant procedure, underscoring differences among state Medicaid officials concerning the therapeutic status of each procedure. Kidney transplants and bone marrow transplants are covered by the majority of states, mirroring Medicare coverage policies.

In the future, it is possible that Medicaid policies will change as states attempt to deal with growing Medicaid expenditures and a limited resource base. Both Arizona and Oregon have attempted to constrain Medicaid expenditures by eliminating coverage for selected organ transplant procedures, including heart, liver, and bone marrow transplants.[3]

Private Insurers

Private insurers fall into four major categories: (1) the Blue Cross and Blue Shield plans, (2) the commercial insurers, (3) health maintenance and pre-

Table 1. Medicaid Coverage of Transplants

Transplant procedures	Number of states covering		
	1985	1986	1988
Kidney transplants	48 + DC	48 + DC	50 + DC
Heart transplants	24 + DC	32 + DC	34 + DC
Liver transplants	32 + DC	40 + DC	42 + DC
Heart-lung transplants	13 + DC	15	20
Pancreas transplants	4 + DC	8	9
Bone marrow transplants	41 + DC	45 + DC	46 + DC

ferred provider organizations, and (4) self-insured plans. Few attempts have been made to canvass private insurers about their policies concerning organ transplant coverage.[8,22,23] Table 2 summarizes the results of survey data made available to the National Task Force on Organ Transplantation in 1985. Not surprisingly, liver and heart transplants were covered by many Blue Cross and Blue Shield plans and by many plans represented by the HIAA.

Virtually no data exist on the coverage policies of self-insured plans. Perhaps this is because coverage policies are tailored to meet the needs of specific employers. At any rate, there is simply no way of gauging how liberal or conservative such plans may be.

Clearly, the foregoing are rather old data, given the rapidity with which change has taken place among insurers. Today, it is likely that a larger percentage of private insurers cover both heart and liver transplants, although it is unlikely that there has been much change in coverage policies pertaining to heart-lung and pancreas transplants. Moreover, it is likely that HMOs continue to be fairly conservative in their coverage of transplants.

CONDITIONS OF ACCESS

Having now established that ability to pay is a very real concern of at least one in four Americans, it is worthwhile considering how the general public views the selection of transplant recipients.

In January 1987, the Battelle Human Affairs Research Centers was contracted by the United Network for Organ Sharing (UNOS) to conduct a national survey of Public Opinion Concerning Organ Donation, Procurement, and Distribution.[23,24] In an introduction to the survey, people were made aware of the fact that there were simply not enough donor organs to meet the need for transplantation. It is interesting to note that over 88.0 percent of the population agreed with the following statement:

Table 2. Private Insurer Coverage of Transplants

	Percent covered by transplant			
Insurer	**Heart**	**Liver**	**Heart-Lung**	**Pancreas**
Blue Cross and Blue Shield	80	84	72	53
Commercial Insurers (HIAA)	85	80	69	57
Group Health Association of America (HMOs)	30	74	23	18

(From references 11 and 33.)

> Regardless of how patients are selected for transplant operations, I am most concerned that donor organs are distributed as fairly and equally as possible.

Moreover, over 80.0 percent of the people surveyed agreed with the following statement:

> Medical need, not social or economic factors, should be the only criterion used to select transplant recipients.

Clearly, the public is very concerned about the process used to distribute donor organs, as well as the criteria used to select transplant recipients.

To assess more precisely public opinion concerning the use of a whole range of social criteria, we asked the following question in our survey:

> Recognizing there are not enough organs to go around, and difficult choices must be made in deciding who will get them, how strongly do you agree or disagree with each of the following statements?

The most significant criteria in order of importance are the following[24]:

Criterion	*% Agreeing*
Patient will survive and benefit	83.3
Patient able to return to work and regular activities	71.9
Sickest patients should have preference	71.1
Younger patients over older patients	56.8
US citizens over all other patients	51.7
People who live a "healthy" lifestyle	40.7
People who do not smoke	26.3
People who do not drink alcohol	19.4
People who can afford them	8.2
People with a religious background	5.4

It is obvious that people strongly object to the use of an economic criterion. Ability to pay is not viewed favorably. People seem to acknowledge some role for social criteria but no role for economic criteria in the selection of transplant recipients.

DISCUSSION

To what conclusion does the foregoing lead me? Should ability to pay ever be a consideration in gaining access to transplantation? In the final analysis, I think that one must be realistic and distinguish among three separate questions regarding ability to pay as an access barrier to transplantation: (1) Should ability to pay ever be a consideration in gaining access to transplantation? (2) Will ability to pay ever be a consideration in gaining access to transplantation? (3) Is ability to pay ever a consideration in gaining access to transplantation? The answer to the first question is an emphatic "No"! Since the answer to the third question is "Yes," the answer to question 2 is a foregone conclusion as well—"Yes." Let me elaborate.

First, I do not think that ability to pay should be an obstacle to transplant. I find the entire practice of rejecting patients for transplant based on their ability to pay distasteful, as well as morally and ethically wrong. In a nation such as ours, people deserve better. However, this brings me to my second point. Although accounting is inadequate, we know that some people are being denied access to transplantation because of their inability to pay. In this regard, I would suggest that our health care delivery system operates in an insidious manner, similar to the British system so well described by Aaron and Schwartz. In their book, *The Painful Prescription,* Aaron and Schwartz describe the delivery of dialysis in the United Kingdom.[25] They note that patients are simply not referred by general practitioners to nephrologists for dialysis if the patients are not considered to be suitable candidates (e.g., they may be too old). Thus, when a nephrologist is asked if they deny patients dialysis, their response is "No." However, the screening has already occurred at the level of the general practitioner without the knowledge of the nephrologist. By analogy, I suspect that some patients in the United States who could benefit from a heart or liver transplant are not referred to a transplant center by a cardiologist or hepatologist because of financial and insurance considerations, even if the patient could have benefited from a transplant. Other patients without the appropriate financial means who are referred are forced to engage in public fundraising efforts. Although the failure to refer a patient for transplant is deplorable and efforts to raise public funds an unacceptable solution, perhaps, oddly, the failure to refer is a more humane and publicly tasteful course of action.

Unfortunately, it is possible that more patients will be denied access to transplantation based on ability to pay. Gradually, legal concerns related to the failure to refer may lead physicians to make prompt referrals, even though a patient may lack the economic resources for transplantation. We know that more and more patients are being referred for transplant, since the waiting lists have grown. This will further increase the burden on transplant centers to make appropriate patient selections. However, as our data have shown, people do not readily accept discrimination based on economic factors.

As I have thought about the ability-to-pay issue, I remain puzzled. There is no clear-cut solution because the problem we face is generic to the delivery of health care services in the United States. Although one can argue that patients should have access to transplantation regardless of their ability to pay, their inability to pay creates special demands on the health care system that many other patients are unable to make. Is it fair to create a payment source for transplants that is not available to patients with other health care needs?

I recognize that patients who are well-insured and have considerable wealth have access to health services and providers to which other economically disadvantaged patients do not have access. For example, the local county hospital may not provide the same quality of health services as the private hospital frequented by the wealthy. Wealthy patients are free to pick and choose as they see fit, and it is ridiculous to assume that constraints can be imposed on their choice of providers simply to ensure that people have equal access to equal care.

Also, I wonder about parallels between access to transplantation and access to experimental and innovative therapy.[26,27] For example, cancer clinics are now operational that cater to the needs of patients who apparently have exhausted all therapeutic options and are willing to pay to receive experimental therapy. Clearly, indigent patients are not able to gain access to such services because they lack the financial resources. Is this unfair in the same way that denial of a transplant on economic grounds is unfair? Is the argument that donor organs are a public resource sufficiently persuasive to give everyone an equal claim to them?

Finally, I believe that innovation in health care is going to be threatened by restrictive coverage policies. Gradually, the focus of attention may not be on the coverage of procedures that are marginally therapeutic but on procedures that are effective yet costly. In effect, we are working the margins of what is an acceptable price to pay for effective medical care. For example, if a totally viable mass-produced artificial heart became available tomorrow, are we capable of generating the resources required to provide it to those patients in need? If we are not, I suspect that we are beginning to realize that life has a price, but one that is not worth paying, given limited resources. If this should be the case, perhaps we should better target our research and development efforts by proceeding with medical research (not medical care) that can be predicted a priori to be cost-effective. In other words, we should target for development those technologies that have the potential to save the most lives at the least cost. Following this approach, we would radically alter the scientific enterprise in the United States as we now know it. Grant research would be replaced by contract research, and basic research would take a back seat to applied research.

Ultimately, I must say that I am hard-pressed to justify economic discrimination in access to transplantation.[28] Yet at the same time, I am sympathetic to the concerns of both public and private insurers, as well as those who argue that at some point we must draw a line with regard to the level of medical care that we can provide, given competing health and social needs.[29-33] If the public insists that everyone should have equal access to transplantation, it must also recognize that this cannot be accomplished without increasing health care expenditures. To meet these rising expenditures, the public must be willing to live with increased taxes to fund public insurance programs or higher insurance premiums to fund private insurance benefits. Since most private insurance is provided as an employer benefit, employees may be faced with higher deductibles and copayments. Alternatively, employees may negotiate for better health benefits and lower wage increases. In the end, it is apparent that we all pay one way or another and that insurers essentially serve as prudent stewards of the resources they command on behalf of the individuals they represent.

We must ask ourselves what are we willing to pay in order to avoid making decisions about medical treatment based on an ability-to-pay criterion. Elsewhere, I have argued that the ESRD Program came into existence as a mechanism by which to avoid the problems attendant to the selection of dialysis patients.[34] By making more funds available, the same approach could be used to resolve the transplant dilemma. It appears, however, that our actions are beginning to speak louder than our words—we seem willing to deny people access to treatment, given recent health care policy decisions, even though we claim that economics should not be a consideration in determining who gains access to transplantation.

REFERENCES

1. Englehardt HT: *N Engl J Med* 311:66, 1984.

2. Baily MA: In: Mathieu D (ed): *Organ Substitution Technology.* Boulder, CO, Westview Press, p 198, 1988.

3. Welch HG, Larson EB: *N Engl J Med* 319:171, 1988.

4. Evans RW: *Issues Sci Technol* 2:91, 1986.

5. Short PF, Monheit A, Beauregard K: *Uninsured Americans: A 1987 profile.* Paper presented at the Annual Meetings of the American Public Health Association in Boston, MA. November 13-18, 1988.

6. Caplan AL: *Circulation* 75:10, 1987.

7. Aday LA, Flemming GV, Anderson R: *Access to Medical Care in the U.S.: Who Has It, Who Doesn't.* Chicago, Pluribus Press for the University of Chicago, 1984.

8. National Task Force on Organ Transplantation: *Organ Transplantation: Issues and Recommendations.* Rockville, MD, Office of Organ Transplantation, Health Resources and Services Administration, Department of Health and Human Services, 1986.

9. President's Commission for the Study of Ethical Problems in Medicine and Biomedical and Behavioral Research: *Securing Access to Health Care.* Washington, DC, U.S. Government Printing Office, 1983.

10. Health Insurance Association of America: *Organ Transplants and Their Implications for the Health Insurance Industry.* Washington DC, Public Relations Division, HIAA, 1985.

11. Evans RW: In: Ginzberg E (ed): *Medicine and Society: Clinical Decisions and Societal Values.* Boulder, CO, Westview Press, p 61, 1987.

12. McKinlay JB: *Milbank Mem Fund* Q 59:374, 1981.

13. Chalmers TC: *N Engl J Med* 319:1228, 1988.

14. Schaeffer LD: In: McNeil BJ, Cravalho EG (eds): *Critical Issues in Medical Technology.* Boston, MA, Auburn House Publishing, 1982.

15. Greenberg B, Derzon RA: *Med Care* 19:967, 1981.

16. Evans RW: *Int J Technol Assessment Health Care* 2:425, 1986.

17. Olivari MT, Antolick A, Kaye MP, et al: *J Heart Transplant* 7:258, 1988.

18. Miller LW, Vitale-Noedel N, Pennington G, et al: *J Heart Transplant* 7:254, 1988.

19. Intergovernmental Health Policy Project: *Medicaid Coverage and Payment Policies for Organ Transplants: A Fifty State Review.* Washington, DC, George Washington University, 1985.

20. Gornick M, Greenberg JN, Eggers PW, et al: *Care Financing Review 1985 Annual Supplement,* p 13. Washington, DC, US Government Printing Office, 1985.

21. Wilensky GR: *Health Affairs* 7:133, 1988.

22. Hellinger FJ: *Int J Technol Assessment Health Care* 2:563, 1986.

23. Evans RW, Manninen DL: *Transplant Proc* 20:781, 1988.

24. Evans RW, Manninen DL: *Public Opinion Concerning Organ Donation, Procurement, and Distribution: Results of a National Probability Sample Survey.* Seattle, WA, Battelle Human Affairs Research Centers, 1987.

25. Aaron JH, Schwartz WB: *The Painful Prescription: Rationing Hospital Care.* Washington, DC, The Brookings Institution, 1984.

26. Antman K, Schnipper LE, Frei E III: *N Engl J Med* 319:46, 1988.

27. Goldworth A: *Hastings Cent Rep* 17:8, 1987.

28. Monaco AP: *Transplantation* 43:1, 1987.

29. Evans RW: *JAMA* 249:2047, 1983.

30. Evans RW: *JAMA* 249:2208, 1983.

31. Colen BD: *Hard Choices: Mixed Blessings of Modern Medical Technology.* New York, Putnam, 1986.

32. Daniels N: *N Engl J Med* 314:1380, 1986.

33. Daniels N: *N Engl J Med* 315:1297, 1986.

34. Evans RW, Blagg CR, Bryan FA Jr: *JAMA* 245:487, 1981.

25. Comment: Ability to Pay and Access to Transplantation

Norman Daniels

Ability to pay now is and probably will remain a factor determining access to transplantation, as Evans shows.[1] In this article, I address the following moral issues: (1) Is ability to pay a morally acceptable criterion for rationing health care services in general? (2) Is it either more or less acceptable to ration transplantation by ability to pay than other health care services?

I agree with Evans that, in general, distributing health care by ability to pay is unjust. As I argue elsewhere,[2,3] health care (I include nonmedical health services) is of special moral importance. Its function is to maintain, restore, and compensate for losses of normal species functioning, and departures from normal functioning have a significant impact on the range of opportunities open to an individual. Since a society is just only if it assures fair equality of opportunity, health care systems should be designed so that they optimally protect opportunity, given the limits of resources and technology. This fair equality of opportunity account implies that there should be no discriminatory barriers to whatever system of services optimally protects opportunity. Still, individuals have rights or entitlements only to those services that are part of the design of such a system. They do not have rights to any or every technology that can in some way provide them with a benefit. Rather, technologies must be assessed before being incorporated in a system so that we include only these services that optimally protect opportunity, given fixed or reasonable limits on resources.

When ability to pay determines access to effective medical treatments, the distribution of opportunity depends in an unacceptable way on inequalities in wealth and income. We should not, then, ration health care in general by ability

Originally published in *Transplantation Proceedings* 21, no. 3 (June 1989): 3424-25. Reprinted by permission of Appleton & Lange, Inc.

to pay—yet we do! The fact that our system is, in general, unjust complicates what we should say about access to transplantation in particular. Is the special concern we often hear about economic barriers to transplantation warranted? Is transplantation exceptional? Is rationing transplantation by ability to pay either more or less acceptable than so rationing other health care services?

Two arguments suggest that it is even worse to ration transplantation by ability to pay than some other medical technologies. The first is the claim that there is an inconsistency between encouraging the free, public donation of organs and then allowing only those who can pay to get them. This point has some initial plausibility, but it is ultimately not persuasive. For one thing, much of the rest of the body of medical knowledge and technology is the result of public support and subsidy, so, despite public donation, organs are not really that exceptional. If we should not ration organs by ability to pay because they are a public resource, we should not ration much else in health care that we do so ration.

A second problem with this argument is that there is nothing strictly inconsistent about asking for free, public donations of organs that will benefit only some people, namely, those who can pay for the costs of having them implanted. The poor have less access than the rich to many of the goods in the common domain. Many of our public parks, for example, are open only to those who pay the fees and can afford to drive or fly to them. Moreover, we have at least some reason for accepting public gifts even under these conditions. Suppose our only choices were (1) to ask for no public donation of organs because we could only make them available to those who could pay or (2) to ask for them knowing that they will go only to those who can pay. We would do more good than harm by at least getting them to those who can buy them and benefit from them. Maybe we should insist on equality of access, but it may cost us in aggregate use to do so. I think what is troublesome here is not the public nature of the organs nor that we encourage a gift that some will not be eligible to receive, but the consequences of the inequality of access, and that is a different point.

A second argument for thinking that rationing transplantation by ability to pay is less acceptable than rationing other health care services turns on the high visibility of denials of transfers. Perhaps more than with other medical services, explicit rationing by ability to pay affects identified rather than merely statistical victims. We face the child in the well with the cameras running, not the invisible teenage mother who fails to receive prenatal maternal care. (In her case, we prefer to wait for her low birthweight child, now an identified victim, to show up in our neonatal intensive care unit!) Although there is some symbolic value to pouring resources into rescuing identified, visible victims, and it is brutalizing for us not to do so, I have never heard an argument that shows me that it is morally correct to prefer the consequences of pricing the value of life of identified victims higher than that of statistical victims. Indeed, depending on perspective, we can easily convert one kind of victim into the other. Finally, there seems to be something especially hypocritical about refusing to ration by ability to pay for identified, poor victims yet doing so all the time for the many more invisible ones. "Out of sight, out of mind" is hardly a fundamental moral principle.

One important argument might incline us to think transplantation is exceptional in the other direction, that is, that it might be better to ration by ability to pay for transplants than for other kinds of health care. The primary reasons for thinking transplants exceptional in this way have to do with their (1) very high costs and (2) problematic opportunity costs. Compared to many other medical treatments (though not all, as Evans argues[1]), transplants deliver a significant benefit to relatively few people at relatively high cost. More to the point, transplant technologies tend to fall at the high end of the opportunity-cost scale: the health care dollars spent on transplantations could be more effectively used to promote normal functioning and thus opportunity in other ways.

It is just this point that apparently motivated Oregon to adopt its policy of noncoverage for transplants. This policy choice rests on the belief that Oregon can do more for the health status of Medicaid recipients by funding services other than transplants, given politically imposed limits on state spending. Their policy seems to rest on this claim: it is better to accept the (visible) inequality of access between Medicaid patients denied transplants and others who can pay for them than it is to accept the even greater (but invisible) inequality that results when Medicaid pays for transplants but fails to provide other, more cost-effective services. In effect, the policy says that it is better to ration transplants by the ability to pay than it is to ration more cost-effective services by ability to pay, given that we have to ration something by ability to pay.

Dividing cases will help us think about this argument.

CASE ONE

Suppose the health care system is otherwise just: it does not ration by ability to pay, and it effectively allocates resources to promote fair equality of opportunity (i.e., we are not talking about Oregon). Suppose that adding transplants would mean adding a technology beyond the resource limits of the sphere of social obligation. Then transplantation is a technology to which people do not have clear entitlements. Is it permissible to allow transplants on an ability to pay basis? If we believed that no economic inequalities should exist that would enable some people to buy more health care than others, we could tax away any ability to buy transplants. If we accept significant economic inequalities, however, it is hard to see why we should prohibit people from purchasing transplants, e.g., through a deluxe insurance scheme, given that we are meeting our social obligations to protect opportunity, unless this private sphere undermined the public sphere of health care delivery.[2]

Nevertheless, I want to protect the principle that ability to pay should not be a criterion for rationing services that have some impact on opportunity. Consequently, I would advocate a cross-subsidy in this private sphere to create an insurance pool for those who could not afford the deluxe insurance (we might also insure children against the imprudence of their parents). We might then let those adults appeal to charity who could have purchased the insurance but did not want to. Still, this is a high price for imprudence.

CASE TWO

This is the real world case, at least in the United States. Ability to pay is a rationing criterion, and resource allocation does not optimally protect opportunity. Should we accept the inequality involved in rationing transplants by ability to pay in order to reduce the inequalities that result from other ability to pay rationing, as in Oregon? Or should we refuse in principle to ration transplants by ability to pay? The correct answer depends on what the effects of the choice we make will be. Specifically, do we reduce injustice in the system as a whole? If our visible affirmation of the principle that it is wrong to ration transplants by ability to pay leads to more general elimination of such rationing elsewhere in the system, we should stand by the principle, contra Oregon. If allowing the rationing of transplants by ability to pay reduces the need elsewhere in the system for more damaging forms of such rationing, or if it brings public protest that increases funding for Medicaid or brings even more substantial reform of the system, the Oregon policy may be acceptable. What is not acceptable, however, is to insist that we should not ration by ability to pay when the only consequence of such scruples is that we turn a blind eye to even more damaging inequalities in access to beneficial services. Such selective appeal to principle is not appeal to principle at all.

REFERENCES

1. Evans R: *Transplant Proc* 21:1989.
2. Daniels N: *Just Health Care.* Cambridge, Cambridge University Press, 1985.
3. Daniels N: *Am I My Parents' Keeper? An Essay on Justice Between the Young and Old.* New York, Oxford University Press, 1988.

PART FOUR

Allocation and Rationing

In light of the great shortage of transplantable organs in the United States, the transplant community has been faced with many seemingly unanswerable questions. In the first chapters of this book, we looked at supply-side questions of organ procurement; from whom can we retrieve organs? and How can we maximize the efficiency of organ collection? Yet, some of the most complex issues in transplantation ethics surround the distribution and allocation of the organs that are available. The resolution of the terrifying dilemma of who lives and who dies when shortage is a reality is an omnipresent ethical challenge in transplantation. It also means that transplantation has much to teach about how Americans respond to situations where rationing is inevitable as well as about how we might defend certain policies and practices when not all lives can be saved.

Two prevailing principles of organ distribution divide the transplant community. The first, maximize efficiency, would favor recipients for whom a transplant would ensure the highest chance of living a long and high quality life. The second, urgency of need, favors allocating organs to those who are the sickest and most likely to die. Both systems represent ethical positions but they lead to very different consequences in terms of who ultimately would live. Those who are younger, relatively healthier, have fewer complicating diseases and conditions and who have not undergone a transplant would be favored by a policy driven by efficiency in the use of donor organs. Those who are older, are at death's door due to the failure of a previous transplant or artificial organ or even a previous xenograft would go to the head of the waiting list on a policy sensitive to medical urgency and patient need.

Our current system relies more on medical urgency then it does efficacy—a system supported by members of the Pittsburgh Transplant Institute.

247

They doubt that the data exists to enable physicians to predict who will do well with a transplant and believe that it would be immoral for doctors not to try and rescue those in the most dire straits. Furthermore, they cite a long tradition in medicine of not abandoning patients no matter how sick or ill they may be thereby justifying a strong allegiance to the "urgency of need" model. However, Peter Ubel and colleagues concluded that the urgency of need model is unfair for recipient selection. They examined the balance between urgency and efficiency in their analysis of retransplantation: transplants for patients whose prior transplants failed. This was done by examining three differences between primary transplantation and retransplantation: (1) the obligations that transplant teams feel not to abandon transplanted patients, (2) the fairness of allowing some individuals to have multiple transplants while other individuals die waiting for a chance at a first transplant, and (3) the differences in medical efficacy between primary transplants and multiple transplants. They state that given the shortage of organs, a moral duty exists to save the most lives with reasonable quality and this points toward a policy based on efficacy and not medical urgency.

In addition to retransplantation, there are a host of other factors that many believe should be considered in organ allocation. Currently, only blood and tissue type, urgency of the patient's condition, time spent on the waiting list, and distance between the donor and the transplant center are supposed to be considered. However, what if a patient is directly responsible for his or her organ failure? What if a person has abused drugs or alcohol and thereby caused organ failure? What if they smoke or are morbidly obese or have a criminal record? What role does fault play in the allocation of scarce resources?

Fault takes on a whole new dynamic when considering end-stage liver disease, a condition principally caused by alcoholism. Alvin Moss and Mark Siegler propose that patients who develop end-stage liver disease through no fault of their own should have higher priority for receiving a liver transplant than those with end-stage liver disease resulting from failure to obtain treatment for alcoholism. The authors justify their position by asserting that transplanting alcoholics may actually lead to a decrease in the overall supply of organs available for transplant since the public may become angry at treating those who abuse themselves as equals to those who lead healthy lifestyles but become sick through no fault of their own. In response to Moss and Siegler's article, Carl Cohen and Martin Benjamin conclude that there are no good reasons, either moral or medical, precluding alcoholics as candidates for liver transplantation. They dismiss the arguments used against transplanting livers into alcoholics by asserting that alcoholics are not morally blameworthy and can exhibit satisfactory rates of post-transplant survival.

Despite beliefs to the contrary, the rich and famous do not get preferential treatment with respect to access to organ transplantation when they are on waiting lists. Such practice would contradict the fundamental principle held by the medical community that physicians distribute treatment based solely on potential medical benefits without regard to nonmedical factors. While it is true that only those who can pay or have insurance are put on waiting lists in the United States, once listed, physicians try to allocate organs with little attention to wealth or social standing. However, is it ever justified for a society to say that not all people on waiting lists are equal. If a president or a senator or a distinguished scientist were to need an organ should they be considered by the same standards as convicted felons; a population that many believe forfeited their entitlement to the same level of medical care simply by being convicted of a serious crime. Lawrence J. Schneidermann and Nancy S. Jecker believe this to be true, especially when considering dire organ shortages.

It is not always obvious what is fair when allocating scarce medical resources. Our desire to rescue the sick conflicts with our desire to do the greatest good for the greatest number of persons with scarce resources. Our moral drive to treat all persons as equally worthy is challenged when persons with a history of drug abuse, criminal activity, or antisocial behavior are pitted against others in the competition for scarce organs. It is not even clear how to weigh factors such as mental illness, disability, and impairment into the equation if quality of life as well as quantity of life are to be factors in deciding who should live and who should die. In transplantation there is no avoiding these issues because scarcity is a simple fact of day-to-day life. In making life-and-death decisions, whatever they are, it is imperative that we be clear, consistent, and honest about the basis for them if they are to secure continued professional and public support.

Arthur L. Caplan
Daniel H. Coelho

26. Prioritization and Organ Distribution for Liver Transplantation

Oscar Bronsther, John J. Fung,
Andreas Izakis, David Van Thiel,
and Thomas E. Starzl

The current policies for cadaver kidney distribution were recently discussed in *The Journal*.[1] Questions about liver allocation are even more important, because there is not the option of artificial organ support.[2] Two principles of liver deployment have been advocated: efficiency of organ use and urgency of need.

THE EFFICIENCY PRINCIPLE

Single Disease Studies

Primary Biliary Cirrhosis

Patients with this disease have been stratified retrospectively into low-, medium-, and high-risk categories, and their actual survival after liver transplantation has been compared with the outcome expected without such intervention.[3] This comparison depended on a Mayo hazard prediction model of the natural history of primary biliary cirrhosis (Table 1).[4] Before the National Institutes of Health Consensus Development Conference of 1983,[5] we reserved liver transplantation candidacy for patients with chronic disease whose life expectancy was a few months.[6] The effect of this restrictive policy could be seen in liver recipients' treated for primary biliary cirrhosis between March 1980 and June 1987. Even in the low-risk group, the bilirubin level

---

Originally published in *JAMA* 271, no. 2 (January 12, 1994): 140-43.

Table 1.—Mayo Cox Proportional Hazard Model for Primary Biliary Cirrhosis*

Risk Factor	Low	Middle	High
Age, y	47	49	54
Bilirubin, μmol/L (mg/dL)	205 (12)	410 (12)	480 (28)
Albumin, g/L	30	27	25
Prothrombin time, s	13.5	15	20
Edema score	0.4	0.8	0.9

*From Markus et al.[3]

averaged 205 μmol/L (12 mg/dL), and in the high-risk group, it averaged 480 μmol/L (28 mg/dL). All three cohorts had hypoalbuminemia (Table 1).

The 75 percent one-year patient survival rate after transplantation was a 30 percentage point gain over the 45 percent rate predicted with medical treatments Because one-year survival rates were 83 percent, 75 percent, and 58 percent in the low-, medium-, and high-risk categories, respectively, the results have been used to demonstrate the inefficient use of organs when they are transplanted to high-risk recipients. Viewed from a different perspective, the gain of survival in the first postoperative year relative to projected outcome without transplantation was actually highest (58 percentage points) in the high-risk patients, next highest (55 percentage points) in the medium-risk group, and lowest (only 14 percentage points) in the low-risk group, whose one-year survival rate without intervention would have been 69 percent (Fig 1). The life survival slope and degree of rehabilitation after one year were the same in all groups.[5]

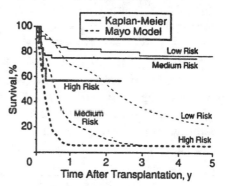

Fig 1.—Actual (Kaplan-Meier) survival after transplantation and estimated survival without transplantation (Mayo model) in patients with primary biliary cirrhosis at low, medium, and high risk (from Markus et al.[3]).

Sclerosing Cholangitis

Similar but more pronounced trends were seen with sclerosing cholangitis[7] using a second Mayo hazard prediction model that factored in age, bilirubin level, splenomegaly, and histopathologic stage.[8] The gain in one-year survival rate with transplantation vs the predicted outcome without this procedure was only 7 percentage points in low-risk cases, a gain relative to the sur-

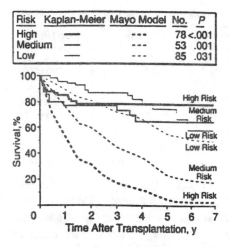

Fig 2.—Actual (Kaplan-Meier) survival after transplantation and estimated survival without transplantation (Mayo model) in patients with primary sclerosing cholangitis at low, medium, and high risk (from Abu-Elmagd et al.[7]).

rogate control that did not increase in the succeeding seven years (Fig 2). In the medium-risk patients, the one-year survival dividend from transplantation was zero, but this steadily increased thereafter. In contrast, the high-risk group achieved a stunning 40 percentage point life survival gain by twelve months, an improvement that had grown to nearly 80 percentage points at seven years, by which time all patients without transplantation were long since projected dead. By seven years, the best absolute survival rate belonged to the patients who originally had been the most ill (Fig 2).

Heterogeneous Diseases: Risk Factors and Cost

At the New England Medical Center, Boston, Mass, 124 adults and children who had a full spectrum of diagnoses and medical urgency were given 142 livers between 1984 and 1992. These cases illustrated the relationship between the severity of pretransplant illness, patient survival, and cost of treatment.[9] Urgency of need was determined with the five-tier scale (called the United Network for Organ Sharing [UNOS] score) that was used nation-

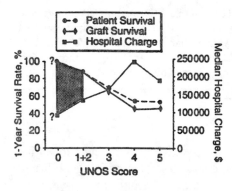

Fig 3.—Survival rates and costs after liver transplantation by United Network for Organ Sharing (UNOS) severity score at the New England Medical Center, Boston, Mass. UNOS severity score: (1) working, (2) at home (many still working) but requiring close medical supervision and/or sporadic hospital care, (3) hospital-bound continuously, or most of the time, (4) in the intensive care unit, usually with ventilator support, and (5) UNOStat, a life expectancy of only a few days without transplantation, often because of fulminant hepatic failure. The "zone of absurdity" (shaded area) has been added to illustrate the folly of going too far toward the use of liver transplantation for clinically well patients (data from Muto et al.[9]).

Table 2.—Kamofsky Scores by Risk Stratification, 1 Year After Transplantation*

Risk Stratification†	Karnofsky Score
Blue Cross/Blue Shield	
Elective patients	82
High-risk patients	82
APACHE II	
Elective patients	82
High-risk patients	82
UNOS score	
1	85
2	83
3	79
4	83
UNOStat	84

*Data obtained from Muto et al.[9]

†APACHE II indicates Acute Physiology and Chronic Health Evaluation II; and UNOS, United Network for Organ Sharing.[3]

ally through 1990 (see legend of Fig 3). UNOS 1 and 2 candidates (the least ill) had the highest rates of posttransplant survival (Fig 3). The poorest results were with the UNOS 4 and 5 recipients. However, the rescue of the majority of these patients whose expected survival was essentially zero without transplantation was at least as noteworthy as the fact that the survival curve was degraded by their admission into candidacy. The cost of caring for the UNOS 4 and 5 recipients was high, reaching nearly $250,000 and $190,000 per case, respectively, including the expenditures before transplantation, which can exceed the expenses afterward.

Poorer and more expensive results also were evident when the high-risk patients were identified using the criteria of the Blue Cross/Blue Shield consortium or using the APACHE II (Acute Physiology and Chronic Health Evaluation) score, which expresses pretransplantation need for intensive care.[9] No matter how sick the patients were before transplantation or how high the risk, however, those who lived (the majority in every subgroup) and were tested one year later had the same degree of rehabilitation, as determined by Karnofsky scores, which were satisfactory in all groups (Table 2).

Transplantation versus Options

The fact that extremely sick patients or those with ancillary risk factors have a reduced survival rate after liver transplantation has been used to decry their treatment. The extrapolation of this logic (Fig 3) could be the absurd recommendation that only asymptomatic (well) candidates be offered this service because they will yield predictably good life survival curves and generate

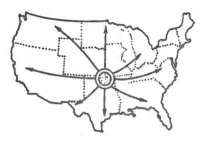

Fig 4.—The United Network for Organ Sharing distribution policy in effect from November 1987 through 1990. This policy emphasized local primacy of organ use but with national distribution thereafter on the basis of urgency (see text). Beginning in 1991, the system was denationalized, wtih each of the 11 United Network for Organ Sharing regions (indicated by broken lines) having the first option to use livers before their release into a national organ pool.

small bills. However, for low-risk patients who still have adequate or restorable liver function, there often are other, safer treatment options short of transplantation.

For example, patients with autoimmune hepatitis frequently are referred as "liver transplant candidates" at a time when consideration of transplantation can be delayed for long periods by treatment with immunosuppression.[10] Henderson et al.[11] recently emphasized the neglected use of distal splenorenal shunt (Warren procedure) for patients with cirrhosis whose principal complication was variceal hemorrhage. The three- and five-year survival rates in this series of patients who still had good (Child's A) or fair (Child's B) parenchymal function were superior to those of the generally sicker transplant recipients (predominantly Child's C) at the same institution, at less than one fourth the cost. The quality-of-life scores one year after both operations were essentially the same.

THE URGENCY PRINCIPLE

A Field Trial (1987 Through 1990)

With the national liver distribution system that was in effect from November 1987 through 1990, livers obtained in a given area could be used locally without regard for urgency status. However, organs not used locally were freely shipped to wherever they were most badly needed (Fig 4). The distribution system used by UNOS was the same as one developed and tested in Pittsburgh, Pa, in the mid-1980s.[12] A report of this field trial was used verbatim in writing the UNOS contract that became operational on October 1, 1987. The plan had two explicit objectives. One was to increase the incentive for organ donation by giving first priority to community recipients. The second was to allow new liver transplant teams to establish credibility by preferentially treating low-risk recipients while referring their gravely ill patients or those with complicated conditions to established programs.

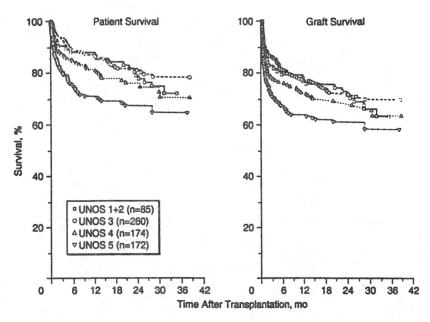

Fig 5.—Patient and graft survival following primary orthotopic liver transplantation in adults, stratified by pre-1991 United Network for Organ Sharing (UNOS) risk categories. The difference between patient and graft survival is accounted for by successful retransplantation.

Transplantation Results During Study

During the last 18 months of this allocation policy, 691 consecutive adult primary liver transplantations were carried out in Pittsburgh. The assessment of treatment efficacy was important in these cases, because two significant improvements had a potential impact on high-risk and all other patients: (1) use of University of Wisconsin (UW) solution beginning in 1988, which extended the safe time of liver preservation from six hours to eighteen to twenty-four hours,[13,14] and (2) use of the immunosuppressive drug, FK 506, which could be used for either primary or rescue treatment.[15]

As expected, the best results were in the low-risk recipients. Few in number (n=12 [1.7 percent]), those in UNOS class 1 survived for one year at a rate of 91 percent; those in combined classes 1 and 2 at 88 percent; those in class 5 (UNOStat [a life expectancy of only a few days without transplantation, often because of fulminant hepatic failure]) at 71 percent; and those in classes 3 and 4 at rates in between (Fig 5, left). The incidence of retransplantation was approximately the same in all cohorts, although it was less frequently successful in the sickest patients, as reflected in the graft survival curve (Fig 5, right). The crucial observation was that the gap in results with

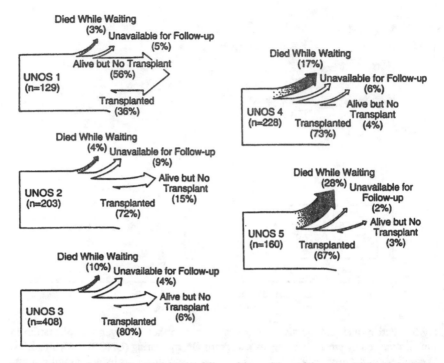

Fig 6.—Increasing incidence of death while waiting with each increase of the United Network for Organ Sharing (UNOS) entry score of liver transplant candidates. The percentage of patients alive who had not received transplants decreased with increasing UNOS score.

different urgency classes had narrowed to the point of nonsignificance except for the UNOStat group, which trailed the low-risk groups by 17 percent. Still, 71 percent of even this highest-risk cohort was alive at one year. After one year, the decline in survival rates was the same in all groups.

Candidate Stability by UNOS Scare

The case flow after evaluation is summarized in Fig 6. At the end of the first year, more than half (56 percent) of the patients who had entered as UNOS 1 candidates remained at this status, while 3 percent had died. As the risk level at entry increased from UNOS 1 to UNOS 3, the population of patients who had transplantations increased, frequently precipitated by worsening status and reclassification. The death rate while waiting was 10 percent for UNOS 3 patients and escalated to 17 percent for UNOS 4 patients and 28 percent for UNOS 5 patients (Fig 6). Of interest, 27 (3.4 percent) of the 796 patients in UNOS categories 3 through 5 improved enough with medical management to leave the hospital. These recoveries were dominated by patients with the entry diagnosis of fulminant hepatic failure.

Termination of Trial

These recipients, including those who were gravely ill at entry or whose condition deteriorated while waiting, could be treated efficiently because of the emphasis on urgency of patient need and the national donor reservoir designed to meet this need. This was changed when a directive from UNOS, effective January 1, 1991, created a functional confederacy in the United States of eleven regions from which the free national movement of organs was discouraged in favor of elective regional use. Urgency of need at a national level was removed as the most pervasive internal principle of the American organ allocation framework.

CONSEQUENCES OF THE UNOS RULES CHANGE

Loss of Patient Choice

Factors that preclude candidacy at any given center, such as age, technical or medical complexity, or advanced illness, frequently are not contraindications in other centers to which rejected candidates can go for a second opinion. Under the new system, such patients no longer have easy access to a national reservoir of organs after leaving their region. Even livers donated in their home community encounter an administrative barrier at the regional boundary. This significantly impairs patient choice of center.

A particularly troubling example of organ flow restriction developed in the Veterans Affairs hospitals, among which two liver transplantation centers were designated to which referrals from all fifty states were directed. Most of the organs available to the veterans, however, were expected to come from the local procurement areas in which the national veteran centers were placed.

Loss of Dispersal Autoregulation

Because urgency of need was a magnet for organs not used electively in their local procurement areas, allocation until 1991 tended to be autoregulatory. Urgent cases surfaced most frequently in centers where large numbers of patients waited and drifted toward greater illness, as described above. It was a patient-driven system. The new system is center-driven, in that the administrative control of a liver has become as much of a factor as the medical indication in recipient selection.

Proliferation of Centers

The development of new centers, which had proceeded in an orderly manner before 1991, turned into a stampede, particularly in organ-rich regions. The concern of existing programs that had been focused on preventing organs from leaving their region was superseded by the threat to their organ supply posed by new teams nearby. In this competitive interface, a syndrome of entry triage was encouraged when government agencies established minimum life survival curves as a measure of medical competence, without an attempt to stratify disease severity using the criteria of UNOS, Blue Cross/Blue Shield, APACHE II, or some other system.

The consequence of denying candidacy to sick patients or those with complicated conditions by the argument of "inefficient organ use" cannot be assessed from the data accrued in this recent period and used in 1993 congressional hearings to defend the probity of current allocation practices. Because many such patients die without being listed, the numbers reported as "died while waiting" are understated. Omitted from the record are patients who were not permitted to wait so that organs could be used for elective recipients. Except for those who are medically sophisticated or wealthy, such disenfranchised potential candidates can neither find treatment within nor escape from their regions. The result has been uneven quality of and access to liver transplantation throughout the United States. This heterogeneity also applies to the standards used for donor acceptance in different regions.

Effect on Donor Procurement

A predictable sobering consequence will be shrinkage of the donor pool. Livers with minor functional or anatomic imperfections or from older donors will be systematically discarded and never offered from regions with an excess of donor organs where recipient candidacy is limited to elective patients. Even if they were procured, organs pronounced not good enough to be used locally would be accepted reluctantly elsewhere.

CONCLUSIONS

Liver transplantation services should be offered at hepatology centers where the requisite medical support and hepatobiliary surgical procedures are also available. In individual cases, it is necessary first to determine whether a meaningful quality of life can be restored using a full armamentarium of therapeutic options, second to decide in what setting health care can best be provided, and third to establish the degree of urgency.

With nonhepatic or hepatic disease, we do not ordinarily pronounce the condition of a patient to be hopeless when it is merely grave and then withhold or impede treatment under the pretense that it would be better invested in patients who are less ill. If patient need dictates liver allograft flow from a national reservoir rather than allowing this to be center-driven, with piecemeal policies from region to region, the national liver graft shortage may not be as great as we repeatedly tell one another. Even if it is, our activities will be self-regulated in a genuinely ethical order.

Part of the self-regulation will involve wise decisions about what constitutes a hopeless condition. Such judgments presumably would be most discriminating in centers of excellence where they are made and audited frequently with direct knowledge of the needs of other candidates. Otherwise, livers could be wasted by being transplanted into moribund recipients who have no chance of recovery or, alternatively, into candidates who do not need this drastic therapy.

REFERENCES

1. Gaston RS, Ayres I, Dooley LG, Diethelm AG. Racial equity in renal transplantation: the disparate impact of HLA-based allocation. *JAMA*. 1993;270:1352-1356.

2. Delmonico FL, Jenkins RL, Freeman R, et al. The high-risk liver allograft recipient: should allocation policy consider outcome? *Arch Surg*. 1992;127:579-584.

3. Markus B, Dickson ER, Grambsch P, et al. Efficacy of liver transplantation in patients with primary biliary cirrhosis. *N Engl J Med*. 1989;320:1709-1713.

4. Dickson ER, Grambsch PM, Flening TR, Fisher LD, Langworthy A. Prognosis in primary biliary cirrhosis: model for decision making. *Hepatology*. 1989;10:1-7.

5. National Institutes of Health Consensus Development Conference on Liver Transplantation. *Hepatology*. 1984;4(suppl):1S-110S.

6. Starzl TE, Iwatsuki S, Van Thiel DH, et al. Evolution of liver transplantation. *Hepatology*. 1982; 2:614-636.

7. Abu-Elmagd K, Malinchoc M, Dickson ER, et al. Efficacy of liver transplantation in patients with primary sclerosing cholangitis. *Surg Gynecol Obstet*. 1993;177:335-344.

8. Dickson ER, Murtaugh PA, Grambsch PM, et al. Primary sclerosing cholangitis: refinement and validation of survival model *Gastroenterology*. 1992; 103:1893-1901.

9. Muto P, Freeman RB, Haug CE, Lu A, Rohrer RJ. Liver transplant candidate stratification systems: implications for third-party payors and organ allocation. *Transplantation*. In press.

10. Van Thiel D, Wright H, Carroll P, et al. FK 506: a treatment for autoimmune chronic active hepatitis: results of an open label preliminary trial. *Am J Gastroenterol*. 1994;57:306-308.

11. Henderson JM, Gilmore GT, Hooks MA, et al. Selective shunt in the management of variceal bleeding in the era of liver transplantation. *Ann Surg*. 1992;216:248-255.

12. Starzl TE, Gordon RD, Tzakis A, et al. Equitable allocation of extrarenal organs: with special reference to the liver. *Transplant Proc*. 1988;20(suppl 1):5131-5138.

13. Kalayoglu M, Sollinger HW, Stratta RJ, et al. Extended preservation of the liver for clinical transplantation. *Lancet*. 1988;1:617-619.

14. Todo S, Nery J, Yanaga K, Podesta L, Gordon RD, Starzl TE. Extended preservation of human liver grafts with UW solution. *JAMA*. 1989;261:711-714.

15. Starzl TE, Todo S, Fung J, Demetris AJ, Venkataramanan R, Jain A. FK 506 for human liver, kidney and pancreas transplantation. *Lancet*. 1989;2:1000-1004.

27. Rationing Failure: The Ethical Lessons of the Retransplantation of Scarce Vital Organs

Peter A. Ubel, Robert M. Arnold, and Arthur L. Caplan

Vital organ transplantation has captured the attention of the medical community and the public in part because of the tragic choices the transplant community must make every day. The demand for vital cadaver organs far exceeds the supply, forcing the transplant community to decide who should get available life-saving organs. At the end of 1991, over 1,500 people were on waiting lists seeking cadaver livers and over 2,000 were seeking hearts[1]; of those patients, 9.9 percent awaiting livers and 16.7 percent awaiting hearts were removed from the waiting lists because they died before transplant organs be came available.[1] Because of this unavoidable shortage, the transplant community has had to literally decide—by choosing who gets an organ—who lives or dies.

Despite the great amount of attention focused on transplant allocation, few have remarked at length about the special issues raised by the allocation of organs to retransplant candidates. This made some sense initially, both because retransplantation was a rapidly progressing field, with uncertain efficacy in many patient groups, and because many were hopeful that enough organs could be procured to reduce the scarcity of available organs.[2-5] But this inattention is no longer justifiable. The shortage of cadaveric transplant organs has grown with time rather than decreased.[1] Meanwhile, retransplantation has become a large part of transplant practice, accounting for 20 percent of all liver transplants (written communication, Steven Belle, PhD, United Network for Organ Sharing [UNOS]/University of Pittsburgh [Pa] Liver Transplant Registry, December 14, 1992) and 10 percent of heart transplants, excluding heart-lung transplants (written communication, Tim Breen,

Originally published in *JAMA* 270, no. 20 (November 24, 1993): 2469-74.

PhD, UNOS Heart Transplant Registry, September 25, 1992). And experience with retransplantation has accumulated to the point where its relative efficacy is clear: retransplant candidates do not do as well as primary transplant recipients[6-9] (written communications, Steven Belle, PhD, December 14, 1992, and Tim Breen, PhD, September 25, 1992).

In cases of unavoidable scarcity, many believe that there is a moral obligation to distribute the scarce resources to those most likely to benefit from them. Yet, present transplant policy seems to violate this maxim. The allocation system distributes 10 to 20 percent of available hearts and livers to retransplant patients, a group of individuals who have not only received the resource already, but who are also less likely to benefit from a new organ. At first glance, it appears that the allocation system, by offering retransplantation to so many patients, risks being both unfair and ineffective.

In this article, we explore how a just allocation system ought to distribute scarce hearts and livers among primary transplant and retransplant candidates. First, we describe how the present system allocates organs to primary transplant and retransplant candidates. Then, we examine three differences between primary transplantation and retransplantation that may affect the priority that retransplant candidates should receive in vying for available organs: (1) the special obligations that transplant teams have not to abandon patients on whom they have already performed a transplant, (2) the fairness of allowing a few individuals to get multiple transplants while some die awaiting their first, and (3) the magnitude of difference in efficacy between primary transplantation and retransplantation. We conclude that because of this last difference, we ought to reassess the way we distribute organs among primary transplant and retransplant candidates. We argue that the present allocation system should be changed so that retransplant candidates no longer get the same access to transplant organs as those awaiting their first transplant.

THE SYSTEM TO ALLOCATE HEARTS AND LIVERS

The system that allocates cadaver hearts and livers to primary transplant and retransplant candidates is coordinated by UNOS, which supervises the procurement of organs and the formulation of patient waiting lists, monitors the conduct of surgeons and transplant centers in utilizing cadaver organs, and distributes cadaver organs among transplant centers.

To enter the system, patients must first be diagnosed as having end-stage heart or liver failure. Patients who may need a transplant are then referred to a transplant center. At the center, patients are evaluated by a transplant team. These transplant teams, made up of physicians, nurses, social workers, and others, decide whether potential candidates meet medical standards of organ failure while remaining healthy enough to survive and adapt to a transplant.

TABLE 1. RULES FOR DISTRIBUTING CADAVER LIVERS

Order of Liver Allocation
    Local, status 4
    Local, all other
    Regional, status 4
    Regional, all other
    National, status 4
    National, all other
Point System for Liver Allocation
    ABO blood group compatibility

Identical match	10 points
Compatible	5 points
Incompatible	0 points

    Time waiting

Longest waiting time	10 points
Others	Percentile of line position × 10†

    Degree of medical urgency

Status 7 (inactive)	0 points
Status 1 (normal)	6 points
Status 2 (ill outpatients)	12 points
Status 3 (hospitalized)	18 points
Status 4 (intensive care unit)	24 points

*Distributed within each group according to number of points, in descending order.
†Example: 50th percentile = 5 points.

Thus, for example, transplant teams may reject a patient with end-stage heart disease who also has a serious, chronic infection. Transplant teams must also decide whether the patient has enough family support, money, competency, and personal stability to manage the complicated posttransplant regimen. These considerations are given significant weight in evaluating patients, as 5.6 percent of patients undergoing evaluation for a cardiac transplant are turned down for psychosocial reasons.[10]

Once deemed to be suitable transplant candidates, patients are placed on a waiting list where they compete with other patients for available organs. Based on the UNOS Articles of Incorporation of June 27, 1991, cadaver livers are allocated according to a point system, which ranks candidates according to degree of ABO blood group compatibility (an immunologic measurement), extent of medical urgency (with critically ill candidates denoted as status 4), and amount of time on the waiting list (Table 1). In addition, priority is given to potential recipients in the same locality or region as the harvesting site. Distribution follows the order shown in Table 1.

Unlike cadaver livers, cadaver hearts are not allocated according to a

TABLE 2.—ORDER OF HEART ALLOCATION*

Local, status 1
Local, status 2
Regional, status 1
Regional, status 2
Zone A, status 1, heart recipients
Zone A, heart-lung recipients
Zone B, status 1, heart recipients
Zones B and C, heart-lung recipients
Zone A, status 2, heart recipients
Zone B, status 2, heart recipients
Zone C, status 1, heart recipients
Zone C, status 2, heart recipients

*In order of descending amount of waiting time, with preference in each category for blood group-compatible (A, AB, B, O) candidates. Zones indicate the following distances between the recipient hospital and the donor: zone A, less than 800 km; zone B, 800 to 1600 km; and zone C, more than 1600km.

point system. However, in other ways the systems are quite similar. Like liver candidates, heart transplant candidates are ranked according to ABO compatibility, medical urgency (with critically ill candidates listed as status 1), time on the waiting list, and local and regional priority. In addition, because hearts cannot be preserved over long distances as effectively as livers, hearts are also allocated according to the distance between the recipient hospital and the donor. Thus, distribution follows the order listed in Table 2 (UNOS Articles of Incorporation, June 27, 1991).

By ranking the candidates according to these criteria the transplant community is attempting to balance fairness, efficacy, and urgency. By factoring waiting time into allocation decisions, the lists resemble an egalitarian, "first come, first serve" allocation approach.[11] All else equal, it seems fair to give organs to those who have been waiting the longest. However, this egalitarianism is balanced by attention to important measures of transplant effectiveness. Thus, the waiting lists distribute organs according to ABO matching and for hearts, cadaver organ ischemic time, because these criteria are important predictors of transplant success. Finally, the waiting list gives great weight to the preoperative medical condition of the candidate. The emphasis on giving organs to those most urgently ill arises from a sense that, all else equal, we ought to give the organs to those who will die soonest without them.

One other fact is important to know for our purposes. Once on the list, primary transplant and retransplant candidates are treated identically. No points are awarded to or deducted from liver candidates because they have already received a transplant, nor are heart retransplant candidates given any special position on the waiting list.

SPECIAL OBLIGATIONS TO RETRANSPLANT CANDIDATES

There are reasons to question whether retransplant candidates should be accorded the same treatment as primary transplant candidates. While most theories of justice would hold that equals should be treated equally, retransplant candidates differ from primary transplant candidates in several important ways. Do these differences merit changing the relative priorities of those needing primary transplants or retransplants?

There are several reasons some might argue that retransplant candidates should be given higher priority in receiving available organs. First, one might claim that the transplant system owes these patients another chance at receiving a transplant to make up for the suffering caused by the failure of their previous transplant. But this claim fails. Decisions to transplant or retransplant would be very hard to base on a scale of comparative misery. To begin with, it would be impossible to calculate how much different candidates had suffered. Even if this could be measured, allocation based on the amount of suffering would raise important moral problems. Should stoic transplant candidates receive lower priority because they have suffered less than other candidates?

Second, some argue that transplant teams have a special duty not to abandon their patients (written communication. Thomas E. Starzl, MD, PhD, University of Pittsburgh, January 28, 1993). In general. health care workers are expected to protect the best interests of their patients.[12-15] This duty persists even when the chances of success seem remote.[16] Surgeons feel an even stronger duty to help patients on whom they have operated. This is likely to affect how transplant teams feel about transplant candidates on whom they have previously performed a transplant.

While these factors understandably create a sense of obligation among some who work on transplant teams, such feelings should not alter allocation priorities. It is not immoral for transplant teams to want their patients to do well. Nor can or should transplant teams avoid emotional attachments to their patients. But if such commitments determined how organs were allocated, we would end up favoring patients who are better at forming relationships with transplant teams. Those who are less likely to become close to team members, whether because of personality, appearance, race, language skills, or socioeconomic background, would be less likely to receive organs. In matters of unavoidable scarcity, health care workers' advocacy duties must be balanced by attention to justice.[17-19]

This conclusion stands even if members of the transplant team feel responsible for the failure of the previous transplant. While most failed transplants do not result from transplant team error, transplant team members may nonetheless blame themselves. This is a very human reaction to an unfortunate event. But although transplant failures are unfortunate, it would be unfair to respond by penalizing others who await transplant organs. Those whose organs fail due to natural causes are no less deserving of a transplant than those few whose illness is iatrogenic.

Is RETRANSPLANTATION FAIR?

Those who would argue that we should give higher priority to retransplant candidates are unconvincing. Allocation priorities should not be affected by how much one has suffered or how well one has bonded to a transplant team. On the other hand, others might argue that retransplant candidates should get lower priority in receiving organs, because they have already had their chance at getting a transplant. Is it fair for some to receive more than one transplant while others die waiting for their first organ?

'It's My Turn': A Hypothetical Case

Imagine two individuals who have equally dire need of a new liver to survive. Both reach the point of needing the liver at the same time, and are coincidentally placed on the transplant waiting list. They are judged, as best as can be determined, to have an equal chance of surviving and benefiting from a new liver. An organ becomes available equally suitable for either candidate. Should their names be placed in a hat and one selected? What if one were to learn of the lottery and complain: "She has already received a liver transplant. I should get a crack at one liver before she gets a second!"

Theories of Just Allocation

In order to evaluate this claim, we need to examine some common views of justice. Theories of justice are developed, at least in part, to find criteria to determine fair ways to distribute scarce goods. Some of the more common allocation criteria include utility, need, merit, age, social worth, ability to pay, personal responsibility, and quality of life. None of these criteria would favor the primary transplant candidate. For example, utilitarian theories hold that goods should be allocated in ways that maximize total happiness or utility.[20] Because our hypothetical case assumes that the two patients would have similar benefit from a transplant (in length and quality of life), utilitarianism would direct us to toss a coin. Similarly, a needs-based theory of just allocation would find each patient in equally desperate need. Those who think we should allocate goods according to age, social worth, personal responsibility, or ability to pay also would not look on the number of previous transplants as a relevant allocation criterion.

Theories of justice based on what a rational planner would choose behind a veil of ignorance could be used either to support or to penalize retransplant candidates.[21-22] It would be rational to choose a system that gives preference to those who have already received a transplant, assuring that once a patient has received a transplant he or she would have a better chance of staying alive. But it would also be rational to choose a system that allows more people to get a chance at transplantation at the expense of decreasing the opportunity for retransplant candidates to get organs. These theories are therefore not much help in deciding how to treat retransplant candidates.

Some might respond that these theories of justice do not capture the real issue. A more commonsense view of justice dictates that we all deserve an equal slice of the health care pie. That is, all else equal, we should not be giving out scarce pieces of pie to those who have already had some, while others await their first piece. This argument has an intuitive appeal. We do not have enough hearts and livers to go around, so we should not let anyone hog those that are available. However, this analogy breaks down. It asks us to base allocation of organs on a very narrow view of the health care pie—the pie of transplant organs—while ignoring other medical services and social goods that can affect health, such as income, education, and access to primary care. The primary transplant candidate in the hypothetical case may have grown up with all of life's advantages while the retransplant candidate has had to struggle to overcome poverty, absent parents, and inadequate access to health care. Fairness may just as well dictate that we should allocate organs according to how many health care goods one has had access to. If so, then primary transplant candidates would no longer have moral priority over retransplant candidates. Fairness based on an idea of a "fair slice of the pie" does not favor either candidate.

In summary, if retransplantation were as likely to succeed as primary transplantation, then theories of justice or ideas about what is a fair slice of the health care pie could not be used to favor primary transplant candidates over those needing retransplantation.

EFFICACY DATA: POSTTRANSPLANT SURVIVAL

There is one other important difference between primary transplant and retransplant patients that might support an argument to give retransplant candidates lower priority. Retransplant patients are less likely to live 1 year after their transplant. Should this decreased efficacy have a bearing on the priority that ought be given to retransplant candidates?

Before we discuss this question further, we must look at the data on retransplant survival. We have chosen to look at one-year survival because it is an important, although minimal, measure of transplant success. In addi-

TABLE 3. LIVER TRANSPLANT PATIENT SURVIVAL RATES
OCTOBER 1, 1987, THROUGH DECEMBER 31, 1991*

Transplant No.	No. Receiving Transplants	1-y Survival, percentage
All Transplants		
1	8539	76.5
2	1226	54.0
3	155	43.3
On Life Support		
1	1158	60.1
2	710	46.7
3	93	35.3

*Data from Steve Belle, PhD, United Network for Organ Sharing Scientific Registry.

tion, there are good data on one-year survival of retransplant patients, and there is not much information on other measures of retransplant success, such as quality of life.

Liver Retransplantation

Data on the survival of patients receiving primary, secondary, and tertiary liver transplants have been compiled by UNOS (written communication. Steven Belle, PhD, December 14, 1992). The data show a significant one-year survival advantage for primary transplant recipients (Table 3). The data continue to show a 10 to 30 percent one-year survival advantage for primary transplant recipients when primary transplant and retransplant recipients are stratified according to the severity of their medical condition preoperatively, as shown in Table 3 for status 6 recipients (on life support prior to transplant). This survival advantage increases another 10 percent when primary transplant recipients are compared with tertiary transplant recipients (76.5 percent one-year survival for primary transplant recipients versus 43.3 percent for tertiary recipients).

The survival advantage for primary transplant recipients holds at even the most experienced transplant centers.[6,7] For example, the largest reported experience with liver retransplantation in the cyclosporine era comes from the University of Pittsburgh, which has published data on sixty-nine retransplant operations.[6] They compared one-year survival in primary transplant and retransplant patients. For adults, primary transplant recipients had a statistically significant survival advantage, with 63.5 percent surviving vs 42.3 percent of retransplant recipients ($P=.026$). In children, primary transplant recipients had a similar advantage, with 76.8 percent surviving vs 56.5 percent of retransplant recipients ($P=.042$).

TABLE 4. HEART TRANSPLANT PATIENT SURVIVAL RATES
OCTOBER 1, 1987, THROUGH DECEMBER 31, 1991*

Group	No. Receiving Transplants	1-y Survival, %
Primary Transplant vs Retransplant		
First transplant	4830	81.6
Retransplant	86	56.7
All Patients		
Work or school, full-time	93	95.0
Work or school, part-time	142	84.4
Homebound	2176	84.1
Hospitalized	486	81.9
Intensive care unit	1174	83.0
Life support	793	73.8
Unknown	93	75.1
Overall	**4817**	**81.6**

*Data from Steve Belle, PhD, United Network for Organ Sharing Scientific Registry.

Cardiac Retransplantation

United Network for Organ Sharing has also collected data comparing heart transplantation and retransplantation (written communication, Tim Breen, PhD, September 25, 1992). As with liver transplants, the data show a significant survival advantage for primary transplant recipients (Table 4). Retransplant candidates have a 25 percent lower one-year survival rate than primary transplant recipients; UNOS has not stratified these data according to the preoperative condition of primary transplant and retransplant recipients. However, even if all retransplant candidates were in intensive care units (ICUs) preoperatively, their survival rate would still be significantly less than that of equally ill primary transplant candidates. This is so because the one-year survival rate for all ICU patients receiving transplants is 73 percent, compared with a 56.7 percent one-year survival rate for retransplant patients. Thus, even adjusting for preoperative condition, retransplant candidates do not do as well as primary transplant candidates.

The survival advantage for primary transplant recipients holds at even the most experienced transplant center. At Stanford University, one recent study compared the success of 288 patients receiving primary heart transplantation and twenty-three requiring retransplantation.[8] Of these twenty-three patients, fourteen required transplantation because of accelerated graft atherosclerosis and the other nine because of acute allograft rejection. The latter group had a significantly higher perioperative mortality than did primary transplant recipients. The acute allograft rejection group had 44 percent one-year survival versus 81 percent for primary transplant. Patients undergoing retransplantation for accelerated graft atherosclerosis had a similar survival rate as primary transplant recipients (85 percent versus 81 percent), but five-year survival was worse in the retransplant group than in the primary transplant group, with only one of the fourteen patients surviving at that time. In a different study, the same group calculated one-, two-, and five-year graft survival rates of 55 percent, 25 percent, and 10 percent in those undergoing retransplantation for accelerated graft atherosclerosis.[9] This compares with patient survival rates for primary transplantation of 67 percent, 46 percent, and 13 percent, respectively.[8]

JUSTICE AND EFFICACY

The available data show that heart and liver retransplant patients do not do as well as primary transplant recipients. Retransplant patients are 20 percent less likely to survive one year after transplantation. This raises an ethical dilemma: should a moderate difference in survival rates make a difference in how we allocate scarce organs?

Perhaps one way to answer this question is to look at how the present allocation system already uses efficacy data to allocate organs. Both hearts and livers are preferentially distributed to those whose ABO types match the available organs. This preference was built into the liver point system after studies showed improved graft survival in patients who received ABO-identical organs.[23-25] The Pittsburgh transplant group compared all their liver recipients between 1981 and 1986.[23] They found a 15 to 20 percent survival advantage for ABO-identical recipients compared with those who were mismatched or incompatible. This difference was slightly smaller after adjusting for severity of illness and removing those patients whose transplants failed due to technical problems. These findings are consistent with more recent data collected by UNOS, which show a 16 percent decrease in one-year graft survival for ABO-incompatible recipients compared with those with ABO-identical organs.[26]

In cardiac transplantation, ABO matching has an even greater impact on outcome. Despite occasional successes,[27] transplantation of hearts into ABO-incompatible recipients is generally associated with a poor prognosis. A survey of cardiac transplant programs revealed that the majority of such patients experience hyperacute graft rejection, with only a 45 percent chance of gaining long-term survival.[28] The prognosis is better for ABO-mismatched but compatible recipients. In a large study in Houston, Texas, one-year survival for ABO-identical and ABO-nonidentical recipients was 79.5 percent and 62.2 percent, respectively.[29]

Thus, ABO mismatching of heart and liver transplants is associated with moderate to large decreases in one-year survival. The current UNOS system for allocating livers and hearts takes these survival differences into account by favoring ABO-identical recipients. As the Pittsburgh transplant group concluded: ". . . liver transplantation across ABO blood groups is usually successful, but not without risk. We, therefore, continue to give preference to ABO compatibility in the selection of liver transplant recipients."[23] The transplant community thus acts as if justice is best served by distributing available organs to those more likely to benefit from them.

However, the survival advantage for ABO-identical heart and liver recipients over most mismatched recipients is no larger than that seen for primary transplant recipients over retransplant recipients. The transplant community has already factored moderate efficacy differences into the allocation system. It seems inconsistent to ignore similar efficacy differences between primary transplant and retransplant recipients.

Should We Factor Efficacy Into Allocation?

While we have shown that it is inconsistent to treat retransplantation status differently than ABO status (since both have a similar effect on transplant efficacy), we have not established that efficacy is a morally relevant allocation criterion. One might argue that we should not factor efficacy into the allocation scheme. However, a number of theories of justice argue that efficacy should be factored into an allocation system. For example, utilitarianism would urge us to distribute organs to accrue the greatest benefit, which would clearly require us to pay attention to efficacy. In addition, a rational planner, choosing an allocation system behind a veil of ignorance, would plausibly opt for a system that favored those most likely to benefit from a transplant. Rational planners, ignorant as to whether or not they will ever need a transplant or a retransplant, would increase their own chances of benefiting from a transplant by setting up a system that, all else equal, distributed scarce organs to those most likely to gain long-term survival from a transplant. It is hard to imagine any theory of justice credibly asserting that we should transplant scarce organs into people regardless of their chance of surviving. As others have argued at greater length,[30] efficacy is a morally relevant criterion for distributing scarce transplant organs.

Balancing Urgency and Efficacy

A critical question for an allocation system is to find an appropriate balance between urgency and efficacy. Some will argue that the urgency of patients' needs for organs should always take precedence over their likelihood of having good outcomes. To turn a dying patient away because of a lower chance of survival, it is argued, violates our duty to help the most urgently ill patients. This is especially relevant to our discussion of retransplantation because retransplant recipients are sicker, on average, than primary transplant recipients (written communication, Tim Breen, PhD, September 25, 1992).

This objection to the use of efficacy in allocating organs assumes that efficacy and urgency are always at odds, forcing us to choose one or the other. However, this is not always the case. While it is true that urgently ill patients are less likely to gain long-term survival from a transplant (written communication, Steven Belle, PhD, December 14, 1992), they are also less likely to live without a transplant. For example, some candidates on the heart waiting list are healthy enough that their chance of living an additional year will not be significantly improved by a transplant.[31] In contrast, some urgently ill candidates have such high mortality without a transplant that transplantation greatly improves their chance of surviving one year. In these cases, allocating organs to those most urgently ill (who have the most to gain from an early transplant) may potentially increase the number of years of life added by a transplant.[32] Only when the likelihood of surviving a transplant gets very low does priority to urgency decrease the amount of benefit brought by transplant. For example, one study estimates that this would occur when a heart transplant candidate's chance of one-year survival fell below 50 percent.[32]

Balancing our duty to urgently ill patients and our duty to use scarce organs in ways that maximize their benefit depends on the complex interaction between patients' predicted prognoses with and without a transplant and the relative weight one places on performing transplants on urgently ill patients. Luckily, the argument for giving primary transplant patients higher priority for organs does not require making these complex calculations. At any level of urgency, retransplant recipients do not do as well as similarly ill primary transplant recipients (written communication, Steven Belle, PhD, December 14, 1992). As we show in Table 3, retransplant recipients do worse than primary transplant recipients even after controlling for their preoperative status. And this difference increases with each successive transplant. Equally ill patients receiving their third liver transplants do even worse than those receiving their second. Retransplantation is an independent risk factor for poor transplant outcome.

Because these primary transplant and retransplant candidates are of similar levels of illness, there is no greater duty to help one group over the other. Thus, efficacy should determine which group has priority in receiving organs. By giving retransplant candidates equal access to transplantable organs, our present policy does not do all it can to distribute organs efficaciously. We give organs to a group of people who have less chance of gaining long-term survival from a transplant. We ignore our duty to distribute scarce resources in ways that increase the chance that the resources will bring benefit.

CONCLUSIONS

We have looked at several ways that retransplant candidates differ from those awaiting their first transplant to see if any of these differences ought to affect how we allocate organs. Two of these differences do not hold up to close scrutiny. Allocation priorities should not be altered on the basis of any special obligations that transplant teams feel to support patients on whom they have already performed transplants. Nor does any sense of justice support a claim that it is unfair to give patients second or third organs while others await their first.

Only one difference holds up to scrutiny: retransplant candidates do not do as well as primary transplant recipients. The current allocation system factors ABO matching into the allocation scheme based on its moderate effect on transplant outcomes. Consistency demands that other factors that are as, if not more, important in predicting one-year survival should also be included in the allocation system. The system should be revised to separate specific groups of candidates with a significantly lower chance of gaining long-term survival from a transplant.

Retransplantation provides one example of the cutoffs the transplant community should make. Retransplant recipients at similar levels of urgency do significantly worse than primary transplant recipients, a difference that increases with each successive transplant. We need to revise the allocation system in a way that directs more organs to primary transplant candidates instead of retransplant candidates. Reasonable people can disagree about the best way to do this. But some type of change should be made so that we can bring more benefit with the few organs available for transplant.

We think that the waiting lists should be altered so that primary transplant candidates have a better chance of receiving organs than retransplant candidates. In addition, we think those needing a third or fourth transplant should be removed from the waiting lists altogether. Instead, we should only allow them a limited number of experimental transplants, in hopes of improving their future chances of survival, or let them receive organs that are, for various reasons, not appropriate for others. But we should no longer allow them to vie for scarce organs on an equal basis with those who have never received a transplant and whose chances of benefiting from a transplant are much greater.

Health care workers cannot always be expected to recognize when it is time to forgo heroic lifesaving measures. Indeed, their traditional role as patient advocates would seem to compel them to ignore the odds and do whatever they can to help their patients, especially when they have already performed a transplant on the patient. However, when such heroic measures require scarce resources that could be better used to help others, their good intentions can be unjust. A change in the allocation system will reduce the tension physicians feel to balance their duties to patients and society. It is time to change the system to limit the number of times we will offer transplants to patients whose previous transplants have failed.

REFERENCES

1. Evans RW, Orians CE, Ascher NL. The potential supply of organ donors: an assessment of the efficiency of organ procurement efforts in the United States. *JAMA*. 1992;267:239-246.

2. Cohen B. Organ donor shortage: European situation and possible solutions. *Scand J Urol Nephrol*. 1985;92:77-80.

3. Cwiek MA. Presumed consent as a solution to the organ shortfall problem. *Public Law Forum*. 1984;4:81-89.

4. Miller M. A proposed solution to the present organ donation crisis based on a hard look at the past. *Circulation*. 1987;75:20-28.

5. Spital A. The shortage of organs for transplantation: where do we go from here? *N Engl J Med*. 1991;325:1243-1246.

6. Shaw BW, Gordon RD, Iwatsuki S, Starzl TE. Hepatic retransplantation. *Transplant Proc*. 1985;17:264-271

7. Wall WJ, Grant DR, Ghent CN, et al. Liver transplantation: the University Hospital-Children's Hospital of Western Ontario experience. In: Terasaki P, ed. *Clinical Transplants*. Los Angeles, Calif: UCLA Tissue Typing Laboratory; 1988.

8. Dein JR, Oyer PE, Stinson EB, Starnes VA, Shumway NE. Cardiac retransplantation in the cyclosporine era. *Ann Thorac Surg*. 1989;48:350-355.

9. Gao SZ, Schroeder JS, Hunt S, Stinson EB. Retransplantation for severe accelerated coronary artery disease in heart transplant recipients. *Am J Cardiol*. 1988;62:876-881.

10. Olbrisch ME, Levenson JL. Psychosocial evaluation of heart transplant candidates: an international survey of process, criteria, and outcomes. *J Heart Lung Transplant*. 1991;10:948-965.

11. Calabresi G, Bobbit P. *Tragic Choices: The Conflicts Society Confronts in the Allocation of Tragically Scarce Resources*. New York: WW Norton & Co; 1978.

12. Abrams FR. Patient advocate or secret agent? *JAMA*. 1986;256:1784-1785.

13. Angell M. Cost containment and the physician. *JAMA* 1985;254:1203-1207.

14. Cassell EJ. Do justice, love mercy: the inappropriateness of the concept of justice applied to bedside decisions. In: Shelp EE, ed. *Justice and Health Care*. New York: D Reidel Publishing Co; 1981.

15. Hiatt HH. Protecting the medical commons. *N Engl J Med*. 1975;293:235-241.

16. LaPuma J, Cassel CK, Humphrey H. Ethics, economics, and endocarditis: the physician's role in resource allocation. *Arch Intern Med*. 1988;148:1809-1811.

17. Cassel C. Doctors and allocation decisions: a new role in the new Medicare. *J Health Polit Policy Law*. 1985;10:549-564.

18. Daniels N. The ideal advocate and limited resources. *Theor Med*. 1987;8:69-80.

19. Jecker NS. Integrating medical ethics with normative theory: Patient advocacy and social responsibility. *Theor Med*. 1990;11:125-139.

20. Mill JS. *Utilitarianism*. London, England: Collins; 1863.

21. Daniels N. *Just Health Care*. New York: Cambridge University Press; 1985.

22. Rawls J. *A Theory of Justice*. Cambridge, Mass: Harvard University Press; 1971.

23. Gordon RD, Iwatsuld S, Esquivel CO, et al. Experience with primary liver transplantations across ABO blood groups. *Transplant Proc*. 1987;19:184-189.

24. Jenkins RL. Georgi BA, Gallik-Karlson CA, Rohrer RJ, Khettry U, Dzik WS. ABO mismatch and liver transplantation. *Transplant Proc.* 1987; 19:184-189.

25. Steininger R, Muhlbacher F, Hamilton G, et al. ABO incompatibility in liver transplantation: a single center experience. *Transplant Proc.* 1987;190-192.

26. Belle SH, Beringer KC, Murphy JB, et al. Liver transplantation in the United States: 1988 to 1990. In Terasaki P, ed. *Clinical Transplants.* Los Angeles, Calif: UCLA Issue Typing Laboratory; 1991.

27. Caruana RJ, Zumbro GL, Hoff RG, Rao RN, Daspit SA. Successful cardiac transplantation across an ABO blood group barrier. *Transplantation.* 1988; 46:472-474.

28. Cooper DKC. A clinical survey of cardiac transplantation between ABO blood group-incompatible recipients and donors. *Transplant Proc.* 1990;22:1457. 29.

29. Nakatani T, Aida H, Frazier OH, Macris MP. Effect of ABO blood type on survival of heart transplant patients treated with cyclosporine. *J Heart Transplant.* 1989;8:27-33.

30. Kilner JF. *Who Lives? Who Dies? Ethical Criteria in Patient Selection.* New Haven, Conn: Yale University Press; 1990.

31. Stevenson LW, Hamilton MA, Tillisch IH, et al. Decreasing survival benefit from cardiac transplantation for outpatients as the waiting list lengthens. *J Am Coll Cardiol.* 1991;18:919-925.

32. Stevenson LW, Warner SL, Hamilton MA, et al. Distribution of donor hearts to maximize transplant candidate survival. *Circulation.* 1991;84:suppl II-352.

28. Should Alcoholics Compete Equally for Liver Transplantation?

Alvin H. Moss and Mark Siegler

Until recently, liver transplantation for patients with alcohol-related end-stage liver disease (ARESLD) was not considered a treatment option. Most physicians in the transplant community did not recommend it because of initial poor results in this population[1] and because of a predicted high recidivism rate that would preclude long-term survival.[2] In 1988, however, Starzl and colleagues[3] reported one-year survival rates for patients with ARESLD comparable to results in patients with other causes of end-stage liver disease (ESLD). Although the patients in the Pittsburgh series may represent a carefully selected population,[3,4] the question is no longer "Can we perform transplants in patients with alcoholic liver disease and obtain acceptable results?" but "Should we?" This question is particularly timely since the Health Care Financing Administration (HCFA) has recommended that Medicare coverage for liver transplantation be offered to patients with alcoholic cirrhosis who are abstinent. The HCFA proposes that the same eligibility criteria be used for patients with ARESLD as are used for patients with other causes of ESLD, such as primary biliary cirrhosis and sclerosing cholangitis.[5]

SHOULD PATIENTS WITH ARESLD RECEIVE TRANSPLANTS?

At first glance, this question seems simple to answer. Generally, in medicine, a therapy is used if it works and saves lives. But the circumstances of liver transplantation differ from those of most other lifesaving therapies, including long-term mechanical ventilation and dialysis, in three important respects:

Originally published in *JAMA* 265, no. 10 (March 13, 1991): 1295-98.

Nonrenewable Resource

First, although most lifesaving therapies are expensive, liver transplantation uses a nonrenewable, absolutely scarce resource—a donor liver. In contrast to patients with end-stage renal disease, who may receive either a transplant or dialysis therapy, every patient with ESLD who does not receive a liver transplant will die. This dire, absolute scarcity of donor livers would be greatly exacerbated by including patients with ARESLD as potential candidates for liver transplantation. In 1985, 63,737 deaths due to hepatic disease occurred in the United States, at least 36 000 of which were related to alcoholism, but fewer than 1000 liver transplants were performed.[6] Although patients with ARESLD represent more than 50 percent of the patients with ESLD, patients with ARESLD account for less than 10 percent of those receiving transplants (*New York Times*, April 3, 1990:B6[col 1]). If patients with ARESLD were accepted for liver transplantation on an equal basis, as suggested by the HCFA, there would potentially be more than 30,000 additional candidates each year. (No data exist to indicate how many patients in the late stages of ARESLD would meet transplantation eligibility criteria.) In 1987, only 1,182 liver transplants were performed; in 1989, fewer than 2,000 were done.[6] Even if all donor livers available were given to patients with ARESLD, it would not be feasible to provide transplants for even a small fraction of them. Thus, the dire, absolute nature of donor liver scarcity mandates that distribution be based on unusually rigorous standards—standards not required for the allocation of most other resources such as dialysis machines and ventilators, both of which are only *relatively* scarce.

Comparison with Cardiac Transplantation

Second, although a similar dire, absolute scarcity of donor hearts exists for cardiac transplantation, the allocational decisions for cardiac transplantation differ from those for liver transplantation. In liver transplantation, ARESLD causes more than 50 percent of the cases of ESLD; in cardiac transplantation, how ever, no one predominant disease or contributory factor is responsible. Even for patients with end-stage ischemic heart disease who smoked or who failed to adhere to dietary regimens, it is rarely clear that one particular behavior caused the disease. Also, unlike our proposed consideration for liver transplantation, a history of alcohol abuse is considered a contraindication and is a common reason for a patient with heart disease to be denied cardiac transplantation.[7,8] Thus, the allocational decisions for heart transplantation differ from those for liver transplantation in two ways: determining a cause for end-stage heart disease is less certain, and patients with a history of alcoholism are usually rejected from heart transplant programs.

Expensive Technology

Third, a unique aspect of liver transplantation is that it is an expensive technology that has become a target of cost containment in health care.[9] It is, therefore, essential to maintain the approbation and support of the public so that organs continue to be donated under appropriate clinical circumstances-even in spite of the high cost of transplantation.

General Guideline Proposed

In view of the distinctive circumstances surrounding liver transplantation, we propose as a general guideline that patients with ARESLD should not compete equally with other candidates for liver transplantation. We are *not* suggesting that patients with ARESLD should *never* receive liver transplants. Rather, we propose that a priority ranking be established for the use of this dire, absolutely scarce societal resource and that patients with ARESLD be lower on the list than others with ESLD.

OBJECTIONS TO PROPOSAL

We realize that our proposal may meet with two immediate objections: (1) Some may argue that since alcoholism is a disease, patients with ARESLD should be considered equally for liver transplantation.[10] (2) Some will question why patients with ARESLD should be singled out for discrimination, when the medical profession treats many patients who engage in behavior that causes their diseases.[11] We will discuss these objections in turn.

Alcoholism: How Is It Similar To and Different From Other Diseases?

We do not dispute the reclassification of alcoholism as a disease.[12] Both hereditary and environmental factors contribute to alcoholism, and physiological, biochemical, and genetic markers have been associated with increased susceptibility.[13] Identifying alcoholism as a disease enables physicians to approach it as they do other medical problems and to differentiate it from bad habits, crimes, or moral weaknesses. More important, identifying alcoholism as a disease also legitimizes medical interventions to treat it.[14]

Alcoholism is a chronic disease,[12,15] for which treatment is available and effective. More than 1.43 million patients were treated in 5,586 alcohol treatment units in the twelve-month period ending October 30, 1987.[16] One comprehensive review concluded that more than two-thirds of patients who accept therapy improve.[17] Another cited four studies in which at least 54 percent of patients were abstinent a minimum of one year after treatment.[18] A recent study of alcohol-impaired physicians reported a 100 percent abstinence rate an average of 33.4 months after therapy was initiated. In this study, physician-patients rated Alcoholics Anonymous, the largest organization of recovering alcoholics in the world, as the most important component of their therapy.[19]

Like other chronic diseases—such as type I diabetes mellitus, which requires the patient to administer insulin over a lifetime—alcoholism requires the patient to assume responsibility for participating in continuous treatment. Two key elements are required to successfully treat alcoholism: the patient must accept his or her diagnosis and must assume responsibility for treatment.[20,21] The high success rates of some alcoholism treatment programs indicate that many patients can accept responsibility for their treatment. ARESLD, one of the sequelae of alcoholism, results from ten to twenty years of heavy alcohol consumption. The risk of ARESLD increases with the amount of alcohol consumed and with the duration of heavy consumption.[22] In view of the quantity of alcohol consumed, the years, even decades, required to develop ARESLD, and the availability of effective alcohol treatment, attributing personal responsibility for ARESLD to the patient seems all the more justified. We believe, therefore, that even though alcoholism is a chronic disease, alcoholics should be held responsible for seeking and obtaining treatment that could prevent the development of late-stage complications such as ARESLD. Our view is consistent with that of Alcoholics Anonymous: alcoholics are responsible for undertaking a program for recovery that will keep their disease of alcoholism in remission.[23]

Are We Discriminating Against Alcoholics?

Why should patients with ARESLD be singled out when a large number of patients have health problems that can be attributed to so-called voluntary health-risk behavior? Such patients include smokers with chronic lung disease; obese people who develop type II diabetes; some individuals who test positive for the human immunodeficiency virus; individuals with multiple behavioral risk factors (inattention to blood pressure, cholesterol, diet, and exercise) who develop coronary artery disease; and people such as skiers, motorcyclists, and football players who sustain activity-related injuries. We believe that the health care system should respond based on the actual medical needs of patients rather than on the factors (e.g., genetic, infectious, or behavioral) that cause the problem. We also believe that individuals should bear some responsibility—such as increased insurance premiums—for medical problems associated with voluntary choices. The critical distinguishing factor for treatment of ARESLD is the scarcity of the resource needed to treat it. The sources needed to treat most of these other conditions are only moderately or relatively scarce, and patients with these diseases or injuries can receive a share of the resources (i.e., money, personnel, and medication) roughly equivalent to their need. In contrast, there are insufficient donor livers to sustain the lives of all with ESLD who are in need.[24] This difference permits us to make some discriminating choices—or to establish priorities—in selecting candidates for liver transplantation based on notions of fairness. In addition, this reasoning enables us to offer patients with alcohol-related medical and surgical problems their fair share of relatively scarce resources, such as blood products, surgical care, and intensive care beds, while still maintaining that their claim on donor livers is less compelling than the claims of others.

REASONS PATIENTS WITH ARESLD SHOULD HAVE A LOWER PRIORITY ON TRANSPLANT WAITING LISTS

Two arguments support our proposal. The first argument is a moral one based on considerations of fairness. The second one is based on policy considerations and examines whether public support of liver transplantation can be maintained if, as a result of a first-come, first-served approach, patients with ARESLD receive more than half the available donor livers. Finally, we will consider further research necessary to determine which patients with ARESLD should be candidates for transplantation, albeit with a lower priority.

Fairness

Given a tragic shortage of donor livers, what is the fair or just way to allocate them? We suggest that patients who develop ESLD through no fault of their own (e.g., those with congenital biliary atresia or primary biliary cirrhosis) should have a higher priority in receiving a liver transplant than those whose liver disease results from failure to obtain treatment for alcoholism. In view of the dire, absolute scarcity of donor livers, we believe it is fair to hold people responsible for their choices, including decisions to refuse alcoholism treatment, and to allocate organs on this basis.

It is unfortunate but not unfair to make this distinction.[25] When not enough donor livers are available for all who need one, choices have to be made, and they should be founded on one or more proposed principles of fairness for distributing scarce resources.[26,27] We shall consider four that are particularly relevant:

- *To each, an equal share of treatment.*
- *To each, similar treatment for similar cases.*
- *To each, treatment according to personal effort.*
- *To each, treatment according to ability to pay.*

It is not possible to give each patient with ESLD an *equal share,* or, in this case, a functioning liver. The problem created by the absolute scarcity of donor livers is that of inequality; some receive livers while others do not. But what is fair, need not be equal. Although a first-come, first-served approach has been suggested to provide each patient with an equal chance, we believe it is fairer to give a child dying of biliary atresia an opportunity for a *first* normal liver than it is to give a patient with ARESLD who was born with a normal liver a *second* one.

Because the goal of providing each person with an equal share of health care sometimes collides with the realities of finite medical resources, the principle of *similar treatment for similar cases* has been found to be helpful. Outka[26] stated it this way: "If we accept the case for equal access, but if we simply cannot, physically cannot, treat all who are in need, it seems more just to discriminate by virtue of categories of illness, rather than between rich ill and poor ill." This principle is derived from the principle of formal justice, which, roughly stated, says that people who are equal in relevant respects should be treated equally and that people who are unequal in relevant respects should be treated differently.[27] We believe that patients with ARESLD are unequal in a relevant respect to others with ESLD, since their liver failure was preventable; therefore, it is acceptable to treat them differently.

Our view also relies on the principle of *To each, treatment according to personal effort.* Although alcoholics cannot be held responsible for their disease, once their condition has been diagnosed they can be held responsible for seeking treatment and for preventing the complication of ARESLD. The standard of personal effort and responsibility we propose for alcoholics is the same as that held by Alcoholics Anonymous. We are not suggesting that some lives and behaviors have greater value than others—an approach used and appropriately repudiated when dialysis machines were in short supply.[26-30] But we are holding people responsible for their personal effort.

Health policymakers have predicted that this principle will assume greater importance in the future. In the context of scarce health care resources, Blank[31] foresees a reevaluation of our health care priorities, with a shift toward individual responsibility and a renewed emphasis on the individual's obligation to society to maximize one's health. Similarly, more than a decade ago, Knowles[32] observed that prevention of disease requires effort. He envisioned that the next major advances in the health of the American people would be determined by what individuals are willing to do for themselves.

To each, treatment according to ability to pay has also been used as a principle of distributive justice. Since alcoholism is prevalent in all socioeconomic strata, it is not discrimination against the poor to deny liver transplantation to patients with alcoholic liver disease.[33] In fact, we believe that poor patients with ARESLD have a stronger claim for a donor liver than rich patients, precisely because many alcohol treatment programs are not available to patients lacking in substantial private resources or health insurance. Ironically, it is precisely this group of poor and uninsured patients who are most likely not to be eligible to receive a liver transplant because of their inability to pay. We agree with Outka's view of fairness that would discriminate according to categories of illness rather than according to wealth.

Policy Considerations Regarding Public Support for Liver Transplantation

Today, the main health policy concerns involve issues of financing, distributive justice, and rationing medical care.[34-37] Because of the many deficiencies in the US health care system—in maternal and child health, in the unmet needs of the elderly, and in the millions of Americans without health insurance—an increasing number of commentators are drawing attention to the trade-offs between basic health care for the many, and expensive, albeit life-saving care for the few.[9,25,38,39]

Because of its high unit cost, liver transplantation is often at the center of these discussions, as it has been in Oregon, where the legislature voted to eliminate Medicaid reimbursement for all transplants except kidneys and corneas.[9] In this era of health care cost containment, a sense of limits is emerging and allocational choices are being made. Oregon has already shown that elected officials and the public are prepared to face these issues.

In our democracy, it is appropriate that community mores and values be regarded seriously when deciding the most appropriate use of a scarce and nonrenewable organ symbolized as a "Gift of Life." As if to underscore this point, the report of the Task Force on Organ Transplantation recommended that each donated organ be considered a national resource for the public good and that the public must participate in decisions on how to use this resource to best serve the public's interests.[40]

Much of the initial success in securing public and political approval for liver transplantation was achieved by focusing media and political attention not on adults but on children dying of ESLD. The public may not support transplantation for patients with ARESLD in the same way that they have endorsed this procedure for babies born with biliary atresia. This assertion is bolstered not only by the events in Oregon but also by the results of a Louis Harris and Associates[41] national survey, which showed that lifesaving therapy for premature infants or for patients with cancer was given the highest health care priority by the public and that lifesaving therapy for patients with alcoholic liver disease was given the lowest. In this poll, the public's view of health care priorities was shared by leadership groups also polled: physicians, nurses, employers, and politicians.

Just because a majority of the public holds these views does not mean that they are right, but the moral intuition of the public, which is also shared by its leaders, reflects community values that must be seriously considered. Also indicative of community values are organizations such as Mothers Against Drunk Driving, Students Against Drunk Driving, corporate employee assistance programs, and school student assistance programs. Their existence signals that many believe that a person's behavior can be modified so that the consequences of behavior such as alcoholism can be prevented.[42] Thus, giving donor livers to patients with ARESLD on an equal basis with other patients who have ESLD might lead to a decline in public support for liver transplantation.

SHOULD ANY ALCOHOLICS BE CONSIDERED FOR TRANSPLANTATION? NEED FOR FURTHER RESEARCH

Our proposal for giving lower priority for liver transplantation to patients with ARESLD does not completely rule out transplantation for this group. Patients with ARESLD who had not previously been offered therapy and who are now abstinent could be acceptable candidates. In addition, patients lower on the waiting list, such as patients with ARESLD who have been treated and are now abstinent, might be eligible for a donor liver in some regions because of the increased availability of donor organs there. Even if only because of these possible conditions for transplantation, further research is needed to determine which patients with ARESLD would have the best outcomes after liver transplantation.

Transplant programs have been reluctant to provide transplants to alcoholics because of concern about one unfavorable outcome: a high recidivism rate. Although the overall recidivism rate for the Pittsburgh patients was only 11.5 percent, in the patients who had been abstinent less than six months it was 43 percent.[2] Also, compared with the entire group in which one-year survival was 74 percent, the survival rate in this subgroup was lower, at 64 percent.[2]

In the recently proposed Medicare criteria for coverage of liver transplantation, the HCFA acknowledged that the decision to insure patients with alcoholic cirrhosis "may be considered controversial by some."[5] As if to counter possible objections, the HCFA listed requirements for patients with alcoholic cirrhosis: patients must meet the transplant centers requirement for abstinence prior to liver transplantation and have documented evidence of sufficient social support to ensure both recovery from alcoholism and compliance with the regimen of immununosuppressive medication.

Further research should answer lingering questions about liver transplantation for ARESLD patients: Which characteristics of a patient with ARESLD can predict a successful outcome? How long is abstinence necessary to qualify for transplantation? What type of a social support system must a patient have to ensure good results? These questions are being addressed.[43] Until the answers are known, we propose that further transplantation for patients with ARESLD be limited to abstinent patients who had not previously been offered alcoholism treatment and to abstinent treated patients in regions of increased donor liver availability and that it be carried out as part of prospective research protocols at a few centers skilled in transplantation and alcohol research.

COMMENT

Should patients with ARESLD compete equally for liver transplants? In a setting in which there is a dire, absolute scarcity of donor livers, we believe the answer is no. Considerations of fairness suggest that a first-come, first-served approach for liver transplantation is not the most just approach. Although this decision is difficult, it is only fair that patients who have not assumed equal responsibility for maintaining their health or for accepting treatment for a chronic disease should be treated differently. Considerations of public values and mores suggest that the public may not support liver transplantation if patients with ARESLD routinely receive more than half of the available donor livers. We conclude that since not all can live, priorities must be established and that patients with ARESLD should be given a lower priority for liver transplantation than others with ESLD.

REFERENCES

1. Scharschmidt BF. Human liver transplantation: analysis of data on 540 patients from four centers. *Hepatology.* 1984;4:95S-101S.

2. Kumar S, Stauber RE, Gavaler JS, et al. Orthotopic liver transplantation for alcoholic liver disease. *Hepatology.* 1990;11:159-164.

3. Starzl TE, Van Thiel D, Tzakis AG, et al. Orthotopic liver transplantation for alcoholic cirrhosis. *JAMA.* 1988;260:2542-2544.

4. Olbrisch ME, Levenson JL. Liver transplantation for alcoholic cirrhosis. *JAMA.* 1989;261:2958.

5. Health Care Financing Administration. Medicare program: criteria for Medicare coverage of adult liver transplants. *Federal Register.* 1990; 55:3545-3553.

6. Office of Health Technology Assessment, Agency for Health Care Policy Research. *Assessment of Liver Transplantation.* Rockville, Md: US Dept of Health and Human Services; 1990:3, 25.

7. Schroeder JS, Hunt S. Cardiac transplantation update 1987. *JAMA* 1987;258:3142-3145.

8. Surman OS. Psychiatric aspects of organ transplantation. *Am J Psychiatry.* 1989;146:972-982.

9. Welch HG, Larson EB. Dealing with limited resources: the Oregon decision to curtail funding for organ transplantation. *N Engl J Med.* 1988; 319:171-173.

10. Flavin DK, Niven RG, Kelsey JE. Alcoholism and orthotopic liver transplantation. *JAMA.* 1988;259:1546-1547.

11. Atterbury CE. The alcoholic in the lifeboat: should drinkers be candidates for liver transplantation? *J Clin Gastroenterol.* 1986;8:1-4.

12. Mendelson JH, Mello NK. *The Diagnosis and Treatment of Alcoholism.* 2nd ed. New York, NY: McGraw-Hill International Book Co; 1985:1-20.

13. Blum K, Noble EP, Sheridan PJ, et al. Allelic association of human dopamine D2 receptor gene in alcoholism. *JAMA.* 1990;263:2055-2060.

14. Aronson MD. Definition of alcoholism. In: Barnes HN, Aronson MD, Delbanco TL, eds. *Alcoholism: A Guide for the Primary Care Physician.* New York: Springer-Verlag NY Inc; 1987:9-15.

15. Klerman GL. Treatment of alcoholism. *N Engl J Med.* 1989;320:394-395.

16. *Seventh Special Report to the US Congress on Alcohol and Health.* Washington, DC: US Dept of Health and Human Services; 1990. Publication 90-1656.

17. Saxe L. *The Effectiveness and Costs of Alcoholism Treatment: Health Technology Case Study No. 22.* Washington, DC: Congress of the United States, Office of Technology Assessment; 1983:3-6.

18. Nace EP. *The Treatment of Alcoholism.* New York: Brunner/Mazel Publishers; 1987:43-46.

19. Galanter M, Talbott D, Gallegos K, Rubenstone E. Combined Alcoholics Anonymous and professional care for addicted physicians. *Am J Psychiatry.* 1990;147:64-68.

20. Johnson B, Clark W. Alcoholism: a challenging physician-patient encounter. *J Gen Intern Med.* 1989;4:445-452.

21. Bigby JA. Negotiating treatment and monitoring recovery. In: Barnes HN, Aronson MD, Delbanco TL, eds. *Alcoholism: A Guide for the Primary Care Physician.* New York: Springer-Verlag NY Inc; 1987:66-72.

22. Grant BF, Dufour MC, Harford TC. Epidemiology of alcoholic liver disease. *Sem Liv Dis.* 1988;8:12-25.

23. Thoreson RW, Budd FC. Self-help groups and other group procedures for treating alcohol problems. In: Cox WM, ed. *Treatment and Prevention of Alcohol Probles: A Resource Manual.* Orlando, Fla: Academic Press Inc; 1987:157-181.

24. Winslow GR. *Triage and Justice.* Berkeley: University of California Press; 1982:39-44.

25. Engelhardt HT Jr. Shattuck Lecture: allocating scarce medical resources and the availability of organ transplantation. *N Engl J Med. 1984;311:66-71.*

26. Outka G. Social justice and equal access to health care. *J Religious Ethics;* 1974;2:11-32.

27. Beauchamp TL, Childress JF. *Principles of Biomedical Ethics.* 3rd ed. New York: Oxford University Press; 1989:256-306.

28. Ramsey P. *The Patient as Person.* New Haven, Conn: Yale University Press; 1970:242-252.

29. Fox RC, Swazey JP. *The Courage to Fail.* 2nd ed. Chicago, Ill: University of Chicago Press; 1978:226-265.

30. Annas GJ. The prostitute, the playboy, and the poet: rationing schemes for organ transplantation. *Am J Public Health.* 1985;75:187-189.

31. Blank RH. *Rationing Medicine.* New York: Columbia University Press; 1988:1-37, 189-252.

32. Knowles JH. Responsibility for health. *Science.* 1977;198:1103.

33. Moore RD, Bone LR, Geller G, Marmon JA, Stokes EJ, Levine DM. Prevalence, detection, and treatment of alcoholism in hospitalized patients. *JAMA.* 1989;261:403-407.

34. Fuchs VR. The 'rationing' of medical care. *N Engl J Med.* 1984;311:1572-1573.

35. Daniels N. Why saying no to patients in the United States is so hard: cost containment, justice, and provider autonomy. *N Engl J Med.* 1986;314: 1380-1383.

36. Callahan D. Allocating health resources. *Hastings Cent Rep.* 1988;18:14-20.

37. Evans RW. Health care technology and the inevitability of resource allocation and rationing decisions. *JAMA.* 1983;249:2047-2053, 2208-2219.

38. Thurow LC. Learning to say no. *N Engl J Med.* 1984;311:1569-1572.

39. Caper P. Solving the medical care dilemma. *N Engl J Med.* 1988;318:1535-1536.

40. Task Force on Organ Transplantation. *Organ Transplantation: Issues and Recommendations.* Washington, DC: US Dept of Health and Human Services; 1986:9.

41. Louis Harris and Associates. *Making Difficult Health Care Decisions.* Boston, Mass: The Loran Commission; 1987:73-89.

42. Fishman R. *Alcohol and Alcoholism.* New York: Chelsea House Publishers; 1986:27-34.

43. Beresford TP, Turcotte JG, Merion R, et al. A rational approach to liver transplantation for the alcoholic patient. *Psychosomatics.* 1990;31:241-254.

29. Alcoholics and Liver Transplantation

Carl Cohen, Martin Benjamin, and the Ethics and Social Impact Committee of the Transplant and Health Policy Center, Ann Arbor, Michigan

Alcoholic cirrhosis of the liver—severe scarring due to the heavy use of alcohol—is by far the major cause of end-stage liver disease.[1] For persons so afflicted, life may depend on receiving a new, transplanted liver. The number of alcoholics in the United States needing new livers is great, but the supply of available livers for transplantation is small. *Should those whose end-stage liver disease was caused by alcohol abuse be categorically excluded from candidacy for liver transplantation?* This question, partly medical and partly moral, must now be confronted forthrightly. Many lives are at stake.

Reasons of two kinds underlie a widespread unwillingness to transplant livers into alcoholics: First, there is a common conviction—explicit or tacit—that alcoholics are morally blameworthy, their condition the result of their own misconduct, and that such blameworthiness disqualifies alcoholics in unavoidable competition for organs with others equally sick but blameless. Second, there is a common belief that because of their habits, alcoholics will not exhibit satisfactory survival rates after transplantation, and that, therefore, good stewardship of a scarce lifesaving resource requires that alcoholics not be considered for liver transplantation. We examine both of these arguments.

THE MORAL ARGUMENT

A widespread condemnation of drunkenness and a revulsion for drunks lie at the heart of this public policy issue. Alcoholic cirrhosis—unlike other causes of end-stage liver disease—is brought on by a person's conduct, by heavy

Originally published in *JAMA* 265, no. 10 (March 13, 1991): 1299-1301.

drinking. Yet if the dispute here were only about whether to treat someone who is seriously ill because of personal conduct, we would not say—as we do not in cases of other serious diseases resulting from personal conduct—that such conduct disqualifies a person from receiving desperately needed medical attention. Accident victims injured because they were not wearing seat belts are treated without hesitation; reformed smokers who become coronary bypass candidates partly because they disregarded their physicians advice about tobacco, diet, and exercise are not turned away because of their bad habits. But new livers are a scarce resource, and transplanting a liver into an alcoholic may, therefore, result in death for a competing candidate whose liver disease was wholly beyond his or her control. Thus we seem driven, in this case unlike in others, to reflect on the weight given to the patient's personal conduct. And heavy drinking—unlike smoking, or overeating, or failing to wear a seat belt—is widely regarded as morally wrong.

Many contend that alcoholism is not a moral failing but a disease. Some authorities have recently reaffirmed this position, asserting that alcoholism is "best regarded as a chronic disease."[2] But this claim cannot be firmly established and is far from universally believed. Whether alcoholism is indeed a disease, or a moral failing, or both, remains a disputed matter surrounded by intense controversy.[3-9]

Even if it is true that alcoholics suffer from a somatic disorder, many people will argue that this disorder results in deadly liver disease only when coupled with a weakness of will—a weakness for which part of the blame must fall on the alcoholic. This consideration underlies the conviction that the alcoholic needing a transplanted liver, unlike a nonalcoholic competing for the same liver, is at least partly responsible for his or her need. Therefore, some conclude, the alcoholic's personal failing is rightly considered in deciding upon his or her entitlement to this very scarce resource.

Is this argument sound? We think it is not. Whether alcoholism is a moral failing, in whole or in part, remains uncertain. But even if we suppose that it is, it does not follow that we are justified in categorically denying liver transplants to those alcoholics suffering from end-stage cirrhosis. We could rightly preclude alcoholics from transplantation only if we assume that qualification for a new organ requires some level of moral virtue or is canceled by some level of moral vice. But there is absolutely no agreement—and there is likely to be none—about what constitutes moral virtue and vice and what rewards and penalties they deserve. The assumption that undergirds the moral argument for precluding alcoholics is thus unacceptable. Moreover, even if we could agree (which, in fact, we cannot) upon the kind of misconduct we would be looking for, the fair weighting of such a consideration would entail highly intrusive investigations into patients' moral habits—investigations universally thought repugnant. Moral evaluation is wisely and rightly excluded from all deliberations of who should be treated and how.

Indeed, we do exclude it. We do not seek to determine whether a particular transplant candidate is an abusive parent or a dutiful daughter, whether candidates cheat on their income taxes or their spouses, or whether potential recipients pay their parking tickets or routinely lie when they think it is in their best interests. We refrain from considering such judgments for several good reasons: (1) We have genuine and well-grounded doubts about comparative degrees of voluntariness and, therefore, *cannot pass judgment fairly.* (2) Even if we could assess degrees of voluntariness reliably, we cannot know what penalties different degrees of misconduct deserve. (3) *Judgments of this kind could not be made consistently in our medical system*—and a fundamental requirement of a fair system in allocating scarce resources is that it treat all in need of certain goods on the same standard, without unfair discrimination by group.

If alcoholics should be penalized because of their moral fault, then all others who are equally at fault in causing their own medical needs should be similarly penalized. To accomplish this, we would have to make vigorous and sustained efforts to find out whose conduct has been morally weak or sinful and to what degree. That inquiry, as a condition for medical care or for the receipt of goods in short supply, we certainly will not and should not undertake.

The unfairness of such moral judgments is compounded by other accidental factors that render moral assessment especially difficult in connection with alcoholism and liver disease. Some drinkers have a greater predisposition for alcohol abuse than others. And for some who drink to excess, the predisposition to cirrhosis is also greater; many grossly intemperate drinkers do not suffer grievously from liver disease. On the other hand, alcohol consumption that might be considered moderate for some may cause serious liver disease in others. It turns out, in fact, that the disastrous consequences of even low levels of alcohol consumption may be much more common in women than in men.[10] Therefore, penalizing cirrhotics by denying them transplant candidacy would have the effect of holding some groups arbitrarily to a higher standard than others and would probably hold women to a higher standard of conduct than men.

Moral judgments that eliminate alcoholics from candidacy thus prove unfair and unacceptable. The alleged (but disputed) moral misconduct of alcoholics with end-stage liver disease does not justify categorically excluding them as candidates for liver transplantation.

MEDICAL ARGUMENT

Reluctance to use available livers in treating alcoholics is due in some part to the conviction that, because alcoholics would do poorly after transplant as a result of their bad habits, good stewardship of organs in short supply requires that alcoholics be excluded from consideration.

This argument also fails, for two reasons: First, it fails because the premise—that the outcome for alcoholics will invariably be poor relative to other groups—is at least doubtful and probably false. Second, it fails because, even if the premise were true, it could serve as a good reason to exclude alcoholics only if it were an equally good reason to exclude other groups having a prognosis equally bad or worse. But equally low survival rates have not excluded other groups; fairness therefore requires that this group not be categorically excluded either.

In fact, the data regarding the posttransplant histories of alcoholics are not yet reliable. Evidence gathered in 1984 indicated that the one-year survival rate for patients with alcoholic cirrhosis was well below the survival rate for other recipients of liver transplants, excluding those with cancer.[11] But a 1988 report, with a larger (but still small) sample number, shows remarkably good results in alcoholics receiving transplants: one-year survival is 73.2 percent—and of thirty-five carefully selected (and possibly nonrepresentative) alcoholics who received transplants and lived six months or longer, only two relapsed into alcohol abuse.[12] Liver transplantation, it would appear, can be a very sobering experience. Whether this group continues to do as well as a comparable group of nonalcoholic liver recipients remains uncertain. But the data, although not supporting the broad inclusion of alcoholics, do suggest that medical considerations do not now justify categorically excluding alcoholics from liver transplantation.

A history of alcoholism is of great concern when considering liver transplantation, not only because of the impact of alcohol abuse upon the entire system of the recipient, but also because the life of an alcoholic tends to be beset by general disorder. Returning to heavy drinking could ruin a new liver, although probably not for years. But relapse into heavy drinking would quite likely entail the inability to maintain the routine of multiple medication, daily or twice-daily, essential for immunosuppression and survival. As a class, alcoholic cirrhotics may therefore prove to have substantially lower survival rates after receiving transplants. All such matters should be weighed, of course. But none of them gives any solid reason to exclude alcoholics from consideration categorically.

Moreover, even if survival rates for alcoholics selected were much lower than normal—a supposition now in substantial doubt—what could fairly be concluded from such data? Do we exclude from transplant candidacy members of other groups known to have low survival rates? In fact we do not. Other things being equal, we may prefer not to transplant organs in short supply into patients afflicted, say, with liver cell cancer, knowing that such cancer recurs not long after a new liver is implanted.[13,14] Yet in some individual cases we do it. Similarly, some transplant recipients have other malignant neoplasms or other conditions that suggest low survival probability. Such matters are weighed in selecting recipients, but they are insufficient grounds to categorically exclude an entire group. This shows that the argument for excluding alcoholics based on survival probability rates alone is simply not just.

THE ARGUMENTS DISTINGUISHED

In fact, the exclusion of alcoholics from transplant candidacy probably results from an intermingling, perhaps at times a confusion, of the moral and medical arguments. But if the moral argument indeed does not apply, no combination of it with probable survival rates can make it applicable. Survival data, carefully collected and analyzed, deserve to be weighed in selecting candidates. These data do not come close to precluding alcoholics from consideration. Judgments of blameworthiness, which ought to be excluded generally, certainly should be excluded when weighing the impact of those survival rates. Some people with a strong antipathy to alcohol abuse and abusers may, without realizing it, be relying on assumed unfavorable data to support a fixed moral judgment. The arguments must be untangled. Actual results with transplanted alcoholics must be considered without regard to moral antipathies.

The upshot is inescapable: there are no good grounds at present—moral or medical—to disqualify a patient with end-stage liver disease from consideration for liver transplantation simply because of a history of heavy drinking.

SCREENING AND SELECTION OF LIVER TRANSPLANT CANDIDATES

In the initial evaluation of candidates for any form of transplantation, the central questions are whether patients (1) are sick enough to need a new organ and (2) enjoy a high enough probability of benefiting from this limited resource. At this stage the criteria should be noncomparative.[15,16] Even the initial screening of patients must, however, be done individually and with great care.

The screening process for those suffering from alcoholic cirrhosis must be especially rigorous—not for moral reasons, but because of factors affecting survival, which are themselves influenced by a history of heavy drinking and even more by its resumption. Responsible stewardship of scarce organs requires that the screening for candidacy take into consideration the manifold impact of heavy drinking on long-term transplant success. Cardiovascular problems brought on by alcoholism and other systematic contraindications must be looked for. Psychiatric and social evaluation is also in order, to determine whether patients understand and have come to terms with their condition and whether they have the social support essential for continuing immunosuppression and follow-up care.

Precisely which factors should be weighed in this screening process have not been firmly established. Some physicians have proposed a specified period of alcohol abstinence as an "objective" criterion for selection—but the data supporting such a criterion are far from conclusive, and the use of this criterion to exclude a prospective recipient is at present medically and morally arbitrary.[17,18]

Indeed, one important consequence of overcoming the strong presumption against considering alcoholics for liver transplantation is the research opportunity it presents and the encouragement it gives to the quest for more reliable predictors of medical success. As that search continues, some defensible guidelines for case-by-case determination have been devised, based on factors associated with sustained recovery from alcoholism and other considerations related to liver transplantation success in general. Such guidelines appropriately include (1) refined diagnosis by those trained in the treatment of alcoholism, (2) acknowledgment by the patient of a serious drinking problem, (3) social and familial stability, and (4) other factors experimentally associated with long-term sobriety.[19]

The experimental use of guidelines like these, and their gradual refinement over time, may lead to more reliable and more generally applicable predictors. But those more refined predictors will never be developed until prejudices against considering alcoholics for liver transplantation are overcome.

Patients who are sick because of alleged self-abuse ought not be grouped for discriminatory treatment—unless we are prepared to develop a detailed calculus of just deserts for health care based on good conduct. Lack of sympathy for those who bring serious disease upon themselves is understandable, but the temptation to institutionalize that emotional response must be tempered by our inability to apply such considerations justly and by our duty *not* to apply them unjustly. In the end, some patients with alcoholic cirrhosis may be judged, after careful evaluation, as good risks for a liver transplant.

OBJECTION AND REPLY

Providing alcoholics with transplants may present a special "political" problem for transplant centers. The public perception of alcoholics is generally negative. The already low rate of organ donation, it may be argued, will fall even lower when it becomes known that donated organs are going to alcoholics. Financial support from legislatures may also suffer. One can imagine the effect on transplantation if the public were to learn that the liver of a teenager killed by a drunken driver had been transplanted into an alcoholic patient. If selecting even a few alcoholics as transplant candidates reduces the number of lives saved overall, might that not be good reason to preclude alcoholics categorically?

No. The fear is understandable, but excluding alcoholics cannot be rationally defended on that basis. Irresponsible conduct attributable to alcohol abuse should not be defended. No excuses should be made for the deplorable consequences of drunken behavior, from highway slaughter to familial neglect. But alcoholism must be distinguished from those consequences; not all alcoholics are morally irresponsible, vicious, or neglectful drunks. If there is a general failure to make this distinction, we must strive to overcome that failure, not pander to it.

Public confidence in medical practice in general, and in organ transplantation in particular, depends on the scientific validity and moral integrity of the policies adopted. Sound policies will prove publicly defensible. Shaping present health care policy on the basis of distorted public perceptions or prejudices will, in the long run, do more harm than good to the process and to the reputation of all concerned.

Approximately one in every ten Americans is a heavy drinker, and approximately one family in every three has at least one member at risk for alcoholic cirrhosis.[3] The care of alcoholics and the just treatment of them when their lives are at stake are matters a democratic polity may therefore be expected to act on with concern and reasonable judgment over the long run. The allocation of organs in short supply does present vexing moral problems; if thoughtless or shallow moralizing would cause some to respond very negatively to transplanting livers into alcoholic cirrhotics, that cannot serve as good reason to make such moralizing the measure of public policy.

We have argued that there is now no good reason, either moral or medical, to preclude alcoholics categorically from consideration for liver transplantation. We further conclude that it would therefore be unjust to implement that categorical preclusion simply because others might respond negatively if we do not.

REFERENCES

1. Consensus conference on liver transplantation, NIH. *JAMA.* 1983;250:2961-2964.

2. Klerman FL. Treatment of alcoholism. *N Engl J Med.* 1989;320:394-396.

3. Vaillant GE. *The Natural History of Alcoholism.* Cambridge, Mass: Harvard University Press; 1983.

4. Jellinek EM. *The Disease Concept of Alcoholism.* New Haven, Conn: College and University Press; 1960.

5. Rose RM, Barret JE, eds. *Alcoholism: Origin and Outcome.* New York: Raven Press; 1988.

6. *Alcohol and Health: Sixth Special Report to the Congress.* Washington, DC: US Dept of Health and Human Services; 1987. DHHS publication ADM 87 1519.

7. Fingarette H. Alcoholism: the mythical disease. *Public Interest.* 1988;91:3-22.

8. Madsen W. Thin thinking about heavy drinking. *Public Interest.* 1989;95:112-118.

9. Fingarette H. A rejoinder to Madsen. *Public Interest.* 1989;95:118-121.

10. Berglund M. Mortality in alcoholics related to clinical state at first admission: a study of 537 deaths. *Acta Psychiatr Scand.* 1984;70:407-416.

11. Scharschmidt BF. Human liver transplantation: analysis of data on 540 patients from four centers. *Hepatology.* 1984;4:95-111.

12. Starzl TE, Van Thiel D, Tzakis AG, et al. Orthotopic liver transplantation for alcoholic cirrhosis. *JAMA.* 1988;260:2542-2544.

13. Gordon RD, Iwatsuki S, Tazkis AG, et al. The Denver-Pittsburgh Liver Transplant Series. In: Terasaki PI, ed. *Clinical Transplants.* Los Angeles, Calif: UCLA Tissue-Typing Laboratory; 1987:43-49.

14. Gordon RD, Iwatsuki S, Esquivel CO. Liver transplantation. In: Cerilli GJ, ed. *Organ Transplantation and Replacement.* Philadelphia, Pa: JB Lippincott; 1988:511-534.

15. Childress JF. Who shall live when not all can live? *Soundings.* 1970;53:339-362.

16. Starzl TE, Gordon RD, Tzakis S, et al. Equitable allocation of extrarenal organs: with special reference to the liver. *Transplant Proc.* 1988; 20:131-138.

17. Schenker S, Perkins HS, Sorrell MF. Should patients with end-stage alcoholic liver disease have a new liver? *Hepatology.* 1990;11:314-319.

18. *Allen v Mansour A,* US District Court for the Eastern District of Michigan, Southern Division. 1986;86-73429.

19. Beresford TP, Turcotte JG, Merion R, et al. A rational approach to liver transplantation for the alcoholic patient. *Psychosomatics.* 1990;31:241-254.

30. Should a Criminal Receive a Heart Transplant? Medical Justice vs. Societal Justice

Lawrence J. Schneiderman
and Nancy S. Jecker

1. INTRODUCTION

DeWayne Murphy was described in a *New York Times* article as "desperately ill with cardiomyopathy, a progressive weakening of the heart muscle."[1] The story went on to say that under ordinary circumstances he would be a candidate for a heart transplant. But Mr. Murphy's circumstances are not ordinary: he is in a federal prison hospital in Rochester, Minnesota, and the Federal Bureau of Prisons which is responsible for his medical costs refuses to pay for a heart transplant.

The reporter suggested that the case "raises troubling questions about access to health care for those in the criminal justice system"[2] and enumerated them as follows:

> Should the nation provide expensive care and scarce organs to convicted felons? Can it justify a system in which an estimated one in four employed Americans cannot have a transplant because they are uninsured or underinsured, yet ask the Bureau of Prisons to provide them for prisoners? If the Bureau will not pay for a transplant, should it pay for a quadruple bypass? Or looking at it in another way, should a nonviolent criminal like Mr. Murphy get a heart transplant but a murderer or rapist not? What about someone convicted of a white collar crime, like tax fraud? Where, if at all, should society draw the line?[3]

The reporter went to two prominent medical ethicists for opinions on the case. Their comments suggested that from an ethical perspective such

Originally published in *Theoretical Medicine* 17 (1996): 33-44. © 1996 Kluwer Academic Publishers.

detailed questions were entirely out of place. Arthur Caplan, then Director for the Center for Bioethics at the University of Minnesota, responded: "For me, it's open and shut. It is absolutely wrong to make judgments about past behavior, criminal conduct, moral worth, indictments, charges or convictions."[4] Nancy Dubler, the director of the division of bioethics at the Montefiore Medical Center in the Bronx, was quoted as saying that "the clear movement since [the time when citizen committees denied access to renal dialysis] has been to establish rigorously abstract criteria so that the worth of an individual is not factored in" [when deciding who should get organs or other lifesaving medical treatments].[5]

Both experts, therefore, apparently took the position that it was unethical even to consider withholding a treatment of restricted availability to Mr. Murphy on the grounds that he is a convicted criminal. In our view, however, these ethicists gave inappropriately short shrift to the journalist's questions by conflating two fields of justice. Although our phrase, "fields of justice," resonates with philosopher Michael Walzer's term, "spheres of justice,"[6] we distinguish between the two concepts as follows: "spheres of justice" describes the array of *resources,* such as money, professional rewards, leisure time, and education, that a just society would attempt to distribute justly; "fields of justice" indicates the array of *criteria* (medical and social), such as urgency of need, capacity to benefit, value to society, and ability to pay, that a just society considers in distributing a single resource, namely health care.

We will argue in this paper that physicians lack the moral authority to deny beneficial medical treatments on any grounds, but that society can ethically choose whom to deny beneficial treatments, on medical or nonmedical grounds, if the availability of those treatments is limited. Expressed differently: although in the *field of medical justice* it is ethically unacceptable to withhold treatments on the basis of societal worth, since societal worth has no moral relevance in medical decision-making, the same ethical principle does not apply in the *field of social justice.* Therefore, to give Mr. Murphy's case due consideration requires examining separately two fields of justice, medical and societal justice. In our opinion, the ethicists quoted above consider only the field of medical justice and fail to consider criteria of societal justice.

2. MEDICAL JUSTICE

In an episode from his turn of the century autobiography, Hans Zinsser describes the efforts expended to rescue a dying patient named König, who strangled a woman to death then stabbed himself in the abdomen with a bread knife.[7] Although no one doubted that the "blond and stocky ruffian" was a brutal murderer, an eminent surgeon rapidly mobilized his team of expert

assistants and saved the man's life. After three months of hospital convales-
cence, König recovered, was duly put on trial, found guilty and electrocuted.
Zinnser, a medical intern at the time, took a dim view of what he regarded as
wasted effort, but the response of the doctors was clearly in keeping with the
time-honored tradition of medical justice. As a profession, physicians owe
(even if they do not always uphold) the ideal of service to anyone in need
who can benefit from medical treatments—even murderers—without regard
to ethnic, racial, societal or economic factors. And although this ideal may be
compromised when physicians face resource limitations, such as ICU bed
shortages, we would argue that the ideal nevertheless remains.

Haavi Morreim[8] argues that, in this era of soaring medical costs, physicians have acquired a new duty, to exercise responsible stewardship over
medical resources. She states that it is

> simply unrealistic to suppose that physicians *can* wait until society's allocation
> scheme is just, before they begin to participate in serious cost containment. . . .
> [Moreover,] while he cannot assure that resources saved in one instance will be
> devoted to other needier patients, the physician nevertheless can be sure in a
> negative sense that whatever he spends on one patient will *not* be available to
> others. . . . Thus the physician cannot escape a direct role, [in rationing medical
> care.][9]

Despite Morreim's excellent point, we would still argue that the *primary*
obligation of physicians remains to act in the best interests of their patients.
Although as citizens in society, physicians can and should contribute to
social health policy decisions, at the bedside of an individual patient they
should avoid making unilateral rationing decisions.

In support of our account of medical justice, it can be said, first, that bedside rationing by physicians runs the risk of not being thoroughly reasoned,
consistently applied, held accountable to the public, or insulated from arbitrary and unfair manipulation. Second, physician decisions made on the basis
of social factors would have adverse effects, such as undermining trust in the
physician-patient relationship. Third, society at large, not physicians, has the
ethical and political mandate to make allocation decisions. Fourth, rationing
should not occur at the bedside because health professionals do not possess
the knowledge or expertise to do it right. According to a recent survey, only
8 percent of all physicians report receiving formal training in cost containment measures.[10] Finally, it can be noted that requiring physicians to make
medical decisions without regard to the perceived social worth of their
patients accords best with the historical traditions of ethics in medicine. The
Hippocratic Oath, for example, requires physicians to swear allegiance to the
welfare of patients. The Oath states, "I swear . . . to follow the method of
treatment which, according to my ability and judgment, I consider for the
benefit of my patients."

Whenever physicians violate this obligation—as for example when evidence appears that their actions are affected by financial self-interest, such as ownership of laboratory of X-ray facilities—the profession as well as society protests.[11]

Prognostic data systems, such as APACHE and PRISM, now being developed by researchers to guide physicians in decision-making, involve only medical factors, namely physiologic measures and mortality outcomes.[12] In addition to these prognostic systems based primarily on mortality, health care researchers also have developed methods that measure quality of well-being as a way of assessing treatment effectiveness. In these latter approaches, preference-weighted measures of symptoms and functioning provide a numerical point-in-time expression of quality of well-being (QWB).[13] In arguing for the application of these systems, health policy experts make the case that if a particular treatment produces no improvement in QWB then the treatment would have no basis for its use nor for the expenditure required. Or, if two or more treatments are being considered, then the treatment that produces the best improvement in QWB for the least cost has a claim to priority.[14] Once again, medical benefit is the outcome criterion physicians apply. This criterion is appropriate within the field of medical justice.

At this point it is worth noting that Mr. Murphy, albeit limited in his capacity to make full use of his health because of his imposed confinement, would not be disadvantaged by any contemporary prognostic data system, such as APACHE or QWB, since his limitations have nothing to do with medical factors. Thus, from the perspective of *medical justice,* physicians should not deny him a transplant.

Physicians' clinical evaluations of new drugs or techniques also base their conclusions on morbidity and mortality outcomes exclusively. And even those medical journal articles calling for restraint in the use of techniques, such as cardiopulmonary resuscitation in various clinical circumstances, base their recommendations only on factors that influence medical outcomes, such as quality, length, and likelihood of medical benefit.[15] The rare study that draws attention to the age of patients does so only because age seems to influence these medical outcomes.[16]

On those occasions when physicians did attempt to restrict treatments based on societal factors, it was in the belief that such factors had prognostic medical significance. Liver failure secondary to alcoholism, for example, was first assumed to be a contraindication to hepatic transplantation because of the expected increased mortality.[17] Patient compliance, an essential component of successful transplantation, seemed unlikely in those with a history of chronic alcoholism. But when outcomes studies disclosed no empirical difference in outcomes compared with other forms of liver disease, therefore no rationale for such discrimination, medicine itself moved to change that policy.[18]

Sometimes physicians go to great lengths to avoid even the appearance that their medical decisions might be influenced by societal factors. For example, when the physicians caring for Helga Wanglie sought court approval to withdraw her life support, they took into account that she was supported by a combination of public and private insurance, reasoning that treatment withdrawal therefore could not be construed as providing a financial advantage for the hospital. In the same hospital at the same time was another patient in the permanent vegetative state who was a member of a minority group and on welfare. The physicians purposely did not seek court approval to withdraw life support from this latter patient, because they feared that these social factors would create the impression of social bias and therefore taint their arguments.[19]

All the above suggests that there is general acceptance within the medical profession that physicians owe patients consideration based solely on potential *medical* benefits and without any regard to nonmedical factors. Ideally, the field of medical justice would be *noncomparative*, to use Beauchamp and Childress's term.[20] That is, physicians would provide or withhold treatments without comparing the potential medical benefit of treating one patient against the potential medical benefit of treating another patient.

However, realities within the field of medical justice dictate that some treatments, such as heart transplantation, are *comparative* (again to use the term of Beauchamp and Childress) in that their limited availability requires that their provision to specific patients take into account the competing claims of others. Medical justice enjoins physicians to provide the treatment to the patient most likely to benefit, as measured by medical outcomes, such as quality of well-being and lifespan. This would be an ethical requirement of medical justice.

We acknowledge, however, that in the real world medical justice does not exist in a pure form but rather is tainted by societal factors. Obviously, when treatments of limited availability provide more benefit (such as greater reduction in mortality or greater improvement in QWB) to one category of patients over another, members of the more favored category of patients enjoy distinct societal advantages that place them in this category in the first place. Conversely, persons who stand to gain less medical benefit from treatments may owe their medical disadvantage to their impaired access to early preventive care, rapid emergency care, adequate nutrition and sanitation, employment, education, and other provisions. The process of assigning any person's location in society might be just, or morally arbitrary and unjust.

We submit, however, that the different availability of societal resources does not alter the requirements of medical justice. Medical justice continues to require distributing resources based on medical benefit whether it operates within the variations of a just or an unjust society. In our view, ethicists should acknowledge that social variables influence medical benefits, while deploring and calling for the correction of those social variables that are irrational and unjust. Calling all variations in the availability of beneficial medical treatments unjust, however, strikes us as inappropriately avoiding drawing distinctions.

3. SOCIETAL JUSTICE

In contrast to the longstanding tradition of medical justice, societal justice first gained public attention in the 1960s, when renal dialysis became available to a limited number of patients as a life-saving treatment. Physicians recognized that many patients were potential beneficiaries of this new treatment and that unprecedented choices had to be made. To help make these choices, physicians enlisted the formal assistance of lay committees, as representatives of society—soon disparaged as "God Squads." Although this process was roundly condemned, it is probably more accurate to call it the first attempt to confront society with the distressing reality of rationing, without any preparation. Notions of medical justice (some patients will benefit more than others) and societal justice (choices inevitably have to be made) were unfamiliar to those early participants.[21] Later, governmental agencies, as official representatives of society, also had difficulty facing these issues. The Department of Health and Human Services, for example, balked at funding Standford's heart transplant program because potential recipients were excluded on the basis of what were deemed to be social criteria, including "a history of alcoholism, job instability, antisocial behavior or psychiatric illness," while recipients were favored who had "a stable, rewarding family and/or vocational environment to return to posttransplant."[22] Although the Stanford health care providers probably lacked conclusive empirical evidence, almost certainly they were considering their choices from the perspective of medical justice, namely, that in their experience the stormy, complex, emotionally wrenching and tediously difficult course of a transplant patient would more likely be traversed successfully by someone with a "stable, rewarding family" than someone with "job instability" and "antisocial behavior." In any event, it is not clear whether the government agency's resistance was based on the absence of empirical evidence to support such categories, or rather on the disagreeableness of confronting the reality of medical justice and the unwillingness to offer explicit guidance in terms of societal justice.

In a just society principles of distributive justice govern the distribution of burdens and benefits. Societal justice is necessarily comparative, since in every community composed of individuals of varying ages, fortunes, skills, talents, capacities, strengths and weaknesses, unless deliberate redistributive mechanisms are put in place, morally arbitrary apportionment of burdens and benefits will occur. John Rawls has proposed applying the principles of fair equality of opportunity, and the "difference principle," favoring the least advantaged, as the best approach to redistributing primary goods, such as income, wealth, power, and authority.[23] However, rather than attempting to apply such principles to health care distributions, we invoke Rawls' conception of an original position behind a "veil of ignorance" as a prior starting point for deliberating about the requirements of societal justice.

Parties in an original position might first ask: Who should be considered a member of the society in which benefits and burdens are to be distributed? Starting from this position, one might ask: If a person has already taken (or attempted to take) more than his or her just share of society's benefits, or unfairly caused undue burdens to others, should that person forfeit membership in society? The question of whether or not Mr. Murphy is entitled to a heart transplant then becomes generalized as: If I were to enter a society in which certain life-saving, medical treatments were limited, would I want persons who have already taken benefits away from those who have attempted to live justly to be eligible for further benefits, such as these limited treatments? It is hard to imagine that persons in an original position would answer affirmatively.

A counter-argument might be made, of course: But the criminal has already been punished for that act of injustice by being sentenced to prison. Therefore, it would be unfair for society to impose an additional burden of withholding lifesaving treatments accorded to all other members of society.

In response, we ask: What levels of health care are we talking about anyway? If society considers the criminal to be a full member of a just society, then that person should be entitled to at least a "decent minimum," namely, that level of care considered basic to all members of that society.[24] The question would then follow: Does that level of health care include equal access to beneficial heart transplants? But even if criminals are not considered entitled to the same level of medical care afforded all members of a society, that does not mean they are not entitled to receive any medical care at all. For there is actually a lower level of care, a kind of "rudimentary decent minimum," granted to persons on simple humanitarian grounds, even though they are not considered members of our society. We refer, of course, to treatments like emergency care given to illegal immigrants. The question then follows: Does that "rudimentary decent minimum"—which is the entitlement to medical care accorded to anyone, regardless of whether or not they are members of the society, and whose deprivation would constitute an inhumane burden—include access to heart transplants?

To address these questions, we first must consider whether or not society should accord Mr. Murphy the rights and privileges of a full member of a just society, retaining his entitlements, having paid his debts through imprisonment. This question inevitably touches on another debate that sociobiologists and psychologists and policy-makers endlessly engage in, namely: should society hold criminals accountable for their own actions and therefore responsible for whatever befalls them, or are they handicapped and unfortunate in the natural lottery of life in that they are more likely to arise out of disadvantaged populations? Clearly, one's answer to this question will determine one's answer to: Is it morally right or wrong for society to exclude criminals from access to certain kinds of scarce medical treatments? If one takes the position that criminality is an unfortunate consequence of factors beyond a person's control, then depriving the criminal of any chance at limited medical resources would in effect be "blaming the victim." If one concludes that criminals are accountable for violations of the social contract, and therefore should pay a price for these violations, that imprisonment may constitute adequate payment, then they are entitled at least to a "decent minimum." One would still have to decide whether or not such a minimum includes equal access to heart transplants. Finally, if one concludes that criminals are accountable for their violations of the social contract, that certain crimes can never be adequately compensated for by imprisonment, then they may be entitled only to a "rudimentary decent minimum." Such a level of health care would not include heart transplants, if precedents in our society are any guide.

Interestingly, in at least one respect, society regards prisoners as deserving *greater* health protection than the general population. Because they are deemed vulnerable to coercion and exploitation, prisoners are not allowed to be enrolled in voluntary human experimentations.

Although societal justice has gained prominence only recently, the notion that in a just society some individuals should be denied what others receive did not originate with modern medical technology. To the contrary, it is as old as Plato, who discussed different criteria for distributing of benefits and burdens in a just republic.[26] The proposal advanced by Paul Ramsey that society should allocate limited medical treatments by random lottery has never met with the approval one might have expected from this seemingly objective standard.[27] To the contrary, within the field of societal justice, failing to make discriminating judgments in medical matters seems unfair.

Would society accept that a young mother with life-threatening septicemia ought not be given priority for the last remaining ICU bed over a recidivist drug addict with bacterial endocarditis? It should come as no surprise that those in charge of the ICU bed allocation often make such allocation decisions. Are those physicians basing their decisions purely on principles of medical justice, or have societal factors intruded? And are those societal intrusions inappropriate? The answers depend in large part on what are taken to be the goals of society and who is supposed to decide. If society's first goal is self protection—or protection of the state during warfare—the selection ought to be based on utilitarian criteria. If in choosing one life over another, society's foremost criterion should be value of present and future services to society, then a person's social value should be weighed.[28] On the battlefield, combat readiness is the overriding priority and triage physicians routinely decide. If, on the other hand, society's first goal is to uphold the ideal of protecting the interests of individual members according to egalitarian criteria—that is giving everyone equal access to limited medical benefits as an expression of that society's value system, allowing exclusions only under unusual and desperate circumstances—then such utilitarian criteria rationally would be called upon only in unusual and desperate circumstances.

4. CONCLUSION

Let us return to Mr. DeWayne Murphy, the federal prisoner suffering from cardiomyopathy whose life depends on a heart transplant, and to the questions raised by the journalist.

Should the nation provide expensive care and scarce organs to convicted felons? Our answer is: Perhaps not. It depends on how one answers several further questions. If convicted felons are not accepted as full members of a just society because they violated a social agreement regarding the distribution of benefits and burdens, then they are not entitled to deprive other members of society, who did not violate the societal contract, of scarce life-saving organs. Thus, societal justice would impose limits on medical justice by providing convicted felons with only a "rudimentary decent minimum," which almost certainly would not include access to heart transplants.

Can society justify a system in which an estimated one in four employed Americans cannot have a transplant because they are uninsured or underinsured, yet ask the Bureau of Prisons to provide them for prisoners? Our answer is, probably not, because such a system imposes an additional financial burden on members of society in order to bring about a benefit that they themselves are denied. However, if one can make the case that prisoners are more vulnerable than uninsured working members of society, then perhaps the Bureau should fund transplants. This position is in the spirit of Rawls' "difference principle," which requires distributing limited benefits to the maximum advantage of those who are most disadvantaged. We do not support the suggestion that prisoners represent "the most disadvantaged."

If the Bureau will not pay for a transplant, should it pay for a quadruple bypass? Our answer is, since quadruple bypass is not necessarily limited by resource availability, it may represent a "decent minimum" treatment to which all members of society are entitled. Therefore, a criminal should not necessarily be deprived of it as a matter of societal justice, so long as that criminal is considered a full member of society. However, a quadruple bypass is not likely to be available as a "rudimentary decent minimum," and therefore might not be available to a criminal who is considered to have forfeited membership in a just society.

Should a nonviolent criminal such as Mr. Murphy obtain a heart but a murderer or rapist not? What about someone convicted of a white collar crime, like tax fraud? Where, if at all, should society draw the line? Our answer to these related questions is that the answer may depend on applications of both medical and societal justice. Even if Mr. Murphy were imprisoned for life, he would be entitled to the "rudimentary decent minimum" benefits of life-saving treatments in terms of medical justice. However, in the case of any limited medical treatment, such as heart transplants, in which medical justice is comparative, one might argue that if a criminal's incarceration exceeded the length of lifespan expected as a result of a treatment, then the treatment might be denied on the grounds of inadequate (or comparatively less) medical benefits.

In terms of societal justice, if society decides one crime is not so bad as another, and therefore one criminal more deserving to participate in the distribution of social benefits, then this discrimination might allow heart transplants for some criminals and not for others. But, society's act of permanently removing someone sentenced to life imprisonment from membership could be interpreted as indicating that he has violated the contract experienced by all citizens in the sharing of benefits and burdens and is entitled only to the "rudimentary decent minimum" level of care, which almost certainly would not include access to a heart transplant.

In summary, we believe it is important for medical ethicists commenting before the public at large either in the media or at the governmental policy level to distinguish between the fields of medical and societal justice. Although we agree with Caplan and Dubler that medical justice prohibits differential treatment based on nonmedical criteria, we also submit that comparative medical justice, as well as societal justice standards, may require acknowledging differential entitlement in distributing scarce resources.

REFERENCES

1. Kolata G. U.S. refuses to finance prison heart transplant. *New York Times* February 5, 1994, 6Y.

2. Ibid.

3. Ibid.

4. Ibid.

5. Ibid.

6. Walzer M. *Spheres of Justice: A Defense of Pluralism and Equality.* New York: Basic Books, 1983.

7. Zinsser H. *As I Remember Him: The Biography of R.S.* Boston: Little Brown 1940, pp. 149-150.

8. Morreim H. Cost containment: challenging fidelity and justice. *Hastings Cent Rep* 1988;18(6):20-25.

9. Ibid., 23.

10. Morreim H. Fiscal scarcity and the inevitability of bedside budget balancing. *Arch Intern Med* 1989;149;1012-1015.

11. Mitchell JA, Sunshine JH. Consequences of physicians' ownership of health care facilities—joint ventures in radiation therapy. *N Engl J Med* 1992;327:1497-1501; Swedlow A, Johnson G, Smithline N, Milstein A. Increased costs and rates of use in the California workers' compensation system as a result of self-referral by physicians. *N Engl J Med* 1992;327:1502-1506; Reiman A. "Self-referral"—What's at stake. *N Engl J Med* 1992;327-1522-1524.

12. Knaus WA, Wagner DP, Draper EA, Zimmerman JE, Bergner M, Bostos PG, et al. The APACHE III Prognostic system: risk prediction of hospital mortality for critically ill hospitalized adults. *Chest* 1991;100:1619-1636; Pollack MM. Ruttmann UE, Getson PR. Accurate prediction of the outcome of pediatric intensive care. *N Engl J Med* 1987;316:134-139.

13. Kaplan RM. Quality of life assessment. In: Karoly P, ed. *Measurement Strategies in Health Psychology.* New York: Wiley, 1985:115-146.

14. Emery D, Schneiderman LJ. Cost-effectivemss analysis in health care. *Hasting Cent Rep* 1989;19(4):8-13.

15. Kellerman AL, Staves DR, Heckman BB. In-hospital resuscitation following unsuccessful prehospital advanced cardiac life support: "heroic efforts" or an exercise in futility? *Ann Emer Med* 1988;17(6):589-594; Lantos JD, Miles SH, Silverstein MD, Stocking CB. Survival after cardiopulmonary resuscitation in babies of very low birth weight: is CPR futile? *N Engl J Med* 1988;318:91-95; Faber-Langendoen K. Resuscitation of patients with metastic cancer: is transient benefit still futile? *Arch Intern Med* 1991;151:235-239; Gray WA, Capone RJ, Moss AS. Unsuccessful emergency medical resuscitation—are continued efforts in the emergency department justified? *N Engl J Med* 1991;329:1393-1398.

16. Murphy DJ, Murray AM, Robertson BE, et al. Outcomes of cardiopulmonary resuscitation in the elderly. *Ann Intern Med* 1989;111:199-205.

17. Flavin DK, Niven RG, Kelsey JE. Alcoholism and orthotopic liver transplantation. *JAMA* 1982;259:1546-1547.

18. Liver Transplantation. Consensus Conference. *JAMA* 1983;250:2961-2964; Luccy MR. Liver transplantation for the alcoholic patient. *Gastroenterology Clinics of North America.* 1993;22(2):243-256; Kuman S, Stauber RE, Gavaler JS, Basista MH, et al. Orthotopic liver transplantation for alcoholic liver disease. *Hepatology* 1990;11(2):159-164; Cotton P. Alcohol's threat to liver transplant recipients may be overstated, suggests retrospective study. *JAMA* 1994;271:1815.

19. Miles SH. Personal communication.

20. Beauchamp TL, Childress JF. *Principles of Biomedical Ethics.* 2nd Edition. Oxford University Press, 1983 NY, p.1985.

21. Alexander S. They decide who lives, who dies. *Life* Magazine 11/9/62:102-125.

22. Beauchamp TL, Childress JF: 212.

23. Rawls J. *Principles of Justice.* Cambridge, Massachusetts: Harvard University Press, 1971.

24. Beauchamp TL, Childress JF: 203.

25. Beauchamp TL, Childress JF: 195.

26. Plato. In: Grube GM, transl. *Republic.* Indianapolis: Hackett Publishing, 1974.

27. Ramsey P. *The Patient as Person.* New Haven, Connecticut: Yale University Press, 1970.

28. Beauchamp TL, Childress JF: 213.

PART FIVE
Value

Transplantation and the issues surrounding its practice have wider implications that applied to health care in general. During the attempted health care reforms of the Clinton Administration in the early 1990s, many in the transplant community voiced what they saw as important lessons to be learned from transplantation. Among them, were the suggestions that current transplantation practice and policy could serve as a useful model in dealing with issues of scarcity, allocation, and physician advocacy roles. In addition, by meeting the goal of serving both individual and social interests, transplantation could serve as a model of rational policy emulation in health care reform.

In making the claim that transplantation is worthy of emulation it has to be presumed that organs are allocated fairly. However, the truth is that equal access to organ transplantation does not reflect reality. Often, non-medical factors are used to screen out potential transplant recipients. The role of money and the ability to pay in gaining access to transplantation (Evans and Daniels' articles of Part Three) have been noted earlier in this volume. Additional non-medical, non-financial factors include personal health habits, psychological status, and family resources. Furthermore, it has been intensely argued within the literature that serious imbalances exist in access to transplantation with respect to race, gender, and age leading some to believe that transplantation is more a reflection of the health system's failures than a model for guiding the system's reform. Problems of disparate access to health care have long haunted American health care and they are present with respect to transplantation as well.

Despite being disproportionately represented on waiting lists for kidney transplants, African Americans are half as likely as whites to receive them and wait longer for them. Robert S. Gaston and colleagues maintain that differences in access to cadaveric kidneys between whites and blacks can not solely be blamed on genomic differences of histocompatability. Rather, the authors contend that significant biases in organ allocation policy prevent the fair distribution of kidneys. Racial disparity is not the only example of discrimination in transplantation. Women tend to receive heart transplants less often then men although they represent a majority of those in need, and younger people generally move up waiting lines quicker than older people. Some older persons are not considered for transplants at all.

In 1998, the Department of Health and Human Services called for a change from multiple local and regional organ distribution systems to a single national waiting list. Previously, organs obtained in a particular community would go first to those in need in the community if a transplant center was available. This policy meant that those living near transplant centers had an advantage in gaining access to them. It also encouraged the proliferation of transplant centers since local organs would be used locally. Now, those areas with high demand and low supply of organs will benefit if the policy is changed whereas areas with previously high supplies and low demand will suffer. It is an idea that has proven popular with some in the transplant community, but a nightmare for many politicians.

Issues of race, gender, and geography all should play an important role in gauging the fairness of access to transplantation. However, even if agreement were reached on what constitutes fair access, there would still be a larger, arching question requiring an answer in assessing the value of transplantation—what is the value of transplantation in our society? Is it really worth the money invested in it? In 1987 the Joint Ways and Means Committee of the Oregon legislature decided to eliminate public funding of organ transplantation in favor of extending funds for basic health care. The law has subsequently been changed, but the events leading to this unprecedented decision, the public reaction, the subsequent state's response, and the lessons drawn from such a decision are chronicled by H. Gilbert Welch and Eric B. Larson.

Whereas the Oregon decision was based on principles of distributive justice, others in the transplant community have faulted transplantation for what they perceived as gross neglect of other fundamental ethical principles, namely benevolence and non-maleficence. Renee C. Fox and Judith Swazey, the two sociologists who have most extensively studied organ transplantation, decided to leave the field after a combined total of sixty-five years. Fox and Swazey ultimately refused to continue as part of a community that failed to accept the limits to the biological and human condition imposed by the aging process and ultimate mortality. It is a powerful condemnation of what American transplantation has, from their perspective, become.

The successes and shortcomings in American transplantation have much to contribute to overall health care and its reform, but the lessons extend well beyond the boundaries of "health care." Transplantation has been viewed as a model of how society in general functions, the study of which has provided great insight on a variety of important topics to sociologists, philosophers, theologians, and economists. For example, through transplantation, sociologists have been able to better address the meanings of giving and receiving and the dynamic of gift exchange in American life. Philosophers have been able to study the direct application of theoretical principles of equity to clinical reality. Economists have used the model of scarcity to better understand the laws of supply and demand as well as the allocation of scarce resources from a limited commons. Theological analysis of transplantation has provided opportunities to revisit the definitions of life and death, the duty to help others, and the sanctity of the human body.

The academic value of transplantation has proven to be powerful, but the ethical and practical policy issues that must be addressed by the reality of scarcity will occupy center stage in discussion of transplants for years to come. In the face of an imperfect and possibly unfair system of transplantation, society must be ready to realize that the symbolic and social costs of shifting values may come at an ethical price too high to pay. How close we are to that point will be a source of great interest in the twenty-first century.

Arthur L. Caplan
Daniel H. Coelho

31. Racial Equity in Renal Transplantation: The Disparate Impact of HLA-Based Allocation

Robert Gaston, Ian Ayres, Laura Dooley, and Arnold Diethelm

Kidney transplantation from either a living related or cadaveric donor is optimal treatment for most patients with end-stage renal disease (ESRD).[1] However, due to a critical shortage of organ donors, while more than 23,000 Americans await a suitable cadaveric kidney, fewer than 8,000 receive transplants each year.[2,3] Approximately one-third of ESRD patients in this country are African American (black), a proportion threefold greater than the representation of this racial group in the general population (12 percent).[1] Recently, the Inspector General reported that blacks are less likely than whites to receive a transplant, with almost double the waiting time.[4] Currently, cadaveric kidneys are allocated according to a federally mandated system based on quality of HLA matching. This policy is based on evidence that antigenic similarity between donor and recipient may enhance cadaveric graft survival and should be the primary factor influencing distribution.[5] Gjertson and colleagues[6] have proposed that there be even greater emphasis on HLA matching in organ allocation, with all cadaveric kidneys to be placed in a single national pool and distributed to the transplant candidate with the "best" HLA match. In the face of a critical (and growing) shortage of transplantable kidneys, current directives place potential black recipients at a significant disadvantage; extension of HLA-based allocation will magnify racial disparity. We contend that all suitable renal transplant candidates should have equitable access to cadaveric kidneys. To the extent that HLA matching demonstrably improves survival of cadaveric renal allografts, it is an efficient means to effect difficult allocative choices. But, given its documented negative impact on black ESRD patients, the system must be reevaluated to determine whether the cost in equity is truly

Originally published in *JAMA* 270, no. 11 (September 15, 1993): 1352-56.

justified. A recent editorial suggested that "every kidney counts";[7] we submit, rather, that every patient counts.

RACIAL DISPARITY IN ESRD
AND TRANSPLANTATION

Minority populations in the United States (American Indians, African Americans, and Hispanics) are at increased risk of developing ESRD relative to whites.[8] Blacks are numerically the largest of these minorities and also have the highest incidence of chronic renal failure.[2] Since 1972, Congress, under the auspices of Medicare, has funded ESRD therapy for most Americans, in the form of either long-term dialysis or renal transplantations.[9] A successful kidney transplant imparts several advantages to the recipient, who is more likely to avoid hospitalization, experience a greater sense of well-being, return to the workforce, and, perhaps, live longer than with dialytic therapy.[10-12] Additionally, after the first year, the costs of caring for a transplant recipient are roughly one third of those associated with long-term dialysis.[1] According to a review of the favorable impact of transplantation on the Medicare ESRD program, "Trends in transplantation have not yet had much effect on black beneficiaries . . . [who] . . . were receiving transplants at only half the rate of white beneficiaries."[1] Indeed, 1989 figures from the US Renal Data System (USRDS) revealed white dialysis patients to be more than twice as likely as black patients to receive a kidney allograft (8.3 percent vs 3.9 percent).[2] Kidneys from living, usually related, donors constitute 20 percent of all transplants.[2] Blacks desiring transplantation are, for poorly defined reasons, less likely than whites to have a suitable living donor and are relatively more dependent on availability of cadaveric kidneys. However, despite their constituting 31 percent of patients on waiting lists, blacks received only 22 percent of cadaveric kidney transplants in 1990, with a median waiting time of 13.9 months vs 7.6 months in whites.[4,13] Among American Indians, rates of transplantation are comparable to those for whites; data regarding Hispanic patients are incomplete.[14] Thus, the impact of disparity in transplantation is greatest for African-American patients.

Possible causes of racial disparity in cadaveric transplantation are numerous, to be sure, and have been the subject of a recent review.[14] Black patients in the Southeastern United States may be less likely than whites to be referred for transplantation.[15] Although the waiting list at the University of Alabama at Birmingham reflects local ESRD demographics (65 percent African American), national data support this finding: blacks, despite receiving fewer living related transplants, are relatively underrepresented on cadaveric waiting lists.[4] Moreover, when a cadaveric kidney becomes available, socioeconomic circumstances may limit the ability of potential black recipients to communicate with or travel to the transplant center in a timely fashion.[16] Nevertheless, organ allocation policy, a previously unacknowledged factor, plays a key role in perpetuating disparate racial access to cadaveric kidneys and, therefore, to transplantation.

ORGAN ALLOCATION IN THE UNITED STATES

The National Organ Transplantation Act (Public Law 98-507) of 1984 mandated creation of an Organ Procurement and Transplantation Network (OPTN), charged with establishing (1) "a national list of individuals who need organs," (2) a national system "to match organs and individuals included in the list," and (3) "membership criteria and medical criteria for allocating organs."[17] A preexisting entity, the United Network for Organ Sharing (UNOS), was awarded the OPTN contract under the auspices of the Department of Health and Human Services. After 1986, UNOS operated as the OPTN. Under penalty of losing all Medicare funding, the Omnibus Budget Reconciliation Act (Public Law 99-509) of 1986 mandated compliance of organ procurement organizations and transplant centers with UNOS directives.[17] Congress charged UNOS with acquiring and allocating all usable organs "equitably among transplant recipients according to established medical criteria"; accordingly, UNOS developed guidelines affecting kidney allocation at both the local and national levels.

A 1987 UNOS ruling stipulated that if a potential recipient shared all six antigens identified at the HLA-A, HLA-B, and HLA-DR loci with any cadaveric donor, "it is mandatory that the kidney shall be offered for the six antigen patient."[18] Multicenter data had indicated that excellent graft survival could be expected for such recipients; to facilitate outstanding matches, a large donor-recipient pool would be required.[19,20] For the first time, nationwide organ sharing was mandated. Enhanced graft survival for six-antigen-matched recipients (who receive <5 percent of all cadaveric transplants) was determined to outweigh all other claims on a donated organ and to justify the excess cost and effort required to transport kidneys on a national level.[21] Recently, an identical "six-antigen match" was effectively redefined as phenotypically identical ("zero-antigen mismatch"), extending mandatory sharing to a greater number of harvested kidneys.[22] Graft survival has indeed been excellent (88 percent at one year) in 1,004 recipients of mandatorily shared kidneys using both definitions. However, successful engraftment was also achieved in 79 percent of 22,188 recipients of mismatched kidneys during the same time period.[23,24]

If a donated kidney fails to qualify for mandatory sharing (no six-antigen–matched patient exists), organ allocation occurs at the "local" level, as defined by individual organ procurement organizations. The first attempt

United Network for Organ Sharing Point System for Kidney Transplant Recipient Selection (1989)

	Points
HLA matching	
No A, B, DR mismatch	10
No B, DR mismatch	7
No A, B mismatch	6
1 B, DR mismatch	3
2 B, DR mismatches	2
3 B, DR mismatches	1
Presensitization	
Panel reactive antibodies ≥80% (negative crossmatch)	4
Waiting time	
Patient with longest waiting time (proportionate fractions of 1 point to patients waiting shorter periods)	1
Each year on waiting list	0.5
Age of children, y	
0-5	2
6-10	1

to standardize local allocation was the adoption of the "Starzl system" in 1987: "points" were awarded to potential recipients on the basis of quality of HLA match, waiting time, degree of presensitization (presence of anti-HLA antibodies), "medical urgency," and logistic factors such as proximity to the transplant center.[25] The candidate on the local waiting list with the greatest number of points for a particular donated kidney was offered the organ. In 1989, the "Terasaki modification" supplanted the initial algorithm.[26] This revision deleted proximity and urgency as factors and placed greater emphasis on quality of HLA match (Table). Under this system, although other factors (such as age and presensitization) impact the selection process, HLA match is the principal determinant of kidney allocation, with waiting time serving largely as a tiebreaker. For example, a patient with only a single antigen matched could conceivably be given priority for a particular kidney over zero-matched candidates who had waited up to two years longer. In the absence of a UNOS-approved alternative plan (termed a variance), all local entities are required to allocate kidneys on this basis.[5]

Racial Impact of HLA-Based Allocation

Despite striking advances in technology, characterization of the major histocompatibility complex (MHC) in humans remains incomplete. It is clear that profound racial differences exist in antigen expression. Blacks have less well-defined HLA antigenic specificities than do whites, particularly at the DR locus.[27,28] Furthermore, HLA antigens are distributed differently among races.[29] For example, at the A locus, HLA-A1 is found in 23 percent of whites, but only 10 percent of blacks; conversely, HLA-A23 is much less common in whites (6 percent) than blacks (22 percent). Newer histocompatibility approaches, including molecular and epitope matching, by defining more precisely MHC and its products, have demonstrated better correlation of HLA matching with graft survival.[30,31] However, application of these techniques has confirmed the presence of even greater heterogeneity in MHC expression.

When current methodology is considered (ie, serological typing for six A, B, and DR antigens), along with other factors such as linkage disequilibrium, histocompatibility exerts a significant racial impact on organ allocation: the closer the match, the less likely a kidney will cross racial lines.[32,33] Lazda and Blaesing[33] examined the quality of the HLA match between 352 cadaveric donors (86 percent of whom were white) and a waiting list of potential recipients who were 51 percent white. Over 70 percent of potential recipients for whom at least four of six antigens matched were white. These investigators have also noted the rarity of kidneys crossing racial lines with fewer than four mismatched antigens.[34] Emphasis on HLA matching in distribution of cadaveric kidneys disfavors interracial transplantation, a fact acknowledged by proponents of HLA-based allocations.

Accordingly, allocation based on HLA matching promotes racial disparity in access to renal transplantation in the United States. Only 8 percent of cadaveric kidneys come from black donors; whites donate the overwhelming majority of such organs.[2] Lazda and Blaesing[33] concluded that ". . . using HLA matching to allocate kidneys from a predominantly Caucasian donor population favors the Caucasian recipients and places . . . blacks at a disadvantage." The racial consequences of HLA-based allocation are confirmed by data derived from mandatory sharing of six-antigen–matched kidneys. Of true six-antigen–matched recipients, initial reports documented fewer than 2 percent as black.[21] Since the incorporation of a phenotypic definition of six-antigen match, this proportion has increased to 7 percent.[24] At the University of Alabama at Birmingham (with a waiting list that is 65 percent black) only one of thirty-three kidneys shipped or received as part of the six-antigen–match program has been for a black patient.[35] Data from UNOS confirm that blacks receive six-antigen–matched kidneys at one-tenth the rate of whites.[36] Hunsicker and Held[37] have estimated that mandatory national sharing of all kidneys with no HLA mismatches would result in a maximum of 8 percent going to black recipients, with a net overall effect of reducing by three percentage points the number of kidneys available for all black candidates. Further, at the local level, white patients receive the vast majority of kidney transplants with excellent donor-recipient histocompatibility.[33,34,38] It is not uncommon to see white candidates receive transplants within weeks of placement on the waiting list, solely because they demonstrate common HLA antigen specificities. Indeed, black patients' receiving transplants may actually be facilitated by a small waiting list: a larger list may include more potentially well-matched (i.e., white) candidates.

Proponents of HLA-based allocation have suggested further extension of mandatory sharing, with all cadaveric kidneys offered to the candidate with the "best" HLA match on a national basis.[6] They argue that graft survival will be maximized, fewer patients will require retransplantation, and, therefore, more kidneys will be available for those remaining on waiting lists. The potential racial impact of such a policy is not addressed directly, but a "trickledown" benefit for blacks is suggested as white patients, with common HLA antigens receive transplants and are removed from waiting lists. However, in the presence of an organ shortage, with a threefold (and growing) excess of potential recipients, along with racial disparity in MHC expression, there will always be white patients who match the donor population better than black patients. In theory, this discrepancy might be ameliorated by increased organ donation from African Americans.[16,21,33] Blacks may be relatively underrepresented as donors; more African-American donors would mean more well-matched kidneys for black transplant candidates. Although such a solution is attractive, the demographic reality is that, due to overrepresentation of blacks in the ESRD population, there will always be more potential black recipients than donors. Organ donors originate within the general population. In Alabama, blacks make up 24 percent of the population, 21 percent of cadaveric donors, yet 65 percent of those awaiting renal transplants.[39] Nationally, blacks constitute 12 percent of the population, 8 percent of donors, but 34 percent of those with ESRD.[2] To satisfy the demand of African-American candidates for well-matched kidneys, organ donation from blacks must increase by 500 percent, to a standard far in excess of realistic goals and donation rates within the white community. Although we emphatically support efforts to promote organ donation among blacks (and whites), increased donation by African Americans is not the sole solution to racial disparity in renal transplantation. Moreover, the presumed (though difficult to confirm) lack of participation by black Americans in the organ donation process does not justify policies that enhance access for individual white ESRD patients relative to individual black patients.

EQUITY AND EFFICIENCY IN ORGAN ALLOCATION: RACIAL IMPLICATIONS

As we have noted, the original charge to UNOS was to allocate organs "equitably among transplant recipients according to established medical criteria."[17] Current policies stress the latter portion of this charge by emphasizing quality of HLA match in an attempt to improve transplant outcomes: efficiency is the goal. The Inspector General's report, recognizing disparity in the process, recommends that the Public Health Service, in collaboration with the OPTN, ". . . distribute donated organs to those patients on a first-come first-served basis, subject to established medical criteria."[4] Equity is thus restated as a primary objective in organ allocation; however, a pure equity-based system, or queue, risks ignoring factors that may have an impact on success rates in transplantation. In both statements, the tension between equity and efficiency centers on the significance of the term "medical criteria." One must then assess whether the benefit of HLA matching in enhancing efficiency is sufficiently great to override equity concerns.[40]

Allocation based on HLA matching is rooted in evidence that antigenic similarity between donor and recipient may enhance graft survival; thus, the most efficient use of a donated organ requires excluding from transplantation those candidates less likely to have a good result (i.e., those with a poorer match). Clear correlation between HLA match and outcome is well documented in living related transplantation, where phenotypic matching is a proxy for underlying genetic similarity.[19] However, in cadaveric transplantation, with genetically diverse donors and recipients, benefit from matching is less well defined.[41-44] In the cyclosporine era, outcomes appear to be improved for recipients of extremely well-matched cadaveric transplants: a difference in graft survival of ten to fourteen percentage points at two years between best (no mismatches) and worst (completely mismatched) donor-recipient pairs is generally accepted, and confirmed by data from the six-antigen–match program.[44] However, incremental changes in graft survival as one moves from six (completely mismatched) to one mismatch are at most one to three percentage points and are inconsistently documented.[36,44] Indeed, USRDS data, derived from Medicare records, demonstrate little statistical relationship of HLA match to survival of first allografts at five years in the presence of one or more mismatches.[37] For black recipients of first grafts, there is no consistently documented benefit of HLA matching on graft survival.[29,45,46] According to data from the UCLA Transplant Registry, matching may not be a significant prognostic factor for black recipients.[47-49] In a recent review of UNOS data, Cicciarelli and Cho[36] state that "black transplant recipients show little or no matching effect when HLA-A, B, and DR antigens matched." Indeed, subsequent data from the UNOS Registry do not indicate significant improvement in graft survival even for black recipients of phenotypically identical grafts.[24] In retransplantation, which occurs in a more complex immunologic milieu, quality of match may assume greater significance.[37,44,50] Thus, the benefits of allocation based on HLA matching are neither uniform nor unequivocal: its greatest influence occurs in white recipients of phenotypically identical kidneys. Enhanced efficiency for other potential recipients, as well as for the "system," is undocumented.

Moreover, enhanced efficiency is not and cannot be the singular objective of organ allocation. If it were, one could compellingly argue that blacks be completely excluded from cadaveric transplantation. To maximize efficiency, any discount in graft survival may be sufficient for exclusion. An eight- to nineteen-percentage-point decrement in graft survival for blacks relative to whites is well documented[2,45,47] and quite similar to differences in outcome between extremely well-matched and poorly matched transplants. Allocation of kidneys to whites only (as occurs indirectly in the six-antigen–match program) might therefore enhance graft survival equally as well as hierarchical HLA matching. Efficiency also has a financial context. Gjertson and colleagues[6] suggest that hierarchical HLA-based allocation would potentially save Medicare $6.5 million over five years: improved graft survival would more than offset the additional costs derived from matching, preserving, and transporting kidneys nationwide. However, exclusion of blacks from cadaveric transplantation, based on racial differences in graft survival, might save even more money. Extending the analysis of Gjertson and colleagues, with hazard rates derived from Opelz and associates,[51] the estimated five-year average cost of a transplant (including return to dialysis in the event of graft failure) is $98,300 for a black recipient and $90,700 for a white recipient. Reallocating to whites the approximately 1,400 cadaveric kidneys that annually go to black recipients might save an additional $10.6 million. Obviously, direct racial exclusion to enhance efficiency in either cost or graft survival is morally and ethically unacceptable. The drive for efficiency must be tempered by a more sophisticated policy of accommodation in kidney allocation.

EQUITY AND EFFICIENCY: ACCOMMODATION

If there were no effect of variables such as race and matching on transplant outcomes, tension between equity and efficiency would be eliminated. Recent advances in renal transplantation hold the promise of such nonexclusionary efficiency. Data from several centers have shown graft survival for all recipients of first grafts, regardless of HLA match, to equal those reported in multicenter data for only the best matches.[42] These results have accrued with quadruple immunosuppression, a regimen that combines administration of four potent agents (Minnesota antilymphoblast globulin, cyclosporine, azathioprine, and corticosteroids) in a sequential fashion. At the University of Alabama at Birmingham, this protocol has abrogated racial differences in primary allograft survival over three years, despite significantly poorer HLA matching in blacks,[38] a finding confirmed by others.[52] Newer, perhaps more effective and less toxic immunosuppressants (FK506, RS61443, rapamycin, and 15-deoxyspergualin) and monoclonal antibodies (anti-ICAM-1) are on the horizon with the potential to further diminish the impact of HLA matching on graft survival.[53-57]

Despite emphasis on HLA matching to enhance efficiency, current UNOS policies already accommodate equity in some circumstances. A relatively lengthy waiting time for patients of blood type O (universal donor) was thought to reflect the practice of offering kidneys with a better HLA match to an ABO-compatible recipient.[58] As a remedy, UNOS policy was amended to specify that O kidneys be offered only to O recipients (except in the presence of a six-antigen match). Thus, transplant candidates with type O blood are offered equal access to cadaveric kidneys despite the potential of better HLA matches in patients with other ABO types.[22] Furthermore, patients who are highly sensitized to HLA antigens (a situation that limits their ability to accept kidneys from potential donors) receive points to enhance equity, despite the knowledge that presensitization is a risk factor for graft loss.[5] Finally, children, who have poorer graft survival than adults, receive additional points to enhance access to renal transplantation.[59] In each of these situations, some efficiency is sacrificed to achieve greater equity.

Accommodation between the competing goals of racial equity and efficiency, while elusive, is nonetheless attainable. Preference for HLA matching should be given only in proportion to its documented effectiveness in improving graft survival, that is, in extremely well-matched recipients (usually white) and retransplant candidates. Mandatory sharing of phenotypically identical kidneys should continue: its utility is supported by a well-defined dividend in graft survival, and relatively few kidneys (<5 percent) are removed from the overall cadaveric pool.[23] Kidneys not qualifying for mandatory sharing would continue to be allocated locally; partial matching would be deemphasized, with no points awarded when more than one B or DR antigen is mismatched. If no well-matched candidate is identified for a donated kidney, a policy to enhance allocation to black recipients should be implemented.

A local variance that moves toward more equitable allocation is currently undergoing evaluation in Illinois.[60] Points are awarded only for "excellent" HLA matches, and waiting time is given greater emphasis. While this algorithm enhances black patients' access to kidneys and preserves the efficiency of outstanding matches, its implicit race consciousness does not address the disparity in waiting times between blacks and whites. In fact, it may exacerbate the problem: prolonged time on the list is required for black patients to accumulate enough "points" to offset the advantage to whites of better matching. Thus, although data are not yet available, the Illinois variance avoids specific reference to race but may perpetuate inequity in waiting times.

An alternative proposal might recognize more explicitly the racial implications of HLA-based allocation and award points to blacks without requiring excessive waiting time. "Race-conscious points" could be used to compensate for points accumulated by whites on the basis of HLA matching. Such a plan offers reduced racial discrepancy in both frequency of transplantation and waiting times, with maintained efficiency for well-matched recipients. Its principal liability is explicit race consciousness, a factor that may conflict with other social norms: race, a concept based primarily on skin color rather than physiological difference, must be defined.[61] Realizing the arbitrary nature of any definition, we would propose a simple one: allow transplant candidates to define their own racial origin, much as is currently done in collecting USRDS and UNOS data.[2,44] Thoughtful dialogue is necessary to further refine such a radical solution. Nevertheless, an approach that openly confronts racial differences may be required, at least temporarily, if equity is to be achieved.

CONCLUSION

The equitable and efficient distribution of limited resources, such as cadaveric kidneys, requires careful evaluation of all the effects of allocative choices that are made. In this essay, we have focused, perhaps simplistically, on the racial impact of allocation policies: clearly, race is not the sole issue impacting organ allocation. However, HLA-based allocation is equally simplistic in the assumption that universal benefit will result from better matching. The truth is that some will benefit, and others will not. Disproportionate representation of African Americans in the ESRD population dictates that racial considerations cannot be ignored in the distribution of cadaveric kidneys in the United States. Efforts to increase black donation are to be encouraged but will not eliminate disparity. If racial equity in renal transplantation is to be achieved, alternative allocation strategies must be formulated that forthrightly address the interests of all potential recipients.

REFERENCES

1. Eggers PW. Effect of transplantation on the Medicare end-stage renal disease program. *N Engl J Med.* 1988;318:223-229.

2. US Renal Data System. *USRDS 1991 Annual Data Report: The National Institutes of Health, National Institute of Diabetes and Kidney Diseases.* Bethesda, Md: National Institutes of Health; 1991.

3. *UNOS Update.* Washington, DC: United Network for Organ Sharing; 1993;9(4):28.

4. Kusserow RP. *The Distribution of Organs for Transplantation: Expectations and Practices.* Office of Inspector General, Dept of Health and Human Services, 1991.

5. *UNOS Policy 3.5.* Richmond, Va: United Network for Organ Sharing; 1990.

6. Gjertson DW, Terasaki PI, Takemoto S, Mickey MR. National allocation of cadaveric kidneys by HLA matching. *N Engl J Med.* 1991;324:1032-1036.

7. Braun WE. Every kidney counts. *N Engl J Med.* 1992;327:883-885.

8. Feldman HI, Klag MJ, Chiapelia AP, Whelton PK. End-stage renal disease in US minority groups. *Am J Kidney Dis.* 1992;19:397-410.

9. Rettig RA. Origins of the Medicare kidney disease entitlement: the Social Security amendments of 1972. In: Hanna KE, ed. *Biomedical Politics.* Washington, DC: National Academy Press; 1991: 176-208.

10. Evans RW, Manninen DL, Garrison LR, et al. The quality of life of patients with end-stage renal disease. *N Engl J Med.* 1985;312:553-559.

11. Fischel RJ, Payne WD, Gillingham KJ, et al. Long-term outlook for renal transplant recipients with one-year function. *Transplantation.* 1991;51: 118-122.

12. Evans RW. The demand for transplantation in the United States. In: Terasaki PI, ed. *Clinical Transplants 1990.* Los Angeles, Calif: UCLA Tissue Typing Laboratory; 1991:319-327.

13. *1990 Annual Report.* Richmond, Va: United Network for Organ Sharing; 1991.

14. Kasiske BL, Neylan JF, Riggio RR, et al. The effect of race on access and outcome in transplantation. *N Engi J Med.* 1991;VA:302-307.

15. Soucie JM, Neylan JF, McClellan W. Race and sex differences in the identification of candidates for renal transplantation. *Am J Kidney Dis.* 1992; 19-414-419.

16. Sanfilippo FP, Vaughn WK, Peters TG, et al. Factors affecting the waiting time of cadaveric kidney transplant candidates in the United States. *JAMA.* 1992;267:247-251.

17. Blumstein J. Federal organ transplantation policy: a time for reassessment. *Univ Calif Davis Law Rev.* 1989;22:451-472.

18. *UNOS Policy 3.3.3.* Richmond, Va: United Network for Organ Sharing; 1990.

19. Mickey MR. HLA matching effects. In: Terasaki PI, ed. *Clinical Transplants 1987.* Los Angeles, Calif: UCLA Tissue Typing Laboratory; 1987:303-316.

20. Mickey MR, Cook DJ, Terasaki PI. Recipient pool sizes for prioritized HLA matching. *Transplantation.* 1989;47:401-403.

21. Terasaki PI, Takemoto S, Mickey MR, A report on 123 six-antigen matched cadaver kidney transplants. *Clin Transplantation.* 1989;3:301-305.

22. *UNOS Policy 3.3.l.* Richmond, Va:United Network for Organ Sharing; 1990.

23. Takemoto S, Carnahan E, Terasaki PI. Report on 604 six-antigen-matched transplants. In: Terasaki PI, ed. *Clinical Transplants 1990.* Los Angeles, Calif: UCLA Tissue Typing Laboratory; 1991:485-495.

24. Takemoto S, Terasaki PI, Cecka JM, Cho YW, Gjertson DW, for the UNOS Scientific Renal Transplant Registry. Survival of nationally shared, HLA matched kidney transplants from cadaveric donors. *N Engl J Med.* 1992;327:834-839.

25. Starzl TE, Hakala TR, Tzakis A, et al. A multifactorial system for equitable selection of cadaver kidney recipients. *JAMA.* 1987;7:3073-3075.

26. *UNOS Update.* Richmond, Va: United Network for Organ Sharing; 1989;5(8):9.

27. Suciu-Foca N, Reed E, Rohowsky C, Lewison A, King DW. Influence of race on the predictability of mixed lymphocyte culture identity by HLA-DR matching. *Transplantation.* 1983;35:35-39.

28. Johnson AH, Rosen-Bronson S, Hurley CK. Heterogeneity of the HLA-D region in American blacks. *Transplant Proc.* 1989;21-3872-3873.

29. Milford EL, Ratner L, Yunis E. Will transplant immunogenetics lead to better graft survival in blacks? racial variability in the accuracy of tissue typing for organ donation: the Fourth American Workshop. *Transplant Proc.* 1987;19(suppl 2):30-32.

30. Takemoto S, Gjertson DW, Terasaki PI. HLA matching: a comparison of conventional and molecular approaches. In: Terasaki PI, Cecka JM, ed. *Clinical Transplants 1992.* Los Angeles, Calif: UCLA Tissue Typing Laboratory; 1993:413-434.

31. Lau M, Terasaki PI, Park MS. International cell exchange: 1992. In: Terasaki PI, Cecka JM, ed. *Clinical Transplants 1992.* Los Angeles, Calif: UCLA Tissue Typing Laboratory; 1993:457-473.

32. Owen M. Major histocompatibility complex. In: Roitt IM, Brostoff J, Male DK, eds. *Immunology.* St Louis, Mo: CV Mosby Co; 1989:4.1-4.11.

33. Lazda VA, Blaesing ME. Is allocation of kidneys on basis of HLA match equitable in multiracial populations? *Transplant Proc.* 1989;21:1415-1416.

34. Lazda VA. The impact of HLA frequency differences in races on the access to optimally HLA-matched cadaver renal transplants. *Transplantation.* 1992;53:352-357.

35. Barger B, Shroyer TW, Hudson SL, et al. The impact of the UNOS mandatory sharing policy on recipients of the black and white races—experience at a single renal transplant center. *Transplantation.* 1992;53:770-774.

36. Cicciarelli J, Cho Y. HLA matching. univariate and multivariate analyses of UNOS registry data. In: Terasaki PI, Cecka JM, eds. Clinical *Transplants 1991.* Los Angeles, Calif: UCLA Tissue Typing Laboratory; 1992:325-334.

37. Hunsicker LG,Held PJ.The role of HLA matching for cadaveric renal transplants in the cyclosporine era. *Semin Nephrol.* 1992;12:293-303.

38. Gaston RS, Hudson SL, Deierhoi MH, et al. Improved survival of primary cadaveric renal allografts in blacks with quadruple immunosuppression. *Transplantation.* 1992;53:103-109.

39. *1991 Annual Data Report.* Jackson, Miss: Network 8 Inc; 1992.

40. Okun AM. *Equality and Efficiency: The Big Tradeoff.* Washington, DC: Brookings Institution; 1975.

41. Alexander JW, Vaughn WK, Pfaff WW. Local use of kidneys with poor HLA matches is as good as shared use with good matches in the cyclosporine era: an analysis at one and two years. *Transplant Proc.* 1987;19:672-674.

42. Ferguson RM. A multicenter experience with sequential ALG/cyclosporine therapy in renal transplantation. *Clin Transplantation.* 1988;2:285-294.

43. Opelz G. In response to the role of HLA matching in renal transplant patients with sequential immunosuppression. *Clin Transplantation.* 1989;3: 233-235

44. Cecka JM, Terasaki PI. The UNOS Scientific Renal Transplant Registry—1990. In: Terasaki PI, ed. *Clinical Transplants 1990.* Los Angeles, Calif: UCLA Tissue Typing Laboratory;1991:1-10.

45. Barger BO, Hudson SL, Shroyer TW, et al. Influence of race on renal allograft survival in the pre and postcyclosporine era. In: Terasaki PI, ed. *Clinical Transplants 1987.* Los Angeles, Calif: UCLA Tissue Typing Laboratory; 1987:217-234.

46. Ward HJ, Koyle MA. The beneficial effect of blood transfusion and the DRI gene dose on renal transplant outcome in blacks. *Transplantation.* 1991; 51:359-364.

47. Kondo K, Shibue T, Iwaki Y, Terasaki PI. Racial effects on kidney transplants. In: Terasaki PI, ed. *Clinical Transplants 1987.* Los Angeles, Calif: UCLA Tissue Typing Laboratory; 1987:339-350.

48. Yuge J, Cecka JM. The race effect. In: Terasaki PI, ed. *Clinical Transplants 1989.* Los Angeles, Calif: UCLA Tissue Typing Laboratory; 1989:407-416.

49. Takemoto S, Terasaki PI. A comparison of kidney transplant survival in white and black recipients. *Transplant Proc.* 1989;21:3865-3867.

50. Gaston RS, Shroyer TW, Hudson SL, et al. Renal retransplantation: the role of race, quadruple immunosuppression, and the flow cytometry cross-match. *Transplantation.* In press.

51. Opelz G, Pfarr E, Engelmann A, Keppel E. Kidney graft survival rates in black cyclosporine-treated recipients. *Transplant Proc.* 1989;21:3918-3920.

52. Butkus DE. Primary renal cadaveric allograft survival in blacks—is there still a significant difference? *Transplant Rev.* 1991;5:91-99.

53. Macleod AM, Thomson AW. FK506: an immunosuppressant for the 1990's? *Lancet.* 1991;337:25-27.

54. Sollinger HW, Deierhoi MH, Belzer FO, Diethelm AG, Kaufmann R. RS-61443: phase I clinical trial and pilot rescue study. *Transplantation.* 1992; 53:428-432.

55. Knight R, Ferraresso M, Serino F, et al. Low dose rapamycin potentiates the effects of subtherapeutic doses of cyclosporine to prolong renal allograft survival in the mongrel canine model. *Transplantation.* 1993;56:947-949.

56. Tamura K, Okubo M, Damata K, et al. 15-deoxyspergualin rescue therapy against methylprednisolone-resistant rejection of renal transplants as compared with anti-T cell monoclonal antibody. *J Am Soc Nephrol.* 1991;2:819. Abstract.

57. Haug CE, Colvin RB, Delmonico FL, et al. A phase I trial of immunosuppression with anti-ICAM-(CD54) monoclonal antibody in renal allograft recipients. *Transplantation.* 1993;55:766-773.

58. Port FK, Held PJ, Wolfe RA, Garcia JR, Rocher LL. The impact of nonidentical ABO cadaveric renal transplantation on waiting times and graft survival. *Am J Kidney Dis.* 1991;17:519-623.

59. *UNOS Policy* 3.5.10.Richmond,Va: UnitedNetwork for Organ Sharing; 1990.

60. Lazda VA. An evaluation of a local variance of the UNOS point system on the distribution of cadaver kidneys to waiting minority recipients. *Transplant Proc.* 1991;23:901-902.

61. Osborne NG, Feit MD. The use of race in medical research. *JAMA.* 1992;267:275-279.

32. Dealing with Limited Resources: The Oregon Decision to Curtail Funding for Organ Transplantation

H. Gilbert Welch and Eric B. Larson

In the spring of 1987, the Joint Ways and Means Committee of the Oregon legislature faced a painful choice. The Division of Adult and Family Services, charged with administering the state Medicaid program, framed the options for the next two years. During the next biennium—the basic funding period in Oregon—Medicaid could either extend its funding for basic health care to include about 1,500 persons not covered previously, or continue to fund a program of organ transplantation (bone marrow, heart, liver, and pancreas) for a projected thirty-four patients.

In a dramatic example of the type of painful decision necessitated by limited resources, the division advocated the former, and the committee concurred. This report chronicles the events leading to the decision, the public reaction, and the state's response. Finally, we discuss several lessons drawn from the experience in Oregon.

EVENTS THAT LED TO THE DECISION

Still recovering from the recession of the early 1980s, Oregon is one of the few states in which voters have approved limits to state revenues and expenditures. Within the framework of a constitutional mandate requiring a balanced budget, the legislature hoped to improve access to basic health care for low-income Oregonians in the biennium 1987 to 1989. Although some monies were available from savings outside the area of health and from the annual allowed budgetary expansion, other health expenditures had to be forgone.

Oregon's experience with organ transplantation (except for kidneys and corneas) had been marked by considerable expense and limited success among relatively few beneficiaries. The first state-funded transplantation was performed at the end of the 1983 to 1985 biennium, when a girl received two liver transplants at a cost of $150,000 and subsequently died. From 1985 to 1987, nineteen transplantations were funded, at a cost of $1 million; only nine patients still survive.[1] The cost of follow-up care for each survivor was $24,000 per year.

The Division of Adult and Family Services projected that thirty-four patients would require transplants during the period from 1987 to 1989, at an estimated cost of $2.2 million—a cost it expects to see double again in the next biennium. Pointing to federal Medicaid statutes requiring equal treatment for similarly situated patients, the division stressed that there was no way the state could limit its funding to a prescribed number of transplant patients. Although explicit criteria for transplantation had been established, the division warned that individual cases had the potential to become highly politicized if transplants were denied. Division leaders urged the legislature to choose between continuing transplant coverage for a few and investing in more basic health care for many.

With little discussion and no public debate, on June 1, 1987, the Joint Ways and Means Committee unanimously voted to discontinue coverage for organ transplants. It substituted expanded coverage of basic medical services for low-income children and pregnant women in the budget package. Later that month, both the Oregon House and the Senate approved the new budget proposal by wide margins (45 to 7 and 19 to 3, respectively). As he signed the bill into law, Governor Neil Goldschmidt expressed the sentiments of many legislators with his comment:

> We all hate it, but we can't walk away from this issue any more. It goes way beyond transplants. How can we spend every nickel in support of a few people when thousands never see a doctor or eat a decent meal?[2]

PUBLIC REACTION

Reaction to the decision was slow to evolve. The initial media coverage was minimal. The cases of two adults who were denied transplants in the summer and fall of 1937 were reported in the news,[3] with little public response. But in November, media interest was aroused when a seven-year-old boy with acute lymphocytic leukemia was denied a bone marrow transplant. His death in December elicited nationwide reaction. the *Washington Post* ran the headline "Rising Cost of Medical Treatment Forces Oregon to 'Play God.' "[2] "Oregon Cut in Transplant Aid Spurs Victims to Turn Actor to Avert Death," reported the *New York Times,* in a reference to the "performance" required of the boy to raise private funds.[4] In fact, this effort raised three quarters of the funds required by the marrow-transplantation facility.

The new Oregon policy sparked two lawsuits and numerous fund-raising initiatives on behalf of those needing transplants.[5] A boycott of organ donations was organized by some low-income people. The issue focused national attention on Oregon; both ABC's "Nightline" and PBS's "MacNeil/Lehrer Newshour" ran segments on the potential effect nationwide. The impact was more immediate in neighboring Washington State, where, for example, one mother moved her family to Seattle in a trailer so that her child would qualify for marrow transplantations.[6]

The most articulate advocate of transplant funding was Craig Irwin, an insurance agent, whose mother had been denied coverage for a liver transplant. Irwin wrote a sophisticated response to the legislative decision, in which he argued for consideration of the net cost (gross cost minus savings), not the absolute cost of organ transplantation. Conceding that transplantations were expensive, Irwin stressed that the conventional therapies given those who were denied transplants were expensive as well. He calculated the net cost of transplantations in Oregon to be only $1.1 million for the 1987-to-1989 biennium. On the other hand, the alternative investment in prenatal care ought to be offset by a savings in neonatal care. He calculated the net cost of prenatal care at only $150,000 for the same period and concluded that the state could well fund both programs. If additional funds were required, Irwin suggested that there were areas in medicine whose benefit was marginal and whose cost could be forgone:

> If Oregon truly has limited resources, it would make sense to allocate those resources to the individuals that would benefit the most. At the same time, perhaps we should withhold resources from those who would survive without our assistance, and we should also deny resources to those who may soon die even with our help [Irwin CJ: unpublished data].

THE STATE'S RESPONSE

Officials of the Division of Adult and Family Services chose to respond formally to Irwin's criticisms. In their rebuttal they agreed that net costs were the issue, but only if they affected the state. Cost savings accruing from improved prenatal care would not benefit the state's budget, since the affected neonates had not been covered previously. The officials contended that the cost of alternative care for a patient who was denied a transplant was about the same as follow-up care for such a patient after transplantation—approximately $2,000 per month. Thus, the net cost of performing a transplantation was the cost of the procedure itself. They reiterated that such costs would be hard to contain:

> It would be difficult if not impossible to open the transplant door part way. Once coverage is available, it is available to all who qualify and the number cannot be limited to some budgeted level.[7]

But the high visibility of those who were denied transplantation kept the debate in public. Concern grew that, in fact, the services being denied had a high probability of success in selected persons. Others lamented that no such visibility was being extended to those denied basic medical care. As the Senate president, John Kitzhaber, M.D., wrote in an editorial,

> Is the human tragedy and the personal anguish of death from the lack of an organ transplant any greater than that of an infant dying in an intensive care unit from a preventable problem brought about by a lack of prenatal care?[8]

The failure of his medical colleagues to see beyond their narrow interests also disturbed Dr. Kitzhaber:

> It is easy for representatives of the Oregon Health Sciences University to argue that the state should pay for organ transplants while neglecting to mention the $7.6 million in general fund budget increases the university was given during the 1987 legislative session. I do not recall lobbyists for the Oregon Health Sciences University recommending additional funds for heart and liver transplants at the expense of their own program enhancements.[8]

An apparent compromise was reached in late March of this year. The state's access to federal matching funds (sixty-two cents on the dollar) and its ability to negotiate lower rates with the transplantation facilities provided a strong incentive to reinstate coverage for transplantation. Thus, the state would pay about a quarter of what a private person would pay,[5] permitting Oregon legislators to propose a novel, and untested, solution. The state promised to reinstate the transplantation program if sufficient private funds could be raised to support it. These monies could then be used as leverage to obtain federal funds and arrange preferred-provider agreements. A set of guidelines for transplantation was developed in April.

Several concerns remain. First, it is unclear how federal Medicaid officials will react to the use of private donations to qualify for matching funds. The paramount question, however, is whether private donations will be sufficient to sustain the program. Because state funding for transplantation has been discontinued for almost a year, there is concern about the possibility of a sizable "pent-up" demand. Most private donations are made on behalf of specific people, and fund raisers may also hesitate to turn contributions over to the state if they believe their candidates will be rejected. Furthermore, questions have been raised regarding the propriety of one recent fund-raising effort and even about the need for the proposed procedures.[9] Many questions await the convening of the 1989 legislature

CONCLUSION

Oregon is not the only state to limit the Medicaid financing of organ transplantation,[4,5] but the fundamental public-policy questions have been most sharply delineated there. Regardless of one's views on the outcome, the Oregon legislature is to be commended for confronting such a difficult issue. Its decision openly acknowledges limited resources and makes a choice among competing health care wants. We are likely to see more of this kind of decision in the future.

But why were organ transplantations the target? After all, they represent an area in which medical success has captured the public's attention. Four reasons seem especially important. First, organ transplantations represent easily identifiable, large-scale expenses. Second, they benefit relatively few people. Third, they represent a new type of therapy that is more easily forgone than other, longer-established ones. Finally, because coverage for organ transplantations (as for chiropractic and dental benefits) is not mandatory under Medicaid statutes, they constitute discretionary expenditures for each state, and are therefore targets for cost containment.

In summary, the Oregon experience suggests four lessons. First, medical resources are limited. The need for allocation engendered by limited and unlimited wants is the first lesson taught to students of economics. For some in health care field, this has been a hard reality to accept. The Oregon debate over the spending of health care dollars vividly demonstrates this principle. The debate was fueled by a realization of the growing inequity of extensive medical care for some and none for others. The Oregon decision attempted to allocate resources in a more deliberate, rational manner.

Second, the need for acute care is more visible to the public than the need for preventive care. The reaction to the Oregon decision suggests that acute care commands more media attention than preventive care. Specific people benefit from acute interventions, but it is unclear who will benefit from preventive ones. Also, the benefit of acute care is felt immediately, whereas the benefit of preventive care is realized in the future. A named person who is dying now is more visible than an unnamed person dying in the future. Such unidentified future patients need strong advocates in the medical community.

Third, regardless of their effectiveness, new medical therapies are more likely targets for cost containment than those already established. As stated earlier, a major reason for the elimination of funding for organ transplantation in Oregon was that they represented a new expenditure. Basic medical care, on the other hand, is seen as the extension of a long-established expenditure to an additional group of people. Therefore, the choice was between making established therapies more comprehensive and financing new ones. Since the medical community did not suggest that a portion of the established therapy might be forgone, the legislature chose accordingly.

Finally, for new therapies to be widely funded, they must replace older, less effective ones if total health expenditures are to be held constant. The message sent from Oregon is clear: budgetary constraints are real, and they apply to health care. Physicians are welcome to join the debate over choices, but choices must be made.[10-13] We must look beyond our own vested interests and no longer assume that medicine is any more important than schools, roads, safety, water, or other public programs. Policy makers need our views in order to establish sensible priorities for medical care. If organ transplantation is an important therapy, we ought to help make room for it by suggesting other therapies that are less useful and can be forgone.

REFERENCES

1. Adult and Family Services Division, Department of Human Resources, State of Oregon. Oregon Medicaid organ transplant services. For public presentation November 20, 1987. Revised March 6, 1988.

2. Specter M. Rising cost of medical treatment forces Oregon to 'play God.' *Washington Post*. February 5, 1988:A1, A7.

3. O'Neill P. State denies funds for two transplants. *Oregonian*. November 3, 1987:Bl, B6.

4. Egan T. Oregon cut in transplant aid spurs victims to turn actor to avert death. *New York Times*. May 1, 1988:12.

5. O'Neill P. State sets tone for far-reaching transplant fight. *Oregonian*. January 31, 1988:Cl, C6.

6. Paulson T. Leukemia-stricken child brought to state in bid to save life. *Seattle Post-Intelligencer*. April 5,1988:A4.

7. Adult and Family Services Division, Department of Human Resources, State of Oregon. AFS analysis of Craig Irwin's transplant paper. January 1988.

8. Kitzhaber J. Who'll live? Who'll die? Who'll pay? *Oregonian*. November 29, 1987:Bl, B6.

9. O'Neill P. Fund drive questions bring study. *Oregonian*. April 23,1988:Al, A17.

10. Fuchs VR. *Who shall live? Health, economics, and social choice.* New York: Basic Books, 1974.

11. Hiatt HH. Protecting the medical commons: who is responsible? *N Engl J Med* 1975; 293:235-41.

12. Evans RW. Health care technology and the inevitability of resource allocation and rationing decisions. *JAMA* 1983; 249:2047-53.

13. Idem. Health care technology and the inevitability of resource allocation and rationing decisions. *JAMA* 1983; 249:2208-19.

33. Leaving the Field

Renée Fox and Judith Swazey

"Well, imagine you had a great-great-grandson . . . and he lived to see the end of the state. No injustice, no inequality—how would he spend his life, Sancho?"

"Working for the common good."

"You certainly have faith, Sancho, great faith in the future. But he would have no faith. The future would be there before his eyes. Can a man live without faith?"

"I don't know what you mean—without faith. There will always be things for a man to do. The discovery of new energy. And disease—there will always be disease to fight."

"Are you sure? Medicine is making great strides. I feel sorry for your great-great-grandson, Sancho. It seems to me that he may have nothing to hope for except death."

The mayor smiled. "Perhaps we may even conquer death with transplants."

"God forbid," Father Quixote said. "Then he would be living in a desert without end. No doubt. No faith. I would prefer him to have what we call a happy death."

"What do you mean by a happy death?"

"I mean the hope of something further."

(Greene 1983, pp. 72-73)

As journeyers into the field, participant observers, and chroniclers, we have been involved in the development of organ transplantation, the artificial kidney, and the artificial heart throughout most of their contemporaneous medical and social history and for many years of our working lives. Since 1951 (RCF) and 1968 (JPS) we have had the privileged opportunity to watch, from the inside, how dialysis and kidney, heart, and liver transplantation, which began as "desperate remedies for desperate patients," with certain "desperate[ly] hopeless" conditions (Moore 1989, p. 1483), evolved into "nonexperimental," though far from ordinary, interventions to treat a wide gamut of end-stage diseases. During those years we have seen the range and combinations of different organs transplanted, the numbers performed, and the array of artificial organs designed increase dramatically, and we have charted at firsthand the early phases of the drive to replace the human heart with a man-made device.

Our intensive, long-term relationship with these therapeutic innovations and their clinical unfolding has had many of the characteristics anthropologist Margaret Mead identified as inherent to field research, no matter where it is located or what its subject matter may be. Field work, as she described it, entails not just the unique

> but also cumulative experience of immersing oneself [*sic*] in the ongoing life of another people, suspending for the time both one's beliefs and disbeliefs, and of simultaneously attempting to understand mentally and physically this other version of reality. . . .
>
> Immersing oneself [*sic*] in the field is good, but one must be careful not to drown. One must somehow maintain the delicate balance between empathic participation and self-awareness, on which the whole research process depends. . . .
>
> Only very slowly did we [field workers] begin to take into account that we ourselves change with each step of the journey, with each new image presented to us . . . and with each day in the field. . . . (Mead 1977, pp. 1, 7, 15).

Our research did not transport us to geographically and culturally isolated primitive villages, where we lived and worked day after day for months without the respite of returning to our home-world. Yet, in many crucial respects, our field experiences parallel those of Mead. We have journeyed far, horizontally and vertically, in our questing after transplantation, dialysis, and the artificial heart—coast to coast in this country, and to Europe, Hawaii, Majuro, and China; down long corridors into the high technology surgical and intensive care chambers of the modern hospital; and ever more deeply into the corridors and chambers of ourselves. The people we have studied have been our "teachers" as well as our "subjects," helping us to learn their language and their ways. We have risen "at cock crow" to accompany transplant teams, donors, and recipients into operating rooms, and we have stayed up all night to "listen for some slight change" in a patient's or prospective donor's condition and "revel or mourn" with medical professionals, patients, and families. We have "used ourselves as instruments," striving to attain and reattain the "kind of reflexive objectivity that calls for continuous self-scrutiny and self-analysis, along with observing and interpreting the actions and interactions of others." For years, as participating observers and observing participants, we have walked the thin line between detachment and concern and between "belief and disbelief." And like Mead, "only very slowly did we realize" that, as a consequence of our "immersion" in the field, deep and enduring changes were taking place in us (Mean 1977, pp. 1-16).

Foremost among the people whose "reality" we have been allowed to share are the physicians and nurses, patients and families who have been the chief actors in the "experiments perilous" through which organ transplants, dialysis, and the efforts to fashion a viable artificial heart have been advanced. It has kept us in close contact with the grave illnesses and frequent deaths they have mutually faced, with the hope and renewal, the "break-throughs," and the despair and disappointments they have experienced, and with the ways of navigating and coping they have forged. We often have been enriched and energized by the many transplantation- and artificial organ-centered communities we entered and by the professional and personal relationships we have established within them. Our association with the human story of these therapeutic innovations, their scientific and clinical significance, and their social and moral import has never been academically detached. In fact, the process of disengaging ourselves from this field has made us feel at times as though we were getting a divorce, departing from a religious order, or forsaking comrades in crisis.

Our decision to leave the field has been a complex one and a long time in the making. Over the past decade or so, we gradually recognized in ourselves the signs and symptoms of what we diagnosed as "participant-observer burnout"—akin to what we have witnessed over the years in some of the medical professionals immersed in the world of organ replacement efforts. Our burnout has its roots in the fact that there have been aspects of these efforts that we always have found especially troubling. Prominent among them have been some components of the "courage to fail" value system prevalent among transplantation and artificial organ pioneers. This ethos includes a classically American frontier outlook: heroic, pioneering, adventurous, optimistic, and determined. It also involves, however, a bellicose, "death is the enemy" perspective; a rescue-oriented and often zealous determination to maintain life at any cost; and a relentless, hubris-ridden refusal to accept limits. It is disturbing to witness, over and over, the travail and distress to which this outlook can subject patients:

> I have often seen transplant surgeons, confronted with a clinical dilemma, begin to invoke a litany of names, like a litany of Roman Catholic saints [a transplant service chaplain reflects]: "It may be a real long shot," they say, "but remember Vernie and remember Toni and remember Carl and remember . . . and remember . . . and remember. . . . (The litany, which always consists of patients who survived against seemingly impossible odds, is used as an argument for pressing on. There does not seem to be a parallel list that would argue for giving up.) (Reimer 1989, p. 41).

It is sometimes hard to meet the eyes of patients who have improved enough to
have been moved to the regular postop floor and finally become alert enough to
communicate their despair and disappointment. . . . Often, after entering the
experience with such great hope, patients for whom transplantation has been a
series of setbacks clearly articulate their feelings of betrayals "No one ever told
me it could be like this." . . .

Certainly they were told that there would be no guarantees, and that it
would be hard, and that there would be setbacks—but probably not how hard,
or what some of the worst-case scenarios could be. When they were told, "You
have to have a transplant or you're going to die," they were left a very slim
margin for decision making. These people need to know not only what it will be
like not to be dying any more, but what it may be like to not live so well. (Park
1989, p. 31)

Another early source of unease was our conviction that if our society is
to engage in such endeavors, we have a moral obligation to ensure equitable
access to organ replacement. In the absence of such equity, we have observed
again and again how specifically designated individuals have been privileged
to obtain needed organs and funding for transplantation by wielding special
emotional, media, political, and economic resources available to them, including, during the Reagan years, the power and resources of the presidency.

Rather than focusing on conditions that ultimately are defensible in terms of
equality and justice, . . . designated . . . person-specific . . . organ donation . . .
ties access to an organ to the emotional appeal (or lack thereof) of the prospective recipient, the public relations skills of the physicians involved, of the next-
of-kin, and of those who orchestrate the media campaign, and the financial abilities of every-one concerned to mount such a campaign in the first place. . . .
[I]n effect [it] . . . singles out a specific individual and characterizes him or her
as someone to whom an organ may be given independently of the established
means of access. The assumption is that this person is ethically special; that he
or she has some particular quality or characteristic that permits an exemption
from the criteria that would otherwise apply to all. (Kluge 1989, pp. 11-12)

Our decision to leave the field actually occurred in two phases. Our first
attempt to do so turned out to be no more than a brief moratorium. During
1979-82, partly under the aegis of the James Picker Foundation Program on
the Human Qualities of Medicine, we conducted targeted field research for a
book of essays that would be a sequel to *The Courage to Fail*. It was during
the course of this work, as we immersed ourselves once more in the "lived-
in reality" of the world of organ replacement endeavors, that we first seriously discussed leaving this field.

Many people and experiences from those years remain indelibly etched
in our minds. It was the identified cases, relationships, and advances we were
privileged to study first-hand that both powerfully bound us to the field for
so long and, cumulatively, led us to withdraw from it. Among those still vivid

images are the vista of an empty thoracic cavity awaiting the implantation of a heart and lungs from a brain-dead donor at Stanford; the sight of desperate parents and their tiny, dying children with huge eyes, bloated bellies, pale, lifeless hair, and ochre-colored skin, who had made pilgrimages to Dr. Thomas Starzl in Pittsburgh to plead for a liver transplant; and, in both of these settings, the first exuberant discussions about the miracles that were being wrought by the discovery of cyclosporine.

Above all, it was the "identified lives"—the patients and families we came to know, some only slightly and others more intimately—that made us feel sadder and more anxious than we had in the past and filled us with painfully unanswerable questions of "why?" Though we had met him only briefly when he was a heart transplant patient at Stanford Medical Center, for example, we felt true human ties to Talcott (Sam) Poole and real sorrow when we read of his death from renal failure in December 1982 at age 24. We thought also of his family and of his caregivers at Stanford, who were portrayed so vividly in an extraordinarily moving book by Sam's mother, *Thursday's Child*, which chronicled the onset of his incurable heart disease, his transplant and life thereafter, and his at-once joyous and stoical spirit through it all.

Another such experience was with Doris, a close, kin-like friend whose "case" we had both studied and participated in personally and professionally for many years. We had talked many times with her and, after her death, with her family about trying to capture in a written "portrait" all that her story entailed about the worst and best of being a chronic dialysis patient. For she, more than any other person we have known, exemplified the finest elements of the "courage to fail" ethos in her life with progressive renal failure, several humanly and medically' difficult years of dialysis, and then a death that represented some of the worst features of a "House of God" teaching hospital (Shem 1978). There is a sense in which we have vicariously experienced what Thomas Starzl has described as "the sense of personal loss" and "the cumulative weight of grief, that transplant surgeons like himself have undergone in response to the deaths of the "desperately ill" persons for whom they have cared, particularly the deaths of individuals who have come to personify for them the suffering of all their patients and the embodiment of their "determination to make things better" for them through transplantation. "The burnout rate," Starzl has observed, was especially "high in the early days of transplantation. Because of this, and because aging spares no one [he added], only a handful of workers in transplantation have stayed in the field continuously throughout its thirty-year modern history" (Starzl 1990).

Six weeks of field research during the summer of 1981 in the People's Republic of China also had a powerful impact on us (Fox and Swazey 1982, 1984). During that era of the "four modernizations," China's medical workers had a collective commitment to "serving the patient" by progressively "scaling the heights" of modern medicine. It was part of a larger "golden dream" they shared with their compatriots about what science and technology might achieve for their country and its people. As part of this drive for medical modernization, hospitals in Tianjin were making their first forays into organ transplantation and chronic dialysis. As we watched these beginnings, we were vividly reminded of what Dr. Francis D. Moore termed the "black years" of renal transplantation in the United States—complete with the high mortality rate of patients and organs and what would now be considered in our country and in Western Europe excessive doses of corticosteroid immunosuppressive drugs, with all their side effects. Absorbed though we were by many features of our Chinese field experience, we were reluctant to "go through again" what RCF observed forty years ago on the metabolic research ward of the Peter Bent Brigham Hospital in Boston, where renal transplantation and dialysis were pioneered (Fox 1959). We also found ourselves in the peculiar cultural and ideological position of being more preoccupied than our hosts with the allocation of scarce resources dilemma that their dawning interest in transplantation, dialysis, intensive care medicine, and other advanced forms of Western medicine would pose for a country as poor as China, with a population of more than one billion persons and massive public health and primary care needs.

China also provided us with a societal telescope through which, from a great historical, cultural, and physical distance, we were able to connect our thoughts about transplantation and dialysis with our growing sociological and moral concern about the state of American ideas, values, and beliefs, as epitomized by the predominant themes of bioethics a decade ago. In a comparative analysis of "medical morality" in China and bioethics in the United States, we wrote that

> if . . . bioethics is not just bioethics and is more than medical—if it is an indicator of the general state of American ideas, values and beliefs, of our collective self—knowledge, and our understanding of other societies' cultures—then there is every reason to be worried about who we are, what we have become, what we know, and where we are going in a greatly changed and changing society and world. (Fox and Swazey 1984, p. 360)

Although we gathered a great deal of material between 1979 and 1982 we kept postponing the task of turning it into a book. Our problem, we finally admitted to ourselves, was that we had lost much of the detached concern that had enabled us to study and write about this field for so many years. Tellingly, by the end of 1982 we had drafted only the final essay in our unborn volume. It was called, as is this chapter, "Leaving the Field," for we had decided that all the signs and symptoms of our self-diagnosed field worker and writerly malaise indicated that we should withdraw from our work on organ replacement.

In December 1982, as we were completing a draft of "Leaving the Field," newspapers headlined the first implantation of a permanent total artificial heart by Dr. William DeVries and his colleagues at the University of Utah Medical Center. For the next 112 days, we and millions of others followed the drama of Dr. Barney Clark's life and death with a Jarvik-7 heart. However, because of the extensive case study we had made of the total artificial heart implant Dr. Denton Cooley attempted in 1969, the Barney Clark/William DeVries story had a magnetic effect on us, drawing us back into the field despite our resolve to leave it (Fox and Swazey 1978a, ch. 6). And so, in June 1983 we found ourselves en route to Salt Lake City, for what we defined as a brief, one-time period of interviews and observations. However, more than five years passed before, in the fall of 1988, we completed what became a detailed and profoundly disquieting study of the development and use of the Jarvik heart. It was that research project and some of the participant observation experiences associated with it that brought our journeying into this field of medical research and therapeutic innovation to a definitive end.

During the 1980s we also continued to monitor developments and issues in transplantation and dialysis, and our uneasiness about the attributes and side effects of organ replacement endeavors continued to grow. It has become increasingly difficult for us to "suspend [our] beliefs and disbeliefs" and "maintain the delicate balance" between "immersion" and detachment that field work optimally requires (Mead 1977). Through the ongoing process of self-scrutiny and self-analysis that participant observation also entails, we have recognized that our years in the field have made us more, rather than less, emotionally and morally perturbable. For example, we found ourselves responding with stronger negative sentiments than in the past to such *déjà-vu* experiences as hearing some of the same transplanters who proclaimed the "cosmic" significance of cyclosporine now hail the newly discovered experimental immunosuppresive agent FK-506 as a once-in-a-lifetime miracle drug and learning that the Boy Scouts of America are offering a Donor Awareness Patch to induce Scouts to talk to their families about organ donation. We reacted with concern to a proposal by Paul I. Terasaki, a pioneer of transplantation tissue-typing methods, that organ recipients "who are now enjoying a second chance at life, thanks to the compassionate generosity of the families of donors" be organized into "a trained . . . volunteer . . . self-perpetuating advocacy group" that could "take turns being on call to ask grieving families to consider organ donations, . . . visit hospital personnel . . . who . . . have limited personal contact with . . . a person who has been given life and health with someone else's heart, liver, or kidney," and "promote awareness" of the mounting . . . need" for donations of cadaveric organs (Terasaki 1989). When we read about multiple organ transplants, live-donor liver and lung transplants, conceiving children to serve as bone marrow donors, the temporary use of diseased donor hearts, and about the merits of markets in "HBPs," we wondered, as did philosopher Daniel Callahan, "what kind of life" our values are driving us to seek, and if we can accept "limits to medical progress" (Callahan 1989).

We are not therapeutic nihilists, nor do we lack appreciation for the impressive medical, surgical, and technological progress that has been made with transplants and artificial organs over the course of the past three decades, or just in the past ten years. If anything, our in vivo historical relationship to their development has heightened our recognition of just how far they have advanced. Nor have we lost our capacity to respond with empathy to the "stories with happy endings" (Park 1989) and to those that tragically never came to pass:

> For my family and me [a friend wrote us], the pain and grief of losing John was complicated by the bitter disappointment that we did not receive a heart in time to sustain his life. Intellectually, I know this is an incontrovertible fact. Emotionally, I know that we, his family, were his life and all of you are helping to sustain us. Perhaps, John *did* receive a heart. Although few of you knew him, you gave him yours.

But we have come to believe that the missionary-like ardor about organ replacement that now exists, the overidealization of the quality and duration of life that can ensue, and the seemingly limitless attempts to procure and implant organs that are currently taking place have gotten out of hand. In the words of a transplant nurse-specialist, "perhaps the most important issue in a critical examination of transplantation involves the need and criteria for responsible decisions about when to stop, when to say 'enough is enough' to the transplant process" (Park 1989, p. 30).

In our view, the field of organ replacement now epitomizes a very different and powerful tendency in the American health care system and in the value and belief system of our society's culture: our pervasive reluctance to accept the biological and human condition limits imposed by the aging process to which we are all subject and our ultimate mortality. It seems to us that much of the current replacement endeavors represent an obdurate, publicly theatricalized refusal to accept these limitations. Physicians are morally guided by what the late Protestant theologian and ethicist Paul Ramsey called principles of "faithfulness" and "loyalty" not to abandon caring for their patients, particularly those who are dying. Ramsey also argued forcibly, however, that we "need . . . to discover the moral limits properly surrounding efforts to save life" (Ramsey 1970, p. 118). With this conviction, we think that he would have joined us in questioning the enactment of the principle of faithfulness in the unremitting efforts of transplant surgeons to prevent the death of their patients by doing numerous retransplants if the donor organ "fails for any reason," because they believe that "once a patient has had a transplant [they] have made a commitment that cannot be abandoned" (Park 1989, p. 30).

Rereading Ramsey's *The Patient as Person,* twenty years after it was first published, we were deeply impressed by how prophetic it has proved to be with respect to our social and cultural problems in accepting limits on organ replacement and the care of dying patients. Culturally, Ramsey argued persuasively, we need to "recover a religious sense that death is not an evil that ought always to be opposed."

> If it is not possible for modern men, when the one "lone hope" is gone, to believe that this is not the end of hope, perhaps we might share the conviction of Socrates, who said, "Now it is time that we were going, I to die and you to live, but which of us has the happier prospect, is unknown to anyone but God." That outlook, too, might save men and doctors today from the triumphalist temptation to slash and suture our way to eternal life." (Ramsey 1970, p. 238)

Two recollections come to mind. The first is our wry memory of the fact that during the early 1970s, when we were trying to find a title for the first edition of *The Courage to Fail,* sociologist Erving Goffman suggested *Spare Parts* to us as a possibility. Although we appreciated the ironic wittiness of his suggestion, at that time we considered it too cynical for us to adopt. Viewed retrospectively, this Goffmanesque title now seems prescient because we feel it captures some of the essences of the evolution that organ replacement and our relation to it have undergone during the past decade.

The second memory is of a field trip that one of us (RCF) made during the late 1970s to a dialysis center located on a small, 3.5 square mile atoll in the Marshall Islands that was supervised from afar by the Institute of Renal Diseases of St. Francis Hospital in Honolulu, Hawaii. For both of us, that coral atoll symbolizes the antithesis of a palm-fringed tropical paradise. It represents the unromantic specter of a world in which every island, no matter how small or remote, will some day have its own machines and personnel to which all persons in end-stage organ failure will "be given unconditional access, until death releases them from this form of treatment, or they can be airlifted to a medical center such as St. Francis for transplantation.

As we look back, we realize that it is not only we who have been changed by the cumulative effects that our field research has had on us. The field itself has changed, especially during the 1980s, in certain ways that have influenced our decision to exit it. Above all, it is the intensity and expansion of the drive to sustain life and "rebuild people" through organ replacement that has progressively alienated us, particularly the unquestioning and even celebratory way in which the transplanting and retransplanting of virtually every organ of the human body is creating larger and larger numbers of "patchwork men and women," (Altman 1989c) whose quality of life is dubious at best. "Our culture," Ramsey observed, "is already prepared for technocratizing the bodily life into collections of parts in which consciousness somehow has residence for a time" (Ramsey 1970, p. 193).

In addition, the determination to procure organs has become so powerful that we believe there is an almost predatory obliviousness to "where [the] organs come from, and how [the] donors died" (Annas 1989, p. 34). We share George Annas' indignation over what he termed the "denial of reality" that underlies the current policy of avidly promoting organ donation and transplantation without publicly acknowledging the kinds of death—from vehicular accidents, homicides, suicides—on which they are based (Annas 1988, p. 621).

However, we disagree with what Annas goes on to say: namely, that it is not only important and right that "we all should know the stories of donors" (Annas 1988, p. 621), but also that the donor's family, the recipient, and the recipient's family should know each other's identity. In his view, the norm of confidentiality that transplant teams have established does more to protect their own emotional equilibrium than that of donors, recipients, and their families. Here we part company with Annas because, like so many analysts commenting on organ transplants during the 1980s, he has not sufficiently taken into account the importance of the gift-exchange dimensions of organ donation, the stresses and burdens that the obligations of giving, receiving, and repaying it impose on donors and donees, or how the policy of confidentiality developed out of transplanters' desire to reduce the "tyranny" of this unrepayable, symbolically charged gift. It seems to us that what Annas has overlooked is a specific instance of a more general trend during the 1980s that is another factor propelling us out of the field. It is the present tendency to minimize the importance of the "theme of gift" and of the gift relation in organ transplantation and to systematically ignore, forget, or deny what was previously known about them. Such disregard for the dynamics and meaning of the gift exchange involved has characterized most of the live-donor liver, lung, and pancreas transplants conducted during the last few years.

Nowhere is the tendency to discount the gift dimension more patently, (and to us distressingly) apparent than in the movement toward the "commodification" and "marketification" of the organs. This development was one theme in a 1988 symposium on organ transplantation policy, in which proponents of a market economy for human body parts wondered why transplantation has not joined the "mainstream" of American medicine.

> Does the difference in policy prescription in the organ transplantation arena reflect a kind of sub rosa, underground ground rejection of the trend toward greater competition, pluralism, and decentralization in the health care industry, or are there certain peculiar characteristics of the organ transplantation enterprise that suggest the inapplicability of competition, pluralism, and decentralization in this specific industry? (Blumstein and Sloan 1989, pp. 1-2)

Arguing, as this representative passage does, that organ transplantation, like health care in general, is analogous to a commercial industry and product and that its nonconformity to a market model is not only curious but possibly subversive makes it difficult for us to identify with the way that transplants, and medicine more generally, are now being conceived and interpreted.

The "de-gifting" of transplantation that this market approach entails has been accompanied and reinforced by the progressive "biologization" of donated organs that has occurred during the 1980s and early 1990s. Increasingly, organs are being thought of as "just organs," rather than as living parts of a person, offered in life or death to sustain known or unknown others, that resonate with the symbolic meaning of our relation to our bodies, ourselves, and to each other, and with the more than fleshly significance of what has been given and received. We believe that this biological reductionism (which as sociologist Howard L. Kaye pointed out is not confined to transplantation but pervades modern biology) has insidious implications for "how we conceive of ourselves as human beings," of our connectedness with others, "and thus how we conceive of a good and proper life" (Kaye 1986, 1991, p. 13).

We are deeply troubled by the subtle but powerful tendency to redefine ourselves and others "as essentially biological beings" (Kaye 1991, p. 16) that is being displayed in current attitudes toward the transplantation of solid organs, tissues, and other body parts. Not only has this living matter been terminologically reduced to "HBPs," but what we regard as something approaching the plundering of the newly deceased person's body is taking place. In May 1991, when the news surfaced that a young organ donor (twenty-two-year-old William Norwood, who had been fatally shot in a gas station holdup) had been infected with the AIDS virus, and a search was launched for the recipients of his organs and tissues, we were struck by the fact that some fifty-six of his body parts went to people in different regions of the country. On the one hand, we are impressed by the magnitude of such gifts and by the number of persons who could be helped by them. On the other hand, we wonder if our avidness to procure as many organs and tissues as possible is leading us to unreflectively disassemble and dehumanize the body.

One of the most urgent value questions that has emerged from our long professional immersion in the world of "spare parts" medicine is whether, as poverty, homelessness, and lack of access to health care increase in our affluent country, it is justifiable for American society to be devoting so much of its intellectual energy and human and financial resources to the replacement of human organs. We realize that in terms of the ways our society provides, allocates, and expends resources within the "medical commons," the aggregate volume and costs of organ replacements are a relatively small portion of medical care activities and expenditures. Nor, given the benefits that many patients may derive from transplants and artificial devices, do we suppose that all organ replacement endeavors should—or conceivably would—cease. We do believe, however, that all the professional and public consideration given to transplants and pursuits such as a permanent artificial heart and the societal value commitments that organ replacement epitomizes are helping to divert attention and human and financial resources away from far more basic and widespread public and individual health care needs in our society.

We still believe that the ultimate significance of these therapeutic modalities lies in their relation to metamedical themes: uncertainty, scarcity, and generosity; the just distribution of material and nonmaterial resources; solidarity and community; life, death, and meaning; and intervention in the human condition. We also share health policy analyst Emily Friedman's passionate conviction that a "silent, largely invisible epidemic [of] medical indigence" has become the most tragically serious health care problem in the United States; that "the noncoverage of the uninsured poor and their resultant lack of access [to health care] affect every American"; that ignoring or accepting this situation puts us "all at risk," because "a society that forces its most vulnerable and needy members to beg for crumbs of care, or to go without care until they are dying, harms itself [and its moral fabric] even more than it harms the victims of its cruelty" (Friedman 1989). Allowing ourselves to become too caught up in such problems as the shortage of transplantable organs while health care continues to be defined as a private consumption rather than a social good in American society, with the consequence that millions of people do not have adequate or even minimally decent care, speaks to a values framework and a vision of medical progress that we find medically and morally untenable. The predicament of these deprived and fragile members of our society has changed the ethical context of transplantation and artificial organs for us; and it is one of the most morally compelling reasons for our leaving the field.

By happenstance, the time we chose to write about organ replacement during the 1980s coincided with a marked escalation of biomedical and technological developments, and of social attention to them. At first, we thought that the ground swell of activity we perceived in the organ replacement sphere was a kind of optical illusion caused by our heightened awareness of the field from which we were taking leave and our ambivalence about doing so. Sheer "observer effect," however, cannot account for the remarkable concatenation of events that took place from July 1989 to August 1991, when we were writing this book. During that interval, for example, the volume of transplants and the audible concern about the scarcity of organs and tissues, their procurement, and allocation mounted appreciably. An array of cluster transplants gained momentum and prominence; their chief performer and promoter, Thomas Starzl, did the first human heart-liver-kidney multiple transplant in December 1989 in a twenty-six-year-old woman who died in March 1990 of complications from hepatitis. Professional and public debate about the feasibility and ethicality of using anencephalic infants as organ donors flared up in response to the Loma Linda Medical Center's program and their subsequent decision to suspend it. Clinical trials were conducted with the transplantation of cadaver organs from persons generally regarded as too biologically old to be donors and with using "flawed" organs for temporary transplants. In October 1989, FK 506, a powerful antirejection agent, burst on the scene. In December 1989, accompanied by considerable fanfare, the first two American transplantations of liver lobes from live donor parents to infants with biliary atresia were performed at the University of Chicago Medical Center, followed by the first parent-to-child lung lobe transplants and the beginning of professional and public debate about the morality of parents conceiving a baby to serve as a bone marrow donor for another of their children. January 1990 brought the announcement that researchers were preparing for their first human tests of a temporary artificial lung, developed by a company in Salt Lake City (Altman 1990b). Simultaneously, the Jarvik-7 artificial heart made headlines again when the FDA officially withdrew approval of the device's continued experimental use because of deficiencies in its manufacture and quality control and in the monitoring of its clinical use. A year later the artificial heart again began to attract attention, as researchers moved toward their goal of the first human tests with a new generation of electrically powered devices to replace the functions of the human heart on a long-term basis.

In the final analysis, our departure from the field in the midst of such events is not only impelled by our need and desire to distance ourselves from them emotionally. It is also a value statement on our part. By our leave-taking we are intentionally separating ourselves from what we believe has become an overly zealous medical and societal commitment to the endless perpetuation of life and to repairing and rebuilding people through organ replacement—and from the human suffering and the social, cultural, and spiritual harm we believe such unexamined excess can, and already has, brought in its wake.

REFERENCES

Altman, Lawrence K. Tracking a new drug from the soil in Japan to organ transplants. *New York Times*, 31 October 1989.

Annas, George J. Feeling good about recycled hearts. *Second Opinion* 12 (November 1989): 33-39.

Annas, George J. The paradoxes of organ transplantation. *American Journal of Public Health* 78 (June 1988): 621-22.

Blumenstein, James F., and Frank A. Sloan (eds.). *Organ transplantation policy: Issues and prospects.* Durham, N.C., Duke University Press, 1989.

Callahan, Daniel. *What kind of life? The limits of medical progress.* New York, Simon & Schuster, 1989.

Fox, Renée C. *Experiment perilous,* rpt. ed. Free Press, 1959; Philadelphia, University of Pennsylvania Press, 1974.

Fox, Renée C. and Judith Swazey. *The courage to fail: A social view of organ transplants and dialysis,* 2d rev. ed. Chicago, University of Chicago Press, 1978.

Fox, Renée C. and Judith Swazey. Critical care at Tianjin's First Central Hospital and the fourth modernization. *Science* 217 (August 20, 1982): 700-705.

Fox, Renée C. and Judith Swazey. Medical morality is not bioethics: Medical ethics in China and the United States. *Perspectives in Biology and Medicine* 27, no. 3 (1984): 336-60.

Friedman, Emily. The torturer's horse. *JAMA* 216 (March 10, 1989): 1481-82.

Kaye, Howard L. *The social meaning of modern biology.* New Haven, Conn., Yale University Press, 1986.

Kluge, Eike-Henner W. Designated organ donation: Private choice in social context. *Hastings Center Report* 19, no. 5 (1989): 10-16.

Mead, Margaret. *Letters from the field.* New York, Harper & Row, 1977.

Moore, Francis D. The desperate case: CARE (costs, applicability, research, ethics). *JAMA* 261 (March 10, 1989): 1483-84.

Park, Patricia M. The transplant odyssey. *Second Opinion.* 12 (November 1989): 27-32.

Ramsey, Paul. *The patient as person: Explorations in medical ethics.* New Haven, Conn., Yale University Press, 1970.

Reimer, Leslie G. The power of the individual's story. *Second Opinion* 12 (Novemeber 1989): 40-45.

Shem, Samuel. *The house of God.* New York, Dell Books, 1978.

Starzl, Thomas. Comments on the death of Stormie James. Unpublished. 1990.

Terasaki, Paul I. A proposal to increase donations of cadaveric organs. *New England Journal of Medicine* 321 (August 31, 1989): 618-19.

34. What Transplantation Can Teach Us about Health Care Reform

Martin Benjamin, Carl Cohen, and Eugene Grochowski

Organ transplantation has been targeted for elimination or reduction in many proposed schemes of health care reform.[1,2,3] Although recent figures suggest a dramatic increase in cost effectiveness,[4] transplantation is expensive and its exclusion is defended in the name of justice. This is ironic, because no part of the health care system has done more to resolve questions of justice than transplantation. As we try to reform health care, much may be learned from our experience in this area.

DEALING WITH SCARCITY

In response to the limited supply of organs, the transplantation system has developed fair and efficient principles of allocation. It has dealt with the organ shortage rationally, and for the most part justly. Rationing involves an explicit policy of allocating a limited supply of goods or services according to principles of justice and efficiency. The word is derived from the Latin *ratio,* for reason or rationality. A system of allocation is rational if it systematically applies defensible principles. It is therefore misleading to say that the present health care system rations "by default." By definition, a system that allocates arbitrarily does not ration; instead, it is probably quite irrational.

The development of rationality in our transplantation system is instructive. At first the system was painfully irrational, marked by organ brokers, offers to sell kidneys, and families pulling strings. Telegenic children

Originally published in *The New England Journal of Medicine* 330, no. 12 (March 24, 1994).

received special resources with great fanfare. Wealthy foreigners received organs at the expense of Americans suffering from the same diseases.[5]

In response to the need for a more just and uniform system, Congress passed the National Organ Transplant Act of 1984, banning commerce in organs, calling for a national network of organ procurement and transplantation, and establishing a national task force to study related social and ethical issues. The most far-reaching recommendation of the task force was "that each donated organ be considered a national resource to be used for the public good."[6] After this, the social aspects of transplantation could no longer be denied. Since the system depended heavily on the donation of organs by the public, it could not have flourished unless there was a general conviction that it was fair. Rational restrictions on the entrepreneurial spirit were accepted.

The national network for organ procurement and transplantation was implemented in 1987 by the United Network for Organ Sharing (UNOS) under contract with the federal government. A national system with uniform policies of allocation replaced a jumble of procurement agencies. A nationwide list of patients waiting for organs is now maintained by the UNOS computerized point system, which ranks patients. Scarce organs are allocated according to impartial criteria that balance considerations of likely medical success, time on the waiting list, and urgency of need. Policies to ensure the fair, efficient, and medically optimal matching of donors and recipients are continually evaluated and refined. In financing, too, the role of the community has grown. Medicare and many Medicaid programs and private insurance policies underwrite much of the cost of transplantation.

The current practice is not perfectly just, of course. Blacks and women receive transplants at what appear to be disproportionately low rates. But the reasons for these disparities almost certainly extend beyond the transplantation system.[7] Claims of medical urgency are sometimes abused, resulting in repeated transplantation for some patients while others desperately await their first transplant. Such situations involve moral complexities. Physicians' loyalty to their patients is commendable, but when carried to excess it occasionally results in dishonesty and erodes overall fairness. Isolated injustices do not discredit the entire system, however; they highlight the continuing need for oversight and education. Less than a decade has elapsed since the attempt to create a rational system began; given the magnitude of the problems, the achievements have been quite encouraging. Our heightened awareness of shortcomings reflects a general acceptance of the rules and principles now governing the allocation of organs.[8]

The overall lesson is important: the system can cope successfully with scarcity. As we turn to the far more complex task of allocating other types of health care resources fairly, our experience with transplantation can serve as a guide.

OPEN AND CLOSED SYSTEMS OF ALLOCATION

The rationing of health care is widely believed to be unrealistic, because our system (in contrast to the British National Health Service or the Canadian system) is essentially open—that is, there is no fixed budget for health care. Hence, there can be no effective way to allocate resources rationally within the system as a whole.

In the United Kingdom it is easier to say no to care that is costly and marginally beneficial, because resources withheld from one patient may reasonably be supposed to go to another patient who is more rationally selected.[9] American physicians cannot make such assumptions. But the system of organ allocation is closed, because it is a "united network for organ sharing." The participants—physicians, patients, and the public—know that an organ is denied to a potential recipient only for reasons of fairness and efficiency, not because of indifference or prejudice. Saying no to a particular patient is hard, but it means we can say yes to another. And the onus of making the painful judgment rarely falls on a single physician. The criteria for allocation, in which considerations of justice and efficiency are combined, have been developed and ratified by public bodies.[10]

Closing the larger health care system (giving it a fixed budget) will be exceedingly difficult. But experience with transplantation teaches that efforts to limit care, in whatever category, will remain difficult to defend—to justify—as long as we are unwilling to have a closed health care system at least in part.

Critics will rightly observe that the problems presented by rationing in the smaller system of transplantation and those presented in the larger system of health care differ in kind as well as in degree. In transplantation, rationing is mandatory because there is a limited supply of organs. Needs are inescapable, and the rules can be made reasonably specific and understandable. In health care as a whole, rationing appears not to be mandatory in the same sense. Instead, the task will be to determine a decent minimal standard of health care to which everyone is entitled—one that differentiates the kinds of health care and their relative priorities. It will be even harder to weigh the needs of health care against competing demands—for national defense, education, repair of roads and bridges, criminal justice, and so on. In comparison, the rationing of transplants seems to be child's play.

The principles used in transplantation cannot be simply transferred to address the larger problems of justice in health care. It is valuable, however, to realize that some obstacles to a more rational system of health care have been confronted successfully in narrower contexts, and it is useful to see how that was done.

THE PHYSICIAN UNDER TWO MASTERS

Any closed system of health care requires physicians to make bedside decisions.[11] What principles will guide them? If doctors serve as gatekeepers within a system, are they not obligated to make some decisions that affect their own patients adversely? "If this is what is required by a rational system," a concerned physician may respond, "then health care reform be damned."

The ultimate loyalty of doctors is to individual patients, such a physician might argue; no other master may be recognized.[12] Therefore, physicians cannot make decisions involving rationing without betraying their fundamental loyalties. Any system that sometimes obliges them to apply general rules to the disadvantage of their own patients forces them to serve two masters—an ethical difficulty that we impose at great peril.[13,14]

In the field of transplantation, the criteria for allocation are applied by physicians, but they are generally accepted. Indeed, the rules are welcomed by many because in large part they objectify the decisions to be made. Criteria for assigning priority to patients have been established and are applied uniformly. The system has four aims: to apply equitable medical criteria, to serve patients fairly, to maximize the chance of a successful outcome, and to minimize organ wastage and encourage organ donation.[15] The relevant considerations are quantified when feasible, in ways that are widely understood, impartial, and morally defensible.

The system is not inflexible. Professional judgment is not precluded, especially when anomalous medical factors or anatomical abnormalities are involved. Patients on the waiting list may be passed over temporarily, but the reasons for such decisions must be submitted to UNOS.

Physicians who perform transplantation balance their obligations to particular patients with their obligations to the larger patient population. Four features of the system should be noted. First, ultimate decisions based on detailed knowledge of an individual patient remain in the hands of attending physicians. Second, the computerized point system, which is continually studied and refined, reflects the most important medical variables. Third, the system is closed, in the sense that organs are allocated fairly. Although some patients die while they are on the waiting list, all know that the available organs are used justly and efficiently. Finally, the system is marked by integrity—there is general confidence that the criteria for allocation are applied evenhandedly.

The issues raised by transplantation oblige us to take seriously our roles as citizens. Health professionals and patients are united in a body larger than themselves, in which they each have duties transcending those associated with their narrower roles. When the community devises defensible principles for the allocation of limited public resources, we all have a duty as citizens to cooperate.

This situation is not utopian. Organ transplantation teaches that we can reasonably aspire to this level of conduct. In truth, two masters are indeed being served, but serious conflict is limited. Though the role of gatekeeper is difficult, it is not intolerable. Within the limitations of a rational allocation system, physicians engaged in transplantation have been able to balance faithfulness to their patients with responsible stewardship of a precious social resource. These qualities can be extended, we may reasonably hope, to the health care system as a whole.

LESSONS FOR HEALTH CARE REFORM

Community involvement has proved essential in organ transplantation, but there is still excessive fear of such involvement. In particular, there is concern that, if extended to the health care system at large, government regulation will lead to the deterioration of health care. But federal funding and regulation of transplantation have led to the improvement of care, not its deterioration. Public oversight has ensured that surgeons are adequately experienced, that certain risky procedures are undertaken only under appropriate circumstances, and above all that Americans who need a transplant are treated with equal respect in the organ-allocation process. Nowhere else in medicine is there so dramatic an illustration of our mutual interdependence and of the ways in which, with intelligence and goodwill, the members of a community can improve each other's lives. The world of transplantation illustrates the advantages and practicality of a system in which resources are pooled and emphasis is placed on fairness and the needs of the community as a whole.

Even the words and concepts have changed. References to justice and equitable access have become part of the everyday vocabulary of those involved with transplantation. We think this change may soon become equally pervasive in the health care system as a whole.

The success of the national network for organ procurement and allocation has been noteworthy. Issues of scarcity have been confronted, the system closed, and questions of justice squarely addressed. Serving both individual and social interests without betraying either, the system gives appropriate place to the role of the community in health care policy. Experience with organ transplantation may teach us that some of the thorniest difficulties associated with rationalizing medical care are within our power to resolve. In so doing, it may give us heart.

REFERENCES

1. Welch HG, Larson EB. Dealing with limited resources: the Oregon decision to curtail funding for organ transplantation. *N Engl J Med* 1988;319-171-3.

2. Callahan D. *What kind of life: the limits of medical progress.* New York: Simon and Schuster, 1990.

3. Gayline W. Faulty diagnosis: why Clinton's health care plan won't cure what ails us. *Harpers.* October 1993:57-64.

4. Evans RW. *Executive summary: the National Cooperative Transplantation Study.* (BHARC-100-91.) Seattle: Battelle-Seattle Research Center, 1991.

5. The challenge of a miracle: selling the gift. *Pittsburgh Press.* November 3-8, 1985.

6. Patient access to and payment for organ transplantation. In: *Report of the Task Force on Organ Transplantation, April 1986. Organ transplantation: issues and recommendations.* Washington, D.C.: Department of Health and Human Services, 1986:86.

7. Kjellstrand CM. Age, sex, and race inequality in renal transplantation. *Arch Intern Med* 1988;148:1305-9.

8. Department of Health and Human Services, Office of Inspector General. *The distribution of organs for transplantation: expectation and practices.* Washington, D.C.: Department of Health and Human Services, 1991.

9. Daniels N. Why saying no to patients in the United States is so hard: cost containment, justice, and provider autonomy. *N Engl J Med* 1986;314:1380-3.

10. Ethics Committee of the United Network for Organ Sharing. General principles for allocation of human organs and tissues. *Transplant Proc* 1992;24:2226-35.

11. Schwartz WB, Aaron HJ. The Achilles heel of health care rationing. *New York Times.* July 9, 1990:A17.

12. Levinsky NG. The doctor's master. *N Engl J Med* 1984;311:1573-5.

13. Angell M. The doctor as double agent. *Kennedy Inst Ethics J* 1993;3:279-86.

14. Menzel PT. Double agency and the ethics of rationing health care. *Kennedy Inst Ethics J* 1993;3:287-92.

15. Policy proposal statement: liver allocation. Richmond, Va.: United Network for Organ Sharing, January 21, 1991:2.

Bibliography

Part One: Sources

Caplan, AL. "Is xenografting morally wrong?" *Transplantation Proceedings*, 24 (2):722-7, 1992 Apr.

Council on Ethical and Judicial Affairs, American Medical Association. "The use of anencephalic neonates as organ donors." *JAMA*, 273(20):1614-8, 1995, May 24-31.

Garry DJ, Caplan AL, Vawter DE, Kearney W. "Are there really alternatives to the use of fetal tissue from elective abortions in transplantation research?" *New England Journal of Medicine*, 327(22):1592-5, 1992, Nov 26.

Hoffenberg R, Lock M, Tilney N, et al. "Should organs from patients in permanent vegetative state be used for transplantation?" *Lancet*, 350:1320, 1997, Nov. 1.

Levey AS, Hou S, Bush BL. "Kidney transplantation from unrelated living donors: time to reclaim a discarded opportunity." *New England Journal of Medicine*, 314 (14):914-6, 1986.

Nelson JL. "Transplantation through a glass darkly." *Hastings Center Report*, 22(5):6-8, 1992, Sep.-Oct.

Ott BB, "Defining and redefing death." *American Journal of Critical Care*, 4(6):476-80, 1995, Nov.

Robertson JA, "Rights, symbolism, and public policy in fetal tissue transplants." *Hastings Center Report*, 18(6):5-12, 1988, Dec.

Strong RW, Lynch SV. "Ethical issues in living related donor liver transplantation [review]." *Transplantation Proceedings*, 28 (4): 2366-9, 1996, Aug.

Truog, RD "Is it time to abandon brain death?" *Hastings Center Report*, 27(l):29-37, 1997, Jan-Feb.

Shewmon DA, Capron AM, et al. "The use of anencephalic infants as organ sources. A critique [review]." *JAMA*, 261(12):1773-81, 1989, Mar 24-31.

PART TWO: POLICY

Caplan, AL. "Ethical and policy issues in the procurement of cadaver organs for transplanta-
tion." *New England Journal of Medicine*, 311(15):981-3, 1984, Oct. 11.
Funerman LG. "Presumed consent: the solution to the critical organ donor shortage? [review]"
American Journal of Clinical Care, 4(5):383-8, 1995, Sep.
Jarvis R, "Join the club: a modest proposal to increase availability of donor organs." *Journal
of Medical Ethics*, 21(4):199-204, 1995, Aug.
Spital A, "Mandated choice for organ donation: time to give it a try." *Annals of Internal Med-
icine*, 125(l): 66-69, 1996, July 1.
Veatch RM, Pitt JB. "The myth of presumed consent: ethical problems in new organ procure-
ment strategies." *Transplantation Proceedings*, 27(2):1888-92, 1995, April.

PART THREE: COMMODIFICATION

Barnett AH, Blair RD, Kaserman DL. "Improving organ donation: compensation versus markets." *Inquiry*, 29:372-8, 1992, Fall.
Caplan AL, Van Buren CT, Tilney NL. "Financial compensation for cadaver organ donation:
good idea or anathema." *Transplantation Proceedings*, 25 (4):2740-2, 1993, August.
Daniels N. "Comment: Ability to pay and access to transplantation." *Transplantation Proceed-
ings*, 21(3):3424-5, 1989, June.
Evans RW. "Money matters: dhould ability to pay ever be a consideration in gaining access to
transplantation?" *Transplantation Proceedings*, 21(3):3419-23, 1989, June.
Morris PJ, Sells RA. "Paying for organs from living donors." *Lancet*, 1(8444):1510, 1985, June 29.
Pellegrino E. "Families' self-interest and the cadaver's organs: what price consent." *JAMA*,
265(10):1305-6, 1991, March 13.
Peters T. "Life or death: the issue of payment in cadaveric organ donation." *JAMA*,
265(10):1302-5, 1991, March 13.
Radcliffe-Richards J, Daar AS, Guttmann RD, et al. "The case for allowing kidney sales."
Lancet, 352:1950-2, 1998, June 27.

PART FOUR: ALLOCATION AND RATIONING

Bronsther O, Fung JJ, et al. "Prioritization and organ distribution for liver transplantation."
JAMA, 271(2):140-3, 1994, Jan. 12.
Cohen C, Benjamin M. "Alcoholics and liver transplantation." *JAMA*, 265(10):1299-1301,
1991, March 13.
Klassen A, Klassen D. "Who are the donors in organ donation? The family's perspective in
mandated choice." *Annals of Internal Medicine*, 125(l):70-3, 1996, July 1.
Moss AH, Siegler M. "Should alcoholics compete equally for liver transplantation?" *JAMA*,
265(10): 1295-8, 1991, March 13.
Schneiderman LJ, Jecker NS. "Should a criminal receive a heart transplant? Medical justice vs.
societal justice." *Theoretical Medicine*, 17(l):33-44, 1996, Mar.
Smart B "Fault and the allocation of spare organs." *Journal of Medical Ethics*, 20(l):26-30,
1994, March.
Ubel PA, Arnold RM, Caplan AL. "Rationing failure. The ethical lessons of the retransplantation of scarce vital organs." *JAMA*, 270(20):2469-74, 1993, Nov. 24.

PART FIVE: VALUE

Benjamin M, Cohen C, et al. "What transplantation can teach us about health care reform." *New England Journal of Medicine,* 330(12):858-860, 1994, March 24

Fox R, Swazey J. "Leaving the Field," from *Spare Parts: Organ Replacement in American Society.* New York, Oxford University Press, 1992.

Gaston R, Ayres I, et al. "Racial equity in renal transplantation." *JAMA,* 270(11):1352-6, 1993, September 15.

Welch HG, Larson EB. "The Oregon decision to curtail funding for organ transplantation." *New England Journal of Medicine,* 319(3):171-3, 1988, July 21.

TRANSPLANT BOOKS

Durrett, Deanne. *Organ Transplants.* Lucent Overview Series, 1993 Massachussets General Hospital Organ Transplant Team. *Organ Transplants: A Patient's Guide.* 1991.

Fox, Renée C., Swazey, Judith P. *Spare Parts.* New York and Oxford: Oxford University Press, 1992.

Gold, E. Richard. *Body Parts.* Washington, D.C.: Georgetown University Press, 1997.

Radin, Margaret Jane. *Contested Commodities.* Cambridge, Mass.: Harvard University Press, 1996.

Starzl, Thomas E. *The Puzzle People: Memoirs of a Transplant Surgeon.* Pittsburgh: University of Pittsburgh Press, 1992.

Titmuss, Richard M. *The Gift Relationship: From Human Blood to Social Policy.* New York: Pantheon Books, 1971.

Youngner, Stuart J., Renée C. Fox, and Laurence J. O'Connell (Eds.). *Organ Transplantation: Meanings and Realities.* Madison: University of Wisconsin Press, 1996.

BIOETHICS BOOKS

Caplan, Arthur L. *Am I My Brother's Keeper?: The Ethical Frontiers of Biomedicine.* Medical Ethics Series. University of Indiana Press, 1998.

———. *Due Consideration.* New York: John Wiley and Sons, 1998.

———. *If I Were a Rich Man Could I Buy a Pancreas?: And Other Essays on the Ethics of Health Care.* Bloomington: Indiana University Press, 1994.

———. *Moral Matters: Ethical Issues in Medicine & the Life Sciences.* New York: John Wiley & Sons, Incorporated, 1994.

Jecker, Nancy S., Albert R. Jonsen, and Robert A. Pearlman. *Bioethics: An Introduction to the History, Methods, and Practice.* Boston: Jones and Bartlett Publishers, 1997.

Jonsen, Albert R. *The Birth of Bioethics.* New York: Oxford University Press, 1998.

———. *Clinical Ethics: A Practical Approach to Ethical Decisions in Clinical Medicine.* New York: Macmillan, 1998.

Jonsen, Albert R., Robert M. Veatch, and LeRoy Walters. (Eds.). *Source Book in Bioethics: A Documentary History.* Washington, D.C.: Georgetown University Press, 1997.

Munson, Ronald, and Christopher Hoffman. *Intervention and Reflection: Basic Issues in Medical Ethics.* Belmont, Calif.: Wadsworth Publishing Co., 1996.

Reich, Warren T. (Ed.). *Encyclopedia of Bioethics,* 2d ed. rev. New York: Macmillan, 1995.

Shannon, Thomas A. *An Introduction to Bioethics.* New York: Paulist Press, 1997.

INTERNET WEB SITES

United Network for Organ Sharing: http://www.UNOS.org

Centerspan: http://www.centerspan.org
    Centerspan is a collaborative project of the American Society of Transplant Physicians and the American Society of Transplant Surgeons, created to support the practice of transplantation through the creation and application of new educational and communication tools on the Internet.

Transweb: http://www.transweb.org
    Transweb's purpose is to (1) provide a resource for transplant patients and families worldwide with information specifically dealing with transplant issues and problems; (2) to provide an index of sources for transplant-related information available through the Internet and otherwise; and (3) to provide information about donation and transplantation to the general public in order to improve organ and tissue procurement efforts worldwide.

University of Pennsylvania Center for Bioethics: http://www.med.upenn.edu/bioethics